A Guide to Street Survival & Strength

Phil Ross M.S.

It's dark and you're alone walking down a deserted street in a strange city. You hear footsteps behind you. You pick up your pace and the footsteps become faster and louder. You look over your shoulder and...

You are awakened from your slumber to the sound of your windows being jostled. There's a faint crash as the window gets broken and the glass falls to the floor. Then you hear the window creak open and a pair of feet land. The intruder makes his way across the room, and you hear the door to your bedroom open and...

The elevator doors are about to close. An arm reaches in and props the door open, enabling six rowdy youths to enter. They look at you laughing, and the comments begin as the circle closes around you and...

You are at the mall and you have forgotten where you parked your car. Your arms laden with packages, you search in the darkness for your vehicle. Suddenly, you hear a voice break the silence "Are you lost?" You turn around and...

It's date night. You and your companion just had a great dinner, and you decide to go dancing at a local club. You're out on the dance floor and there's a group of guys out there, and they begin to bump into you and start to grind on your girlfriend. The dance floor is crowded and there's no way for you to get out of the circle, nor can you get the attention of security. You see the fear in her eyes, and then...

Your car breaks down on a deserted highway. It's going to take an hour for AAA to arrive. You are traveling with your wife and two small children. You see a pick-up truck arrive and pull up behind you. Three large, scruffy gentlemen get out and approach your vehicle. Two of the large men come to your window and the other goes to your wife's car door. With a tooth-gap grin, the man closest says, "You havin' a little car trouble, er ya?" You see a crowbar in his hand and...

Scary scenarios, aren't they? What would you do? Read this book and you'll be ready to answer this question ...

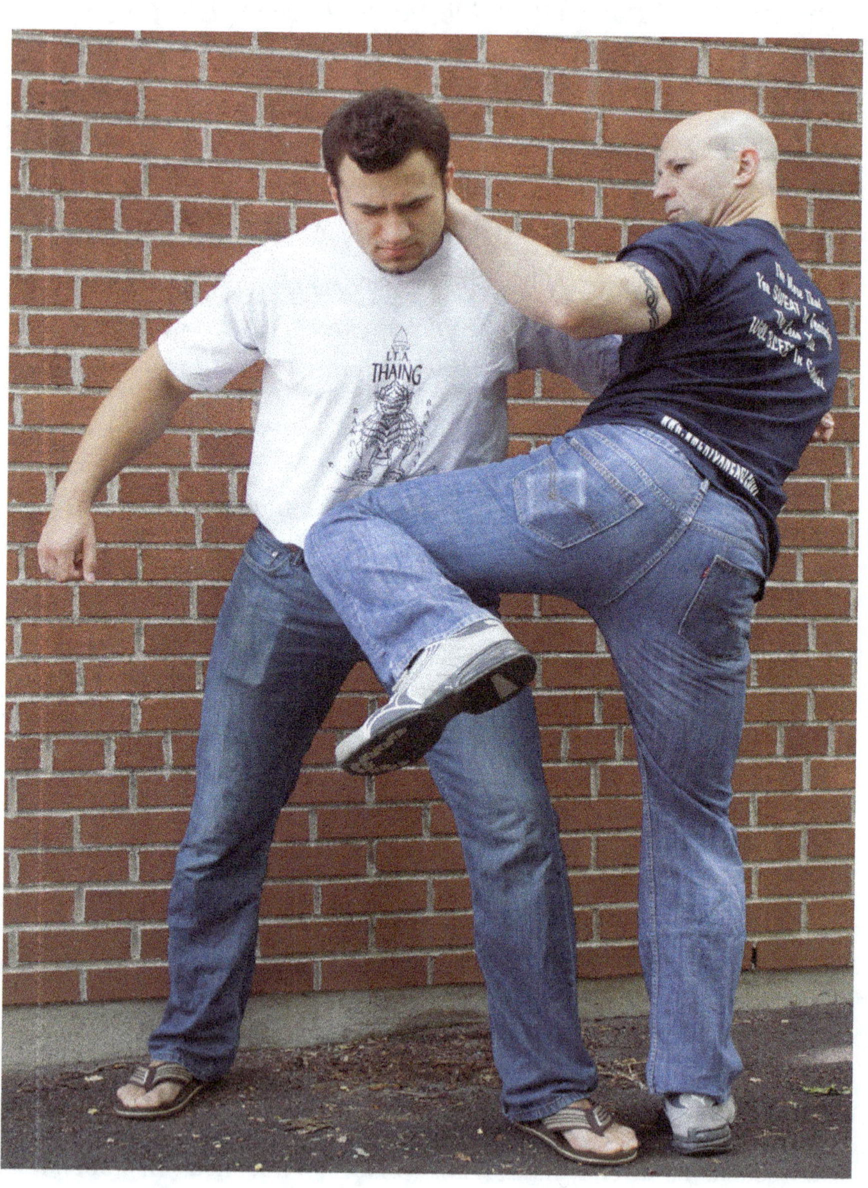

Contents

Prelude   vii

1. Introduction   1
2. Real-World Application   13
3. Mindset   19
4. Physical Fitness and Strength   38
5. Weapons of The Human Body   108
6. Targets of The Human Body   117
7. Generation of Power   130
8. Grips and Locks   135
9. Entry and Single Techniques   155
10. Movement and Zones   188
11. Basic Grappling   193
12. Combinations and Series   199
13. Street Applications and Tactics   202
14. Practice and Training   293
15. Dog Attacks   309
16. Unconventional Weapons: Practice Is Essential   313
17. Conventional Weapons   320
18. Home-Preparedness   324
19. Every-Day Public Places   327
20. Mass Hysteria   331
21. Car Safety   336
22. The Importance of Training   340
23. Breathing and Meditation   345
24. Recommended Training Aids   347
     Epilogue   353

Acknowledgments   357
About the Author   359

Prelude

I will first tell you what I am not. I'm not a retired Navy SEAL, Marine Recon or Green Beret. I wasn't a police officer in a high-crime area. I didn't do any hard time (although I spent a few nights locked up, but was later found not guilty). I was not part of a street gang, motorcycle club or organized crime syndicate. I was not an MMA (Mixed Martial Arts) cage fighter, although I did compete successfully in the arts that comprise MMA.

You may be asking yourself, "If you weren't all of these things, then what qualifies you to write a book on self-defense?"

In the 2002 movie *The Knockaround Guys*, Vin Diesel's character says, "Five Hundred". He then explains to the guy he is squared up with that to be considered a tough guy, you have to have had over 500 fights.

This is where my qualifications come from. If you tally up my list of conflicts, confrontations and competitions, the number far exceeds 500. I was victorious in over 300 martial arts competitions, primarily covering point contact but also a fair number of bare-knuckle karate, kickboxing, full-contact Taekwondo, submission fighting, Brazilian Jiu Jitsu, and Continuous Fighting matches. I fought in some of the toughest areas in the East: Paterson, NJ; Newark, NJ; Camden, NJ; South Plainfield, NJ; Washington, DC: Baltimore, MD: Brooklyn, NY; New York, NY; Youngstown, Ohio; and Philadelphia, PA, to name a few. Then you must add in the over 200 street confrontations I've had, from my time as a bouncer and bodyguard.

Then factor in the additional street fights and living in a high-crime area (Prince George's County, MD). This does not include the hundreds of wrestling matches and the thousands of hours spent in live combat training of various types with another human being trying their darndest to subdue me.

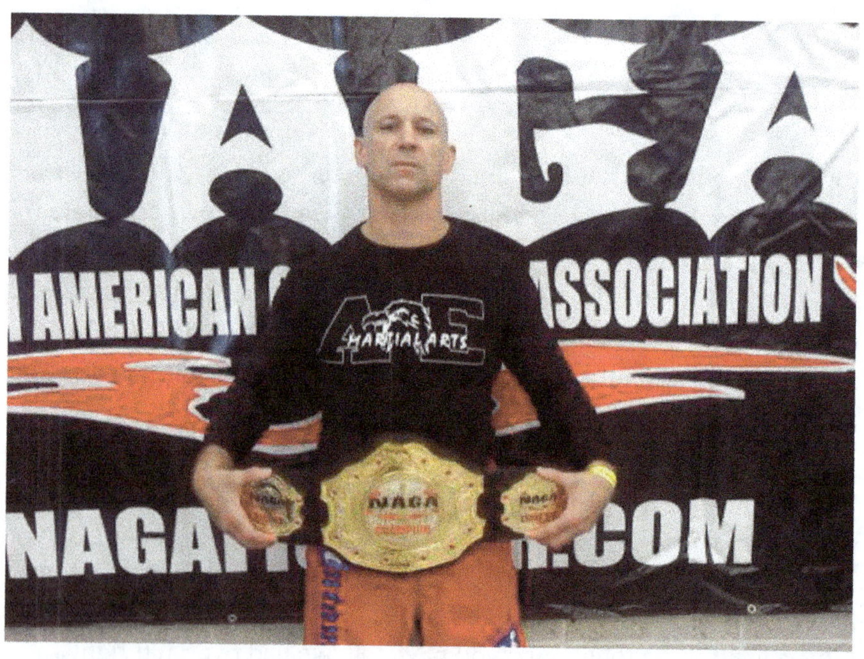

I have been on the wrong end of knives, nunchakus, guns, clubs, chains, bottles, and multiple attackers, and have been in some other extremely precarious situations where I had to rely upon my wits and training to survive. I will be the first to say that I've been extraordinarily fortunate not to have had more serious injuries or met my demise—although I did sustain one heck of a beating once when I fought six guys. Not a smart move, but hey, sometimes those things happen.

I will also tell you that I'd rather be lucky than good. But I am convinced that you create your own luck, whether it be good or bad. As the great coach Vince Lombardi said, "Luck is when opportunity meets preparation." As a street fighter, bouncer or protection specialist, you want to be as prepared as possible so that when the opportunity arises, luck will be on your side!

Victory favors neither the wicked nor the righteous, *victory favors the prepared*. Fail to prepare, prepare to fail.

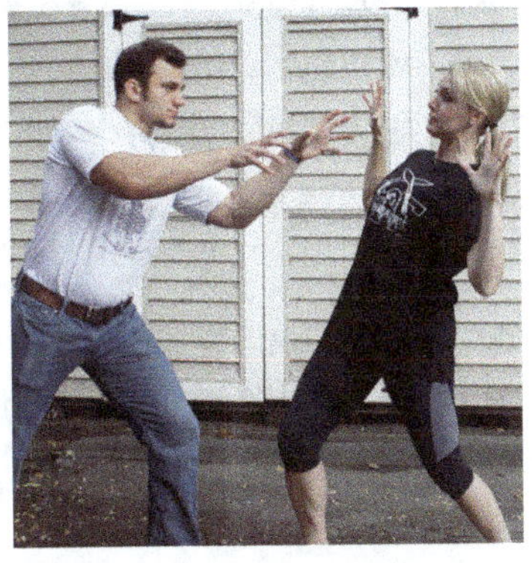

There are endless slogans regarding being prepared for good reason. Being prepared not only has you trained for the situation, and equipped with the proper tools, but it also gives you the confidence and belief in yourself to employ your skills when called upon. The police will be there in minutes when seconds count, leaving you as your only realistic line of defense.

Statistics demonstrate that everyone will be a victim of a violent crime at some point in their lives. Knowing this, you have to ask yourself, what measures have you taken to beat the odds?

Are you prepared to handle the situation when violence comes knocking at your door? How will you react? Will you be able to protect yourself and your family? What will you do in the face of a home invasion? How will you handle a terrorist attack? What would you do if faced with multiple attackers? How will you address the various weapons that you may face? What will you do if you are faced with an execution-type assault?

The most important factors are your mindset and your training. Notice that I put my mindset first. Your mind is your most potent weapon. It is your mind that drives you to train and have the proper attitude to fight back. Meanwhile, your training must be purposeful and regular. It's not enough to think that you "know what to do". I know how to hit a baseball, yet I don't play for the Yankees. You need to practice so you will be able to react instantly and without thinking to any impending threat. IT, or Instinctive Technique, needs to be developed.

There is a Kukri (short sword) recitation in Bando (a Burmese martial art) that states: "Repeat draws, cuts and blocks. Repeat steps, turns and locks until sword frees from thought." In layman's terms, you need to practice so you are able to simply react without hesitation and without thought. If you have to stop to think, it's too late. The time you needed to think has cost you precious milliseconds. Maybe that's all you had. Do not permit yourself to become a statistic.

We need to employ the Four A's and S.I.P.D.E. These two components go hand in hand. They are essential survival skills and should be practiced until they become second nature.

Chapter 1
Introduction

The art of learning how to defend oneself is developed through skills acquired during defensive tactics training. It's not as simple as "how to defend against a choke". There are a multitude of factors and determinants to take into account during your preparation. Not only must we consider mindset and avoidance, but we have to look at various types of technique application.

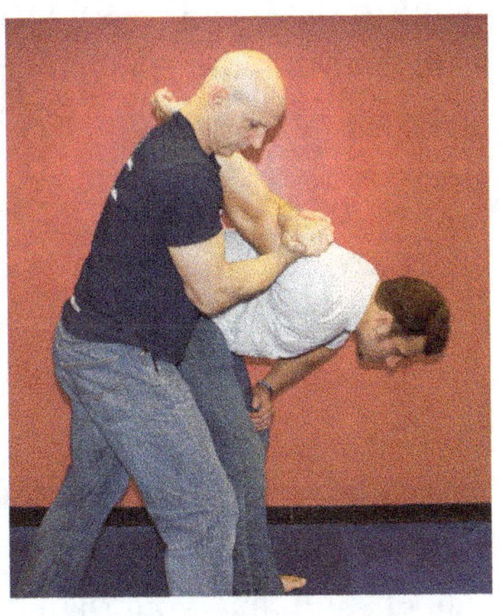

There are different levels of threat, for lack of a better phrase. These are determined by the distance of the offender, the speed of the attack and the circumstances, none of which you will have control over. You can only control how you respond to these situations.

The types of situations you may encounter include:

1. Confrontation with a verbal exchange
2. Confrontation with no verbal exchange

3. Surprise attack when you are caught off guard
4. Hostage situations
5. Intercepting an attack with a preemptive strike

All of these scenarios are addressed in the *Survival Strong Self-Defense and Strength System,* which combines the leveraging of body weight and sound defensive tactics. The system is practical, concise and unmatched. Not everyone has the time, inclination or circumstances to join a full-blown martial arts school and train for hours and hours a week to advance in belt levels. This system can be incorporated into an existing martial arts program, or it can be used as a standalone training regimen that will help you develop great strength and defensive skills with very little or no equipment at all.

The movements and techniques espoused are designed for partners, small groups, and/or solitary practice. If it's inconvenient at times to train with another person, many of the techniques, much of the pad work and the strength and conditioning elements may be practiced alone.

There are certain aspects of the training that do require a partner. *When training for actual combat, there is no substitute for actual human-to-human (man-to-man) action.* Even though bag work and pad work are strongly recommended, the variables of another human body cannot be replicated with any apparatus in your solo training. The bag and pad work are necessary for helping you develop power in your techniques and ensure that your hands and feet are properly positioned when executing striking techniques. Whatever your circumstance is, train often, mix your methods and make your training a regular part of your life.

In self-defense gross motor skills trump small, intricate and complex techniques. You will discover that many of our defensive responses end up in one of a few (seven basic) positions. This is appropriate, since in a stressful situation you will only be able to recall five to nine strategies and/or concepts.

The "Magic Number Seven, plus or minus two" theory was developed by Princeton University cognitive psychologist George Miller. According to Miller, the human mind can only hold seven plus 5-9 objects in its working memory at any given moment. This is referred to as *Miller's Law* and is one of the main reasons that phone numbers and social security numbers have seven and nine digits (minus the area code of course!) Additionally, the more components involved, the greater the chance is for something to go wrong.

There are certain principles to be aware of that must be adhered to when practicing and applying techniques. They include the following:

- Anticipate the worst at all times and always maintain good physical condition.
- Trust no one and always assume that there is more than one attacker
- Operate on the "All or Nothing" principle: either do nothing or completely incapacitate the opponent(s) to ensure your survival and escape
- Always practice vigilance and look for unconventional weapons and escape routes.

As for the actual fighting, your stance is extremely important. You must be able to move quickly, comfortably and with power, taking angles to improve your position in relation to your opponent. Keep your hands up at all times, even when speaking; place your hands up (open palm) and out front and one foot slightly back in a "hidden" fighting stance. Your assailant will not feel threatened or may have no idea that you have already assumed a fighting position. However, your hands are in a "Defend and Counterattack" position and with your one foot back, you have moved your center line out of the direct line of attack plus increased your ability to move and strike. Develop the ability to "Flip the Switch" from being docile to an aggressive, formidable predator!

You can maintain your balance by keeping your nose over your navel, while preserving a good posture and a neutral spine. Don't use force against force; the stronger opponent will always win. The navel points in a power direction, and the hip position is crucial. Never have straight knees when you are facing your opponent, this leaves you immobile and vulnerable to attacks to that area. Point your index finger in the direction that you want to take your opponent, when performing small joint locks.

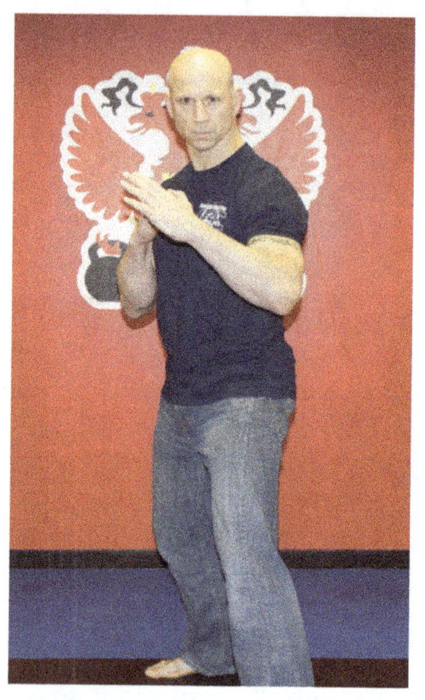

Deliver strikes to hard parts of the body with the soft part of your hand and strike the soft parts with a hard part of your body. The whole notion of yin/yang comes into play here. Dark vs light, good vs evil and hard vs soft. It is better to strike someone with a closed fist to the abdomen rather than punch them in the head. You stand a greater chance of injuring yourself going "Hard to Hard." Soft to Soft is not as effective. Slapping an opponent with an open hand to the stomach may be annoying, but generally will not produce sufficient trauma to put them down. On the other hand a well-placed knee to the stomach, bladder or groin can be extremely effective.

Only trained, seasoned fighters stand a chance of not injuring their hands with a strike to an opponent's face or head. However, many fighters have broken their hands even while gloved in combat or training. Use the soft parts of your body to attack the hard parts of your assailant and vice versa for maximum effectiveness with minimum risk of injury to yourself.

Strike an opponent without chambering your technique or "drawing back to go forward." Doing so will significantly slow down your techniques and "telegraph" your strikes. It is essential to practice delivering your blows from your hips while utilizing full body tension as you lock into the technique.

The incomparable Bruce Lee developed a technique called the "one-inch punch," which encapsulates this wisdom. Starting from a completely relaxed state, move and apply full body tension upon contact. Whether executing a one-inch, three-inch or standard strike, employ this method for maximum power.

Distract your opponent by striking with the closest hand, foot or knee and understand leverage to gain and maintain an advantage. "Vanish" from your opponent's view by always maintaining angles and improving your ability to deliver strikes to exposed and vulnerable areas. Always keep your eyes on the lower center of your opponent's chest during initial contact. Learn basic limb dynamics and their associated reflexive movements. It is important to know how the body reacts to being hit and what the resulting movement will be after you deliver a blow.

Most vital and semi-vital target areas are located centerline. It is crucial to keep yours unavailable as much as possible and focus your strikes on your opponent's. Thus, knowing and working your angles is critical. Your attacks and counterattacks should always attempt to end with a significant strike to these areas. This will increase your rate of success.

Keep the back of your hand facing your opponent (your palm facing you). This will position the back of your hand between you and a possible edged weapon. The back of your forearm is more resilient than the front. Arteries are located on the inside section of your arms (as well as the inside of your legs). Always assume that your opponent is armed even if you don't see a weapon. If he brandishes a weapon, assume he has another. There have been many examples of a victim disarming an assailant only to be attacked by the opponent with a secondary weapon.

When practicing disarming tactics, NEVER hand the weapon back to your training partner. This will create improper muscle memory. Remember, "Perfect practice makes perfect." There have been many occurrences of trained martial artists disarming an assailant, only to hand the weapon back to them as if by reflex! Don't be *that guy!*

To expand on this notion even more, don't help your partner up once you've taken them down. No one is going to help you up in the street, so you better practice how to get up on your own, into a defensive posture. You don't want to knock a perpetrator down and then help them up because you have trained yourself "to be nice" to your training partner. Let them and you both get up on your own accord and you'll be doing both of you a favor.

Take advantage of the element of surprise. In every confrontation, there is one opportunity to make a decisive move. If you are smaller, appear weaker or are unarmed, your perpetrator may not expect you to launch an attack. Use their notion of superiority to your advantage. Do your best to mentally disarm them and then take advantage of the opening.

Getting back to the "All or Nothing" principle, you either "go or you don't go." *Never do anything halfway or hold back at all.* If you are faced with an imminent threat, go all out and completely finish your assailant. You hit and hit as hard as you possibly can until you no longer see movement or you have rendered your opponent helpless enough to secure your escape. Your survival and the survival of your loved ones are dependent upon your ability to act and react swiftly and furiously.

The average street confrontation lasts a mere ten-seconds, but you still need to be in outstanding shape. Yes, most street confrontations last only seconds, but there is a condition that occurs during stressful situations called an adrenaline dump. This occurs when the body goes into *Fight, Flight* or *Freeze* mode. The better condition you are in, the better your body processes stress and the better you'll be able to control your breathing.

Additionally, what if you are tired after a long day of work or travel? What if you are a little sick? What if the fight does last more than a few seconds and you need to contend with multiple attackers?

Also consider that you are quicker and stronger if you are in good physical condition. Did you consider that you may go into cardiac arrest if you are overweight and become stressed?

If you don't want to dedicate yourself to fitness, this book is not for you. Either hire bodyguards or get a gun and a big dog, or just never leave your house.

Meet Phil Ross M.S.

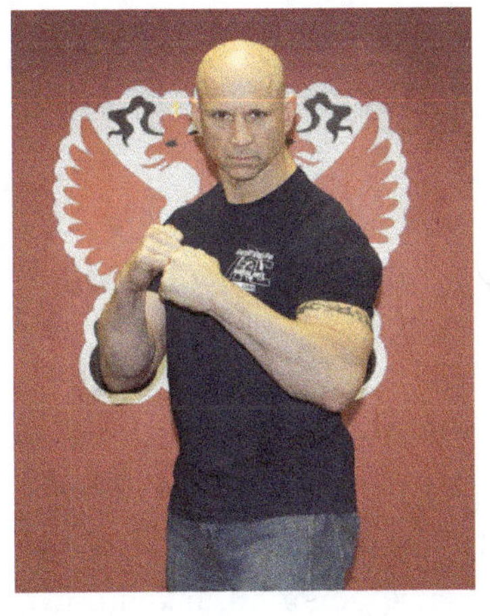

I developed the American Eagle Mixed Martial Arts and Defensive Tactics system from a unique blend of martial arts training and real-world experience.

These martial arts included Burmese Bando, Combat Jiu Jitsu, Brazilian Jiu Jitsu, Korean Taekwondo, Filipino Arnis, Jun Fan, Muay Thai, Western boxing and wrestling, Submission fighting and Shotokan karate. In addition to the formal martial arts, I was an executive protection agent for over ten years, as well as a bouncer in Washington DC, New York City and various establishments in New Jersey for many more years.

The real-life experience that I have had has contributed significantly to the realistic application of techniques I recommend and the tried-and-true theories set forth. I successfully competed on the national level in wrestling, karate, taekwondo, submission fighting, free-fighting and continuous point fighting from 1979 through 2010. Including wrestling, I was victorious in approximately 500 physical contests in the aforementioned disciplines. These numbers do not include the physical confrontations incurred during my employment as a bouncer or bodyguard, as those number in excess of 200 conflicts.

In order to effectively teach a defensive tactics program, you have to have significant experience in either the street, in the ring or on the mat, and I have all three.

The street or "real-life" experience is to be gained from the military, as a police officer, bouncer or bodyguard, from being incarcerated, or from other volatile environments where there are no rules and anything can happen. The ring would include any of the full-contact sports that involve striking. This includes, but is not limited to boxing, kickboxing. Muay Thai, full-contact (or knock-down) karate, Mixed Martial Arts (or cage fighting) or any other type of competition where a knockout is permitted. The last area is on the mat, and this would include wrestling, judo, Brazilian Jiu Jitsu, Pankration, Catch Wrestling and of course Mixed Martial Arts.

Also included on this list is any full contact grappling competition where the controlling, submitting or manipulating of another individual is required for victory. If you are a black belt in a kata-based system or practice self-defense maneuvers learned from a DVD or YouTube video, you are not qualified to develop, provide advice or otherwise present a defensive tactics system. You must have trained, competed, or been faced with situations where bodily harm could have come to you and you must have a measure of experience being hit, taken down or forced to submit. I'm not saying that you have to be a UFC Champion or a Navy SEAL to be able to teach, but you have to have had some real-world experience.

Here are some of my Accomplishments and Credentials:

- 2023: Certified CCW (Concealed Carry Weapons) for New Jersey and Florida
- 2023: Certified USA Boxing Coach
- 2022: Coach/Presenter with The Z-Winning Mindset
- 2022: Outstanding Leadership Award, Education 2.0

- 2021: Full-Time Lecturer at Bergen Community College
- 2021: Nominated as America's Favorite Trainer, BurnAlong
- 2021: APUS/AMU, American Public University System Adjunct Professor
- 2021: P3 Training Group Defensive Tactics and Fitness Instructor
- 2021: Association of College and University Educators (ACUE) Certified
- 2020: UBQFIT Trainer Relations: Virtual Training Platform Consultant
- 2020: Industry Advisory Council member for the Sports & Health Sciences program at APUS
- 2020: Collaborative Institutional Training Initiative IRB member ID# 30892170
- 2020: Featured Blade Wielder in the *Trusted Butcher Chef Knife* infomercial
- 2019: Launched the BodyBell Method
- 2019: Featured Performer on History's Knife or Death
- 2019: Selected as the AMU/APUS Graduate Commencement Speaker
- 2019: Master's Degree AMU: Sports and Exercise Science
- 2018: Our Health is Wealth: Fitness Coordinator
- 2018: Blade Wielder on History's Knife or Death and Forged in Fire
- 2018: Contract Trainer New York Football Giants
- 2017: ACE Certified Personal Trainer
- 2017: Adjunct Professor: Bergen Community College
- 2017: IBJJF Registered Black Belt
- 2016: Authored the book Ferocious Fitness
- 2016: Black Belt in Brazilian Jiu Jitsu, Team CheckMat under Prof. Mitch Coats
- 2016: Principal Actor in the Commando Light commercial
- 2016: Feature Presenter at the 2nd Annual Health & Strength Conference
- 2015: Authored first edition of book SURVIVAL STRONG

- 2015: Featured Presenter at the Health and Strength Conference
- 2014: Developed Survival Strong Certification program
- 2014: Parisi's Speed School Programming Board
- 2014: Expert on Back Health panel aired on local TV
- 2014: Featured Presenter at the ACE Symposium in Orlando, FL
- 2014: Chief Instructor for Survival Strong
- 2014: Kettlebell and Bodyweight Consultant for Parisi's
- 2013: Progressive Calisthenics Certified
- 2012: Promoted to Master RKC Kettlebell Instructor
- 2012: Team Alliance Brazilian Jiu Jitsu Instructor
- 2011: East-West Martial Alliance: Appointed as System Head (Naban)
- 2010: NAGA Battle of the Beach: Expert Level Submission Fighting Champion
- 2010: RKC Team Leader and CK-FMS Certified Movement Specialist
- 2009: Region 2 Wrestling Team of the Year, Head Coach, Mahwah
- 2009: NBIAL Wrestling Champs, Head Coach, Mahwah
- 2008-2012: UFC Fight Trainer, Corner and Coach
- 2008: County Wrestling Champs, Head Coach, Mahwah
- 2008: RKC Certified Level 2 Instructor
- 2008: Asst. Wrestling Coach of the Year, District 5 NJSAAI
- 2007: RKC Certified Kettlebell Instructor
- 2007: Head of Security, NJ All-Star Girls Soccer Team to Brazil
- 2007: NJ Licensed Mixed Martial Arts Trainer and Manager
- 2006: Mahwah HS Wrestling Coach, League Champs, State Sectionals 2005: Certified Shamrock Submission Fighting Level II Instructor
- 2005: Inducted to the Action Martial Arts Hall of Fame
- 2004: Certified Shamrock Submission Fighting Level I Instructor

- 2003: AFPA Certified Personal Trainer
- 2000: Garden State Games Black Belt Heavyweight Sparring Champion
- 2000: Garden State Games Karate Masters' Kata Champion
- 1999: Certified CDT Master Tactical Instructor
- 1998: Medalist in Weapons, Kata and Free-Fighting, Bando Nationals
- 1997: President-Elect of the International Federation of Fighting Arts
- 1997: NRA Certified in Use of Handguns for Protection Purposes
- 1997: Featured in the CDT Police and Bodyguard Manual
- 1996: MVP Award in the New York vs. New Jersey Team Challenge
- 1996: United Kung Fu Federation - Competitor of the Year Award
- 1995: Amateur National Heavyweight Freestyle Fighting Champion
- 1995: Garden State Games Empty-hand and Weapons Dual Medalist
- 1994: World Martial Arts Hall of Fame - "Man of the Year"
- 1994: Instructor, NJ Dept. of Criminal Justice, Defensive Tactics
- 1994: Captain of Garden State Games - Black Belt Championship Team
- 1994: Captain of World Karate Union - Team New Jersey
- 1993: Instructor for the State-of-the-Art Security Training Commission
- 1993: NJ State AAU Taekwondo Chairman
- 1992: Bronze Medalist - AAU Taekwondo Nationals
- 1989: Featured Performer ABC WWS "Oriental World of Self-Defense"
- 1989: Garden State Games, Black Belt Heavyweight Gold Medalist
- 1988: Big Apple Challenge Heavyweight Karate Champion

Phil Ross M.S.

- 1987: Reebok Classic Powerlifting Champion - 181 lbs.
- 1983: Mr. DC - Middleweight Bodybuilding, 3rd Place
- 1982: University of Maryland Olympic lifting Champion - 181 lbs.
- 1981: Empire State Games Karate Champion
- 1981: Mr. Wilkes Bodybuilding Champion
- 1979: AAU Junior Olympic Eastern National Greco- Roman Runner-up

Chapter 2
Real-World Application

When considering self-defense and actual application. There's nothing like hearing it from those who have "Walked the Walk." Many people "Talk the Talk", but what have they really done? I have trained and worked with both of these types of professionals in the field. We have seen each other in action on a multitude of occasions, both in the ring and out. Percy Alston and I were training partners for years and bounced at several bars together. We competed on the same karate team in college. Steve Cirone and I trained together on many occasions and worked a fair amount of security, as well as bodyguard assignments. We also worked together as instructors to teach defensive tactics to law enforcement agents on many occasions.

Read what they have to say and enjoy:

I have known Phil for more than thirty years. When we first met, we were bouncers at a local bar near the University of Maryland. We also trained together at the University of Maryland Bando club. I had also trained in various styles of martial arts, as did Phil. I believe that we were doing what is now called "Mixed Martial Arts". As bouncers, we fought and/17 or engaged with people on a nightly basis.

These fights were rough and sloppy. In the early 1980s, they were also more "honorable." Most of the fights were one-on-one and weapons weren't utilized. This is just what you would expect in a college bar. While working, we never lost a fight. During this time, we both competed in numerous karate tournaments. I did well, but wasn't the best point fighter. I relied heavily on my power. Phil was more successful in the tournaments because of his speed and agility.

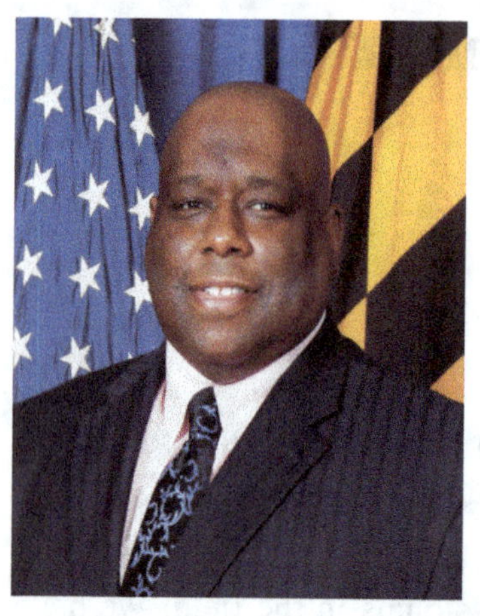

In 1984, I became a Prince George's County Police Officer. PG County is a jurisdiction that borders Washington, DC and Northern Virginia. While it is considered somewhat affluent, there are many pockets that are laced with poverty and riddled with violent crime. Early on and for most of my career, I worked as a narcotics investigator in an undercover capacity. My philosophy about fighting changed from bouncing and competitive fighting to fighting for life or death. Dealing with murderers, robbers and drug dealers, I knew that losing a fight might cost me my life.

While I was a police officer, Phil and I continued to train together until he moved back to New Jersey. Phil started a martial arts gym. I gravitated to and competed in powerlifting. When we had a chance to get together, he would show me new holds, throws and techniques that I was able to apply throughout my career. Even though these techniques weren't taught or approved by my department, I was going to do whatever it took to stay alive. I know that my martial arts training honed my ability to perceive a threat. I was 18 able to use wrist locks, chokes and strategic strikes in order to achieve pain compliance while arresting the bad guys.

Unfortunately, I have seen a lot of police officers receive unwanted scrutiny and criticism because they lost control and used too much force or struck someone too many times while attempting to effect an arrest. Image, appearance and body language definitely play a part in how people size you up. If you project an image of strength and confidence, a potential adversary will take pause before deciding to confront you. On the other hand, if you look weak and vulnerable, you will appear as the perfect victim. Of course, I believe my greatest skill was/is my ability to avoid, and talk my way out of or through violent encounters. All of this comes from maturity and experience.

As a law enforcement officer, I observe people meander through life as what I call "sheeple". These are people who always follow and are not prepared for life's challenges. They present themselves as victims. Unfortunately, in our society there are wolves or predatory criminals who are looking for the "sheeple". In 2014, this is a fact of life. While Phil and I will never prey on the weak, when the wolves see us, they will turn and run or be repelled.

Percy Alston
Retired Prince George's County Police Officer.
Instructor (Criminal Law and Narcotics) Public Safety and
Security Institute
Municipal Police Academy Prince George's Community
College

My name is Steve Cirone. Born (1961) and raised in Hudson County, New Jersey. Across the river from New York City.

I have three tough brothers. Growing up wasn't easy. Fighting with my brothers every day until we were bloody, was normal. Also, I survived many street battles. I've been shot in the knee, stabbed in the arm, hit in the face with bottles, hit in the head with a two-by-four, had my nose broken six times, spent several weekends in jail and much more. Also, the enormous number of devastating tragedies that I have endured throughout my life, hardened me even more. I've been a bouncer, a bodyguard, and a boxer since 1978. A street fighter most of my life. I also worked as a corrections officer. I earned a black belt in a street combative style of martial arts, taught to me by a great instructor (Tom Patire). I was inducted into the International Black Belt Hall of Fame in 1999. I'm a U.S. Army veteran. I'm an instructor of martial arts, boxing, kick-boxing, fitness, and defensive tactics for police and body-guards. I have many other certifications.

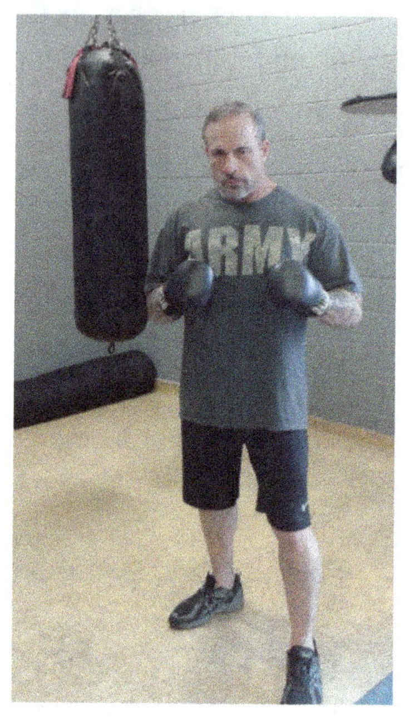

I'm also deeply involved with MMA cage fighting. My resume goes on and on. I'm a highly seasoned and experienced veteran of protecting people, crowd control, defusing volatile situations and confrontation. I'm about to share some real-life situations that I've experienced and how my martial arts training and street knowledge came into play.

First, I'd like to say something about Phil Ross. I've known Phil Ross for a very long time. He is like my brother. We have worked as bodyguards together, as bouncers together, as instructors together, fought back-to-back, and protected people together many times. I trust him with my life. Phil's credentials speak for themselves. I vouch for him one hundred percent.

I've been involved in thousands of dangerous, hands-on, life on the line, take care of business situations. Let me share a few with you.

Several years back, I was hired to work as a bodyguard, protecting a news crew and a news reporter in a rough area of New York City. The neighborhood was volatile and on the verge of a riot because one of the locals had been killed by a cop. I was standing by the news van with the reporter and news crew. The reporter was sitting in the van with the side doors open. A man approached the news van that the reporter was sitting in. I stopped the man by identifying myself and telling him to step back please. He said, "I want to talk to the reporter." I once again said "Step back please." The reporter said, "I'll talk to him."

The man stepped closer to the van and started talking to the reporter. I positioned myself to protect the reporter if needed. The man put his hand in his pocket. He started to pull a knife out of his pocket. I immediately reacted. I took the man down using a martial arts/bodyguard technique, as I disarmed the knife. I held him down using another technique, as I was controlling him on the ground, I looked across the street and noticed that the locals were looking at me and yelling at me with anger, as if I was hurting one of their own. The authorities were informed; they arrived and took the man away. I didn't think of the danger I was in. I was just doing my job. What I did came naturally, thanks to my training.

The next experience I'd like to share with you took place in a night-club on the Jersey shore, where I was the head bouncer at the time. The place was rocking as fifteen hundred people were drinking and dancing and having a wild time. The beer muscles were flexing. A fight broke out on the dance floor. Fists were flying. I signaled my crew of bouncers. I was the first to arrive. I stepped in to break up the fight. The other bouncers soon arrived to help. We had to get rough with some of the participants. We got the fight under control. Ten or so had to be escorted out of the club. As my bouncers escorted the last few out, I was watching the bouncers' backs, when suddenly, a choke hold was applied to my neck from the rear. The choke was very tight. I said, "What are you doing?" The man choking me said, "You threw my friend out, this is what I know how to do."

At that point, I put my body in the position it needed to be in to defend myself. I then said to him, "You better let go." He said, "F*** you." At that point, I went into action. I used a martial arts technique to get myself out of the choke hold, and in one motion I reversed his arm, dislocated his shoulder out of the socket, and took him down to the ground. Then I picked him up, and ran him through the club and out the front door, while controlling his arm with a chicken wing technique and passed him off to the authorities.

My mindset when handling a volatile situation or any situation, is unique. Defusing situations and putting people in their place and standing up for what's right, and trying to keep order, and never backing down, is who I am, and it comes natural to me. Thank you for letting me share with you some of my life experiences. There was another time; Phil Ross and I were working security together at a 600-person private party, which turned into two rival gangs starting a riot, which Phil and I were in the middle of, trying to defuse it. (That was fun.) That story is for another time.

Steve Cirone
Black Belt
Security Expert
VIP Bodyguard
Army Veteran

Chapter 3
Mindset

There are certain defining moments in everyone's life and the one I am about to describe has motivated my quest for street fighting prowess. Previously there were quite a few less severe confrontations, but this one had a significant impact on me and my mindset when it came to defending myself.

I must warn you, it's fairly graphic and what transpired may upset you in some way. If you don't like what I did and how I defended myself, that's too bad. I responded to an attack by an older, larger and more experienced assailant, and I did what I felt I had to do to win and deter any further potential retaliation. There will be others reading this who may not think the incident is a big deal.

I'm OK with that as well. Bear in mind that I was only seventeen years old at the time.

That being said, this is one of the incidents that I can relay without any potential legal ramifications. One, I was only seventeen and the assailants were above the age of majority. Two, I'm writing this book 34 years after the fact. So, I am quite certain that the statute of limitations has long expired. Three, there was a time that the perpetrator relinquished his opportunity to press charges because he was not only involved in an assault on a minor, but also trespassing.

It was June,1980. I believe that it was Friday night for two reasons. I know that I graduated on a Thursday night and the Friday night was June 20th (or at least Google Calendar shows it as the date). We were celebrating my high school graduation and hosting a big shindig with a band and family and friends in attendance. Please note that I had quite a few friends from other towns, and being wrestlers, many of us formed friendships with the area athletes. So there were quite a few young, tough kids at my house.

Three uninvited guests showed up and a couple of my friends that I had assigned to the bouncing duties denied their entrance and subsequently threw them out. They got into their car and drove off, almost hitting me and two other guests, one of them a female (my date). I yelled at them, and they turned their vehicle around. One kid decided to throw an M-80 at me.

An M-80 is a potent firecracker. *It has the power of one-fourth a stick of dynamite. I leaped out of the way as the explosion resounded through the air. They sped off.*

Little did they know that I lived on a circular court, one way in and one way out. They were traveling the long way out. I directed my friends to cut them off with their car. They sped to the intersection and blocked the road. The party emptied behind me as we ran to the corner and engulfed their car.

The driver had his window open, so I reached in, grabbed him by the throat with one hand and pummeled his face with my other, very willing fist. The kid in the back seat got out; one of my friends grabbed him and tossed him across the hood of the car. Another of my friends jumped on the vehicle's hood and started to stomp up and down on it.

Before I ran to the other side of the car, I first stopped to punch dents into the car's trunk. The only guy who had not gotten hit yet was the one who threw the firecracker. I asked him, "You like throwing fire-

crackers?" He received the same treatment as the driver, only worse. We left the three bloodied and battered and headed back to the party "high-fiving" each other and giving each other accolades for administering immediate retribution. Only, it wasn't over yet...

The displaced partiers decided to recruit some muscle and attempt to exact their own vengeance. They were to be met with a surprise.

Five guys showed up at my party as it was winding down. I think it was close to midnight, and nothing good ever happens after this hour. They were older than my friends and me. Some of them had been out of high school for a few years already, others more recently.

Set the stage in your mind now. There were approximately 25 or 30 people left at the party. Mostly close friends and family. We were on my front lawn. My dad was out front and speaking with one of the parents. My father was a former Marine and an ex-All Metropolitan high school football player. He played guard on offense and nose tackle on defense, despite being only 5'8". He did have a fairly short fuse, to say the least.

*The ringleader (let's call him Will Saylor) approached me at the same time my dad directed one of the other uninvited "guests" to get off of our property. The knucklehead said "F**k you!" My dad cracked him in the chest with a forearm shiver and as the guy was off balance, charged him again with the same blow, knocking him into the street. As the "recruited muscle" was sitting on his ass looking up at the world, my dad said, "Now you're off my property."*

Now, the ringleader was about 6'1 or 6'2", 185 pounds or so. He had a rap sheet as long as your arm. He was thrown out of high school for detonating explosives and had apparently done some time. He had the reputation of being the best street fighter in town and I know a couple of rough kids that he had beaten up. At the time I was about 5'9" and tipping the scales at 170 pounds.

Immediately after the confrontation with my dad occurred, I walked up to Will Saylor, put my hand on his shoulder and said, "Get you and your girlfriends the hell out of my party and off of my property now! Or I'll break your NECK!"

Saylor *promptly replied with "Get your F**king hands off of me" and swatted my hand away. With that, I punched him with a devastating overhand right that landed squarely between his eyes. Blood spurted out of his head and traveled over 20 feet. One of my friend's dad was picking him up and he still to this day claims that I owe him a shirt from the blood that he got on it! I told him with a chuckle that it wasn't my blood and to get the new shirt from Saylor.*

After the well-placed right hand, Saylor fell backwards and into his group of friends. They propped him up and he staggered forward. I shot in on a double-leg takedown. At this point I achieved a full mount position with me sitting on his chest. I started raining down punches on him, smashing blow after blow into my barely moving target. I was in a frenzy and consumed with bloodlust. I wanted to inflict more pain. I saw his throat and I sunk my teeth right into his neck and tried to tear his flesh off.

Luckily for Mr. Saylor, my friends pulled me off. They had seen me in confrontations before and knew that I wouldn't stop on my own accord. His limp, bleeding body lay on the ground. What was left of his friends picked him up and took him to the hospital.

A week or so later I was with my cousin uptown. We saw him and a few friends. He saw us. As Saylor was standing on the corner with his friends, I instructed my cousin to drive past them slowly. As I gripped my lead-filled pipe in my hand, my cousin stopped the car at the corner where Saylor and his buddies were standing. He had stitches on his face and neck. Both of his eyes were black from me breaking his nose. I looked at him and said, "Hey kid, how's your nose?" He said nothing and we slowly pulled away. On the surface, you may think that what we did and what I said was the wrong thing, but by establishing that I wasn't afraid, I actually squashed any thoughts that he may have had for retaliation.

Now don't get the impression that I think that this is the best course of action. At the time, it was the only one that I felt I could take. Plus, I was young and wanted to impose my will on anyone that challenged me. So-called "experts" falsely state that insecure people have to fight to "prove themselves." Well, I think that is a hundred percent incorrect. Insecure people bully others and pick on weaker victims. They are insecure and suffer from other issues. I tend to agree with the other studies that demonstrate people with high levels of confidence are open to confrontations to prove that they are right.

I have since modified my outlook on fighting. I know what I can do and what I have done. A true warrior tries his best to avoid confrontation for he knows the ramifications of his actions. I know that if I get into a volatile situation, the results will not be good. So, I tend to avoid them and go home before midnight! I will only get into a physical confrontation if I feel the safety of one of my loved ones or myself is in jeopardy. And if I see a person in need, I know that I'll jump in, it's my nature. So is the manner in which I fight.

Always keep these words in mind: *"Cooler heads prevail."* Whether you are dealing with a road-rage incident, a person screaming and threatening you or a knife at your throat - *keep your cool.* This enables you to take advantage of your opportunities and make your move when the occasion presents itself.

If you are still alive and have not allowed yourself to be tied up or taken from Point A to Point B, you will have an opportunity. If you lose your cool, you may miss your chance. Do your best to keep your cool and look for your chance to make a move.

If you can escape, do so. But I'm not going to teach you how to run. There are a great number of highly qualified track coaches, YouTube videos, and books on running available. I'm here to show you options for tactical defense responses.

As stated previously, your mindset is paramount. You must adopt the "All or Nothing" principle. Let us assume that you have exhausted all avoidance techniques, your verbal entreaties were unsuccessful, and you have no choice but to get physical.

Please note that there generally is very little time between verbal and physical confrontations. You have to be a hundred percent committed to the execution of the technique. DO NOT HOLD BACK! You have to be mentally prepared to hit as hard and as often as you are able until the attack is over and the assailant rendered unable to retaliate.

The target areas for your strikes are extremely important. For instance, if a hundred-pound woman were to hit a two-hundred-pound man in the chest, she may use every ounce of her power yet not produce any result, except a more angered perpetrator. Yet if she pokes him in the eye, knees him in the groin and delivers a kick to his shin, she will most likely gain the upper hand, allowing her time to escape.

Everyone has eyes and throats. Everyone also has a groin; however, groin strikes and grabs are more effective on males. It's your job to attack the vital and semi-vital target areas. Proper positioning and an attack on secondary targets may be necessary before reaching the primary targets. Secondary targets include of the back of the head, temple, ears, back of the neck, floating ribs, kidneys, liver, elbows, wrists, inside of the thighs (femoral artery), outside of the thighs (peroneal nerve), shin, talus and the top of the foot.

As a general rule, primary targets are located on the centerline of a person. The major primary targets are the eyes, nose, throat, solar plexus and groin.

Applying a proper strike to these areas generally results in at least a momentary incapacitation of the assailant. Levying strikes to these areas also bides you time to either escape or deliver additional blows to areas of the head, knees and spine to further render your assailant incapable of causing you harm. You must create a situation that enables you to have time to escape before the assailant can retaliate. Destruction of your assailant's limbs or the administration of a knock-out blow is the best method to ensure your successful escape.

Be mentally prepared to unleash Hell when attacked. The life you save may be your own or more importantly, that of a loved one's. Your mindset and your willingness to do whatever is necessary to win is your only chance to gain an edge. Remember, there is no cheating in a street fight. "Fair fights" do not exist. You have to be prepared to do whatever it takes to emerge victorious.

How can you toughen yourself and develop the mindset that enables you to fight, push yourself, believe in yourself and be triumphant? You have to challenge yourself, there are no shortcuts here. Throughout this book you will witness training that will challenge you physically and mentally.

Here's a challenge that I came across and used to strengthen my resolve. I have heard that this test was used by certain Native American tribes and also by some special forces. I cannot attest to either, as I am not from any of the aforementioned groups.

The challenge is, take a cup of water and drink the contents, but DO NOT SWALLOW. Hold the water in your mouth. Place the cup on the ground and go for a two-mile run. When you return, spit the water back into the cup.

Seems simple enough, right? Try it. You can only breathe through your nose and the temptation to swallow the water is great. I've attempted and accomplished this challenge only a few times in my life. I figured the indigenous braves only had to do it once as a rite of passage, but I wanted to do it more than once.

APPAREL

What are you wearing?

You may be asking, "Why is that important?" If you can't move, you can't fight and that's the bottom line. If you can afford to be driven in a limo and have bodyguards, you don't need to concern yourself with apparel. Most of us don't enjoy that luxury though.

Let's go through your wardrobe and start from the ground up.

<u>Shoes:</u> First, you must begin with your shoes. I recall the response from a female executive at a *S.A.V.E.* corporate workshop that I conducted. When I was speaking about footwear, this fashion plate executive stated that she wasn't "going to give up wearing her $350.00 Prada shoes." Her comment elicited a chuckle from the participants. My reply was, "If you ever have to run, you'll not be able to do so wearing those things." Guess what happened? 9/11. She was in Tower 2 and had to run for her life.

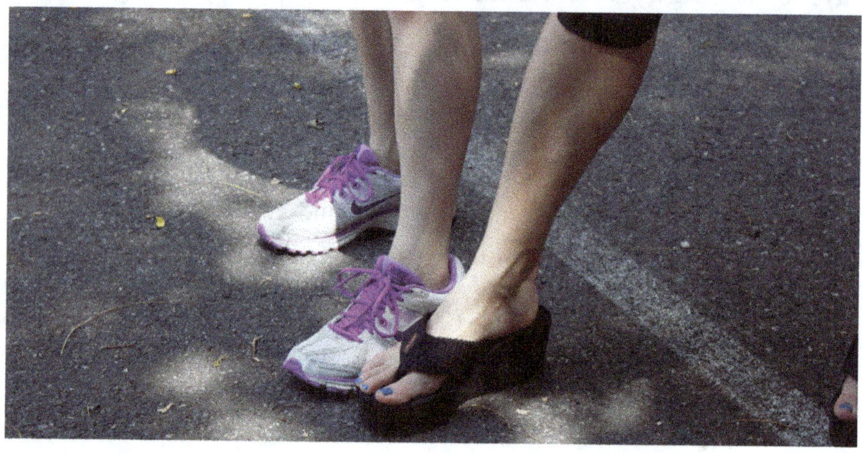

She was forced to kick off her shoes and take off running, subsequently cutting her feet on the fallen debris and shards of glass from the falling towers. Her concern for her expensive footwear went out the window. Isn't it strange how priorities change when one is faced with the reality of life and death?

I will tell you that I got a phone call from her shortly after 9/11, and she asked me to come in for another workshop and to make some recommendations on "fashionable, yet practical footwear." Thank God that she escaped, but had she stepped on something large and sharp, twisted an ankle or injured her knee, she may not have escaped with only minor cuts and bruises.

Examine your footwear. You need to be able to run, kick and climb with it. If you can't, understand the chances that you are taking.

A tight skirt or skin-tight pants do not permit much freedom of movement. Therefore, your ability to run, jump, kick, and stretch is significantly impaired. Your pants or skirt should allow you freedom of movement.

I will not even address those who wear their pants with their underwear exposed. These guys should simply get a knock on the head and be sent home. It's laughable. First of all, no one wants to see your underwear. Secondly, I will not entertain "prison inspired style." Look at the other constraints. How are you going to run or even move with your pants hanging off you like that? It's just plain silly.

Are you wearing a belt? A belt can be used as a great unconventional weapon, especially if it's a sturdy leather one with a sizable buckle. Wrap the belt around your hand and leave a length of six to eight inches free. Wield the buckle end in a Figure 8 motion and keep it between you and your opponent. The leather wrapped around your hand also serves as protection for your knuckles and adds stability to your hand. A belt can also serve as an implement to choke an assailant or as a rope substitute.

The time of year and the weather should dictate your attire. Freedom of movement is hindered if you are wearing a tight jacket. You must be able to throw a punch and move without restrictions due to your clothing.

If you work as a bouncer and are required to wear a tie, use a clip-on. A standard necktie is a great handle for your adversary to grab hold of and yank you around or choke you with. If this does happen, be certain to move with him and deliver a strike to the side of the head of the hand that is gripping the tie. He will be unable to block your strike with that hand while gripping onto your necktie.

I learned this from experience as a nineteen-year-old bouncer.

Luckily for me, I was comfortable at close range. When my necktie got grabbed, I went right into the guy. I was also fortunate that the rest of the bouncers were right there taking care of the others as I grappled with my attacker. I started wearing clip-ons after that incident. The additional upsides are you don't have to spend much time tying a Windsor knot and clip-ons are generally cheaper as well. Two bonus points, and you are also protecting yourself!

What is your adversary wearing? Does he have a heavy jacket on? What is he wearing on his lower extremities? How about his footwear?

You want to consider one aspect, in almost any weather condition, and that is that people tend to not have much clothing on their lower bodies. Generally, there is only a thin layer of cloth between you and the vital and semi-vital target areas. Your initial strikes should be directed to the shins, groin, pubic bone, peroneal nerve (IT band), and femoral arteries of the lower body. The upper-body attacks should be focused on the areas above the throat, including the throat, carotid arteries, eyes, ears, temple, nose, and mandibular process. These areas are generally exposed and readily accessible.

THE FOUR A'S - AWARENESS, AVOIDANCE, ACTION AND AGGRESSION

AWARENESS

Be aware of your surroundings. Where are the escape routes? What are the potential hazards in the room or area? Who is in the vicinity? Where are the "friendlies" and "foes"? Who just walked into the movie theater or restaurant? Who is looking at my child? Why is that guy hovering around the playground? What is that knapsack doing on the floor of the train? Why are there three guys standing in the unlit doorway of that building? Where did you park your car? Who is on the plane, bus or train? Do I have a weapon? What weapons in the environment are available to me? How am I dressed?

This applies a great deal to women. As previously addressed, many women sacrifice mobility for fashion's sake. You should be able to kick, run, and jump in your attire. Know the limitations of your dress and plan accordingly. Know who is in your area and know your escape routes.

You should employ the "Thousand Yard Stare" when walking in populated areas. You look almost through the other people as you pass them. Be aware of them, but direct eye contact is not recommended; neither is "shying" or looking away, though.

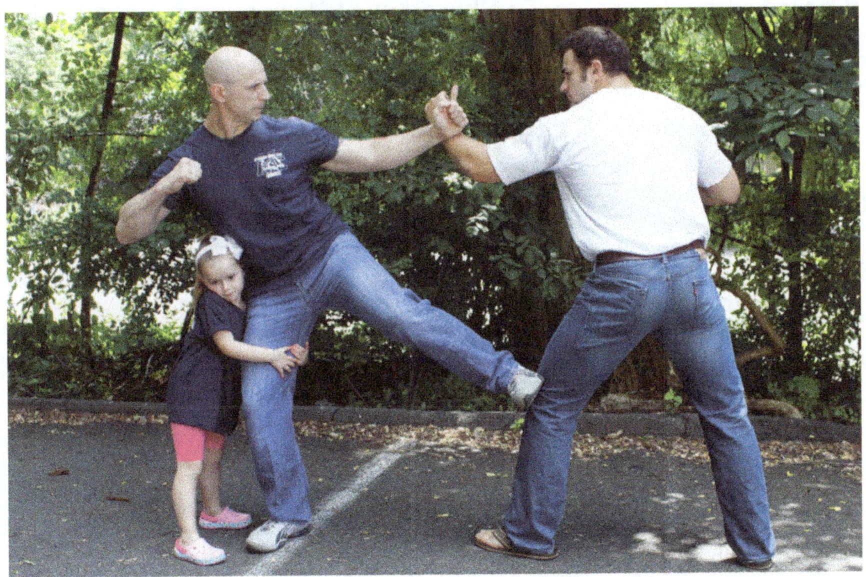

Maintain a neutral disposition and a level head as you scan the area. You should be cognizant of who is in your sight path yet appear unaffected by their presence.

Who am I with? What is my responsibility to them? If you are alone, your immediate responsibility is to yourself. If you have travel companions, what is your responsibility to them? What are the physical limitations and capabilities of my travel companions? My responsibility is different if I am with my wife and children than if I am with my friends, training partners or fellow instructors.

You should have a game plan in place. My wife and children know that if the proverbial "stuff ever hits the fan," they need to take off and get to a safe haven quickly. I'll stay and deal with the imminent threat. I'd rather deal with the assailants alone than have my mind occupied with worry about the safety of my family. Set a designated meet-up place selected prior to traveling, as this is a helpful strategy if you get separated.

Be Alert. Period. If you are walking down the street or in a parking lot and you're texting away or bopping to the music pumping into your ears through a set of headphones, how can you be attuned to your environment? Do yourself a favor—pay attention to what is going on around you.

AVOIDANCE

Most hazardous situations are avoidable. Do not unnecessarily put yourself in harm's way. Perpetrators are predatory, opportunistic creatures who seek the most gain with the least amount of effort.

Does the lion attack the strongest and fastest wildebeest, or does it seek out the weak, slow, old and young targets? Obviously, the lion will take the path of least resistance and the ticket to the easiest meal.

Don't allow yourself to be an easy meal ticket. Avoid potentially harmful situations. It only takes one incident to dramatically change or end your life.

Know where you parked your vehicle. Make sure that it's in a lighted, highly visible area. Know where you are traveling to, and leave ample time to travel—being rushed will cause you to make mistakes. Check your routes prior to your departure. Use your GPS device and have a map and/or a printed route with you as well. Avoid bad or unfamiliar neighborhoods.

Do not get drunk or high! Illegal narcotics should NEVER be used. They should not even be a consideration in the self-preservation equation. Don't take a drink from a stranger. If you need to drink, take it from a bottle that you saw get opened or opened yourself. Keep your hand over the top of the beverage at all times. Don't put your drink down and come back to it. Avoid illegal parties or "secret get togethers."

Listen to the "little voice" in your head and pay attention to your instincts. If you train long enough and focus on your awareness, your survival instincts will develop. If you feel strange or uneasy about an impending situation - DON'T DO IT! There is most likely a good reason that you are feeling apprehensive.

Don't wear excessive or obvious jewelry. Attempt to blend. Be sure that your cell phone has a full charge and that you have a back-up plan. Expect the worst and hope for the best.

When traveling abroad, if you aren't accompanied by a partner who knows the area or if you are not meeting with someone, hire a licensed guide. There are generally bilingual retired or off-duty police officers available in many countries. It's a worthwhile investment. Make certain that you budget for it and have your guide validated by a known and trusted source.

ACTION

Here's where the rubber hits the road! You've taken all of the precautions possible. You've done everything by the book, yet there he is, sticking a gun in your face and demanding your wallet.

So what to do when the inevitable occurs? Look for your opening and make a concise, precise, all-or-nothing relentless action. We have taken into consideration all of the aforementioned variables: if you can run, do so, but if you are coming to your car with your baby in a stroller, you won't be able to get away. You'll have to fight or comply. I cannot and will not preach to you what your personal priorities are. Some people are willing to give up their house, their car and their possessions. Some won't hand over a dime. I'm not here to tell you who is right or wrong. Just know that whatever your position is regarding your choice, you must be comfortable living with it for the rest of your life. You don't want to put yourself in a position of would've, could've or should've.

Focus on a much smaller word - did. What *did* you do to prevent loss, injury or death? Be comfortable with your mindset before a situation occurs. Hindsight is always 20/20. Predict the outcome and minimize the loss. There will always be a potential for loss or harm in an altercation. Oftentimes it's unavoidable, but do your best to keep the losses at a minimum.

AGGRESSION

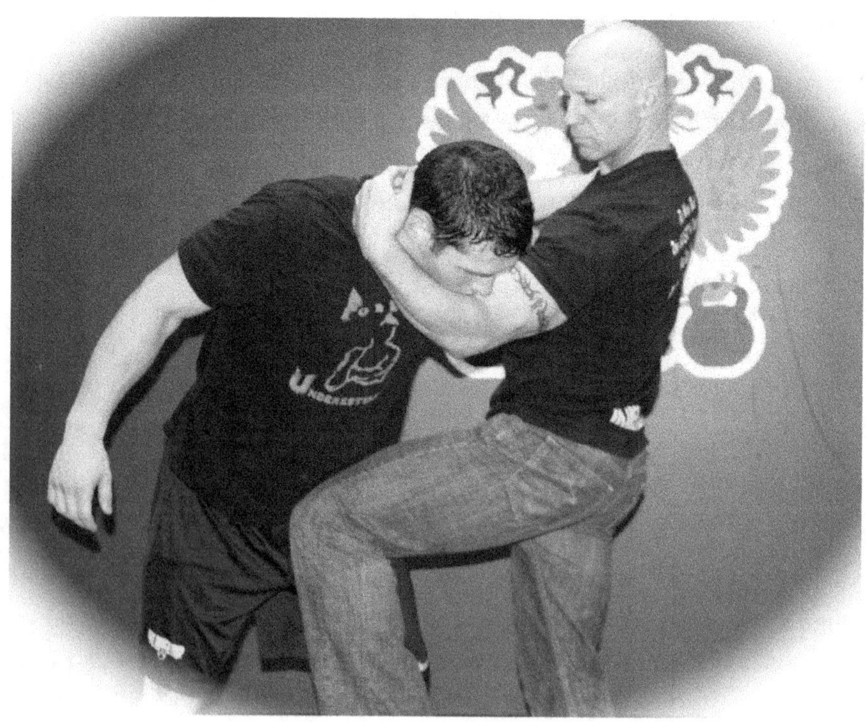

We are all taught from a young age that in modern society, we must be docile and nice to one another. This is all good until it's not good any longer. The people that you face in the street or invading your home or trying to steal your car or abduct you, do not observe these rules.

There are no two ways about it: extreme, focused and relentless aggression is essential to success in a street confrontation. The victim must possess the ability to conjure up all of the power, drive and intestinal fortitude to apply whatever means are necessary to "Flip the Switch" and "Turn the Tables" on the assailant. The Victim must be determined to be the Victor.

For good to triumph over evil, good must be very strong and willingly enlist pure, unadulterated aggression at a moment's notice, directed at the intended target. Aggression bridges the gap and can compensate for lack of size, strength or knowledge. Aggression is your friend in a self-defense situation, so use it.

S.I.P.D.E. - SCAN, IDENTIFY, PREDICT, DECIDE AND EXECUTE

SCAN

Use your ears and ears to scan the area. As with awareness, scan your surroundings looking for potential threats and escape routes. Register who is in the area and take notice of potentially dangerous people.

IDENTIFY

Identify potentially hazardous situations and persons. Recognize the threat(s). Pay attention to how the person(s) is/are standing. What are they wearing? Where are they positioned? Is there a road blocked off? Why are those guys hanging around the street corner? Why is there a burning tire in the middle of the road?

PREDICT

Predict what may occur. Given the assessment of your surroundings, the people, the escape routes, limitations, and other variables; what could happen? These assessments need to be made expeditiously, as time is of the essence. Your safety depends upon you making the right predictions.

DECIDE

Decide what to do. Do I call 911, run, turn around and take a different route, employ verbal contact to determine threat level, attack first, or do nothing? The last option of the normal choice in most instances, but if your senses tell you that something is awry, it most likely is. So whatever action you decide to undertake, make it decisive and complete.

Don't "half" do something. The end result will usually not be good. Unfortunately, you have very little time to make your decision. Things happen fast, *very fast*. You cannot hesitate with whatever course of action you decide to take. Additionally, you must be totally committed.

EXECUTE

Act upon your decision and do so in a concise, precise manner. Some course of action will have to be taken. If you are going to flee, do so, and make it quick. Leave the area and be sure that you are headed to a safe haven. You may avoid an actual physical confrontation by your posturing and verbal response to a potential threat. If you are going to get physical, follow through with full power and intent.

Here's an example from my life that illustrates the importance of execution:

I was in Philadelphia for the weekend. It was late and I was very hungry. I decided to walk down the street and go to an all-night diner.

Maybe not the best choice I could have made, but hunger took over. It was approximately 2:30 AM as I returned to my hotel room. As I rounded the corner, I noticed two other gentlemen across the street. No cars, no other people; just me and the two other guys. I had about a block and a half to walk until I reached my hotel as one of the guys crossed the street toward me.

I noticed them and decided that I was going to take my chances and head toward my hotel. I was too far from the diner and there were no immediate safe havens. I knew that once he crossed the street a confrontation was imminent. I had made my decision and planned to execute it.

As he approached, he asked to "borrow" some money from me. Please note that I did not allow him to get closer than ten feet from me before I aggressively responded with: "Stop right there - I'm in no mood for you or any of your bull#**t! Tell your story walking!" The guy stopped dead in his tracks, turned around and walked back across the street. Had he continued toward me, the first strike would have been a firmly planted low kick followed by axehands, elbows and knees. However, he most likely listened to *his* inner voice and decided to wait for an easier victim.

The whole time I viewed his body language, and posture and watched his hands to see if he was going to pull a weapon and I also kept an eye on his partner across the street. When he left, I did not turn my back on him until he was a reasonable distance away from me. I was also aware of the position his partner had taken. He never advanced.

FIGHT, FLIGHT OR FREEZE

We have all heard of the "Fight or Flight Syndrome."

In real life, more often than not, most people freeze. Fight - you defend yourself. Flight - you run for the hills. However, there has not been much attention dedicated to the *freeze*. Most people have never even been hit, much less attacked. The moment an assailant lays their hands on them or smacks them, they freeze up like a "deer in the headlights" and get bludgeoned. The perpetrators are counting on this.

When the proverbial "*S*" hits the fan, you have to be prepared. There will be an incredible adrenaline dump and your arms and legs will feel very heavy. Things may go in slow motion, and you will experience tunnel vision and what I call the "whirr" in your head. This "whirring" sound occurs right before and during a physical confrontation. This physiological reaction is a result of the infusion of adrenaline, your increased blood pressure and the psychological stressors that the mind undergoes when faced with extreme conditions. The key is to be able to maintain a clear head and allow your body to respond properly.

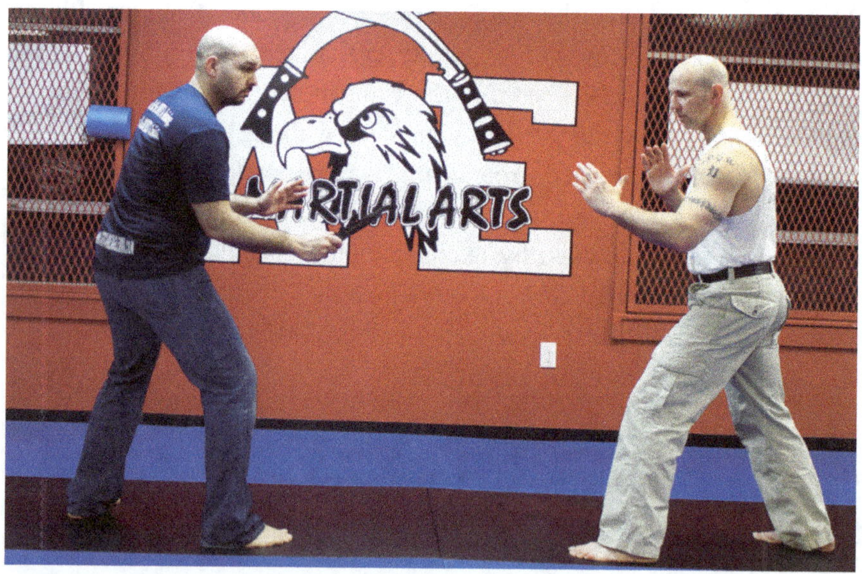

Following our physical training, learning what it feels like to get hit, and undergoing the mental preparation involved will get you prepared. However, until you have been in an actual situation, you will not know how you will react. Please also bear in mind that your reaction may differ from situation to situation, depending upon the circumstances.

One of the best training methods to help the body handle an adrenaline dump is to employ breathing ladders, which you can do using kettle-bells. This type of training has been successfully used by firefighters, police officers and other military and paramilitary organizations to aid in reducing the effects of the adrenaline dump. It involves taking three breaths after completing three reps of a kettlebell exercise, then four breaths after four reps, and so on, making sure not to breathe at all until a set of reps has been completed. This slows breathing down and shows you how to control your breath during a stimulating event.

You need to train and become mentally and physically conditioned to instinctively respond. Thought and emotion have no place here. Concise response and action are required. This ability is acquired through consistent, meaningful training. There are no secrets, beyond diligence and steady effort.

Chapter 4
Physical Fitness and Strength

"To defeat evil, good must be very strong!"

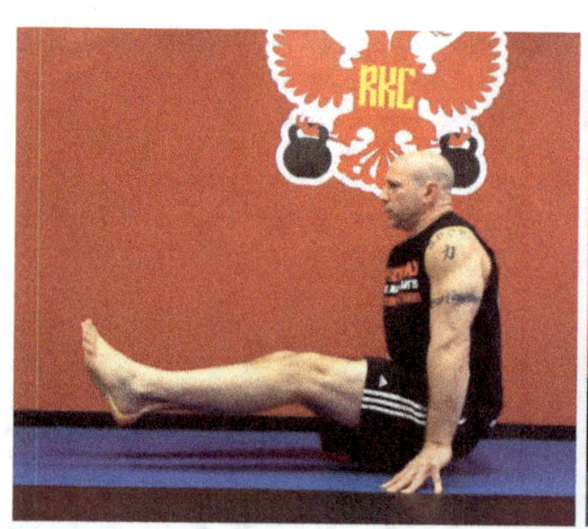
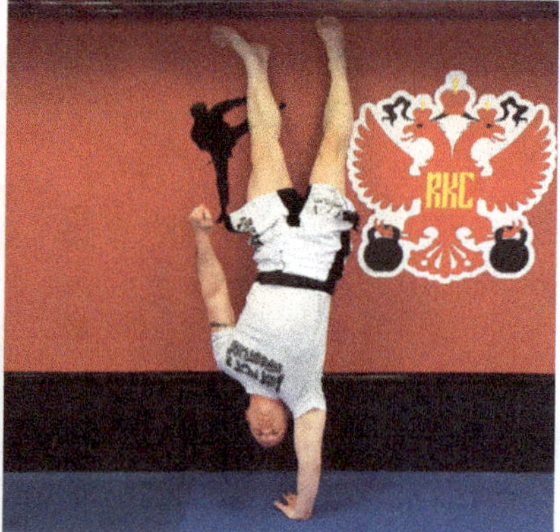

COMPLETE PHYSICALITY

There are certain minimum physical requirements you will need for the proper application of most fighting techniques. For example, you will need flexibility and strength in your hips, shoulders and spine.

It's up to you to forge your body like steel, in order to both withstand a blow and deliver one with maximum effect. If you are conditioned, your chances of survival will be dramatically increased.

POWER DEVELOPMENT

The development of upper and lower body explosive power and general strength is essential to effective striking and throwing. The stronger you are, the easier it will be to impose your will upon another and defend yourself from attack.

KETTLEBELLS, SANDBAGS AND WEIGHT TRAINING

These are excellent methods for developing additional strength. There are many publications dedicated to these training methods. The focus of this book is based on what you are able to do with your body, a partner or very little equipment.

However, if you are using external resistance apparatus, I recommend training three to four times a week. Your workout should be an hour or less. Anything more and you are training for something other than fighting and may actually hinder your performance.

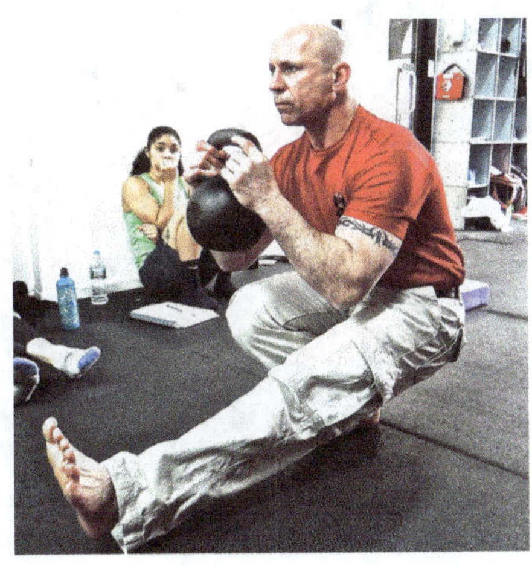

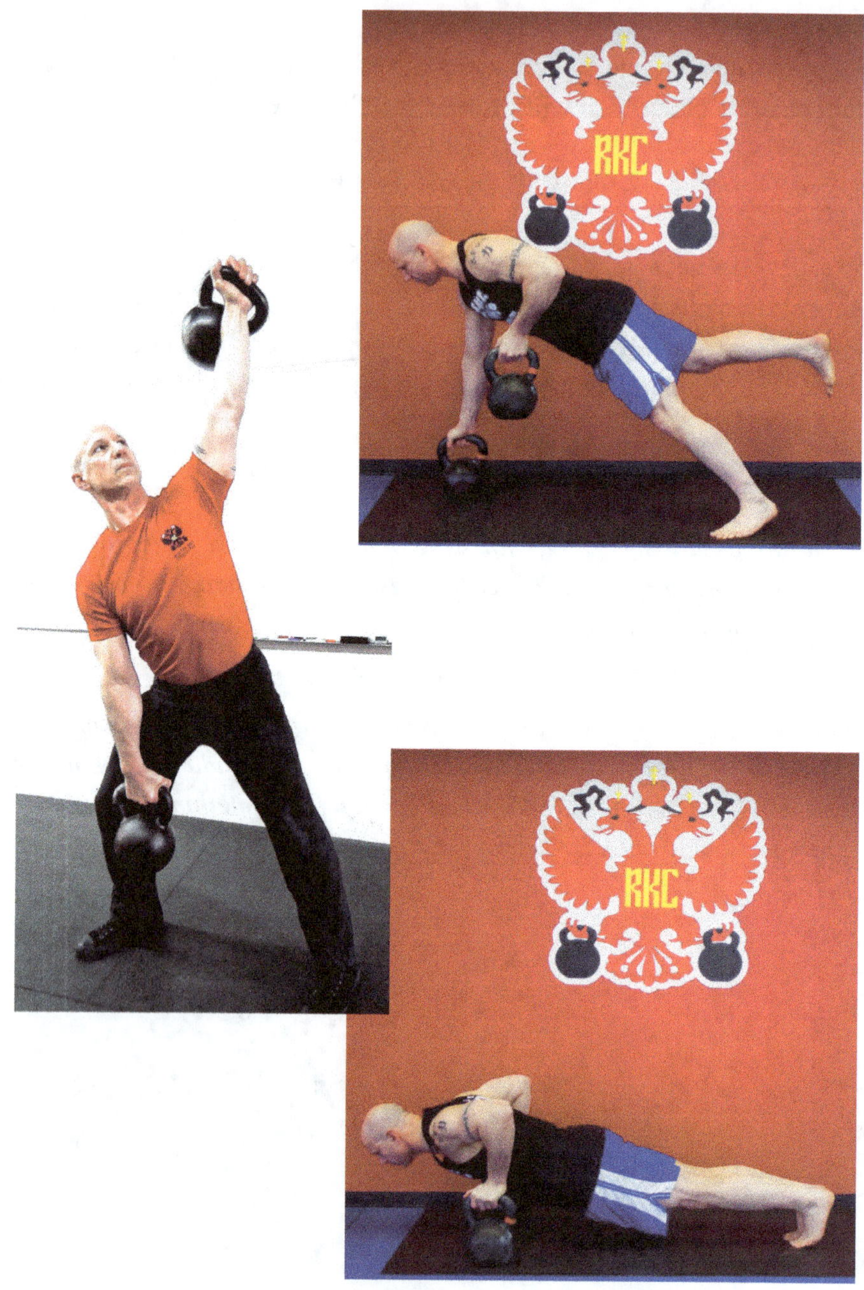

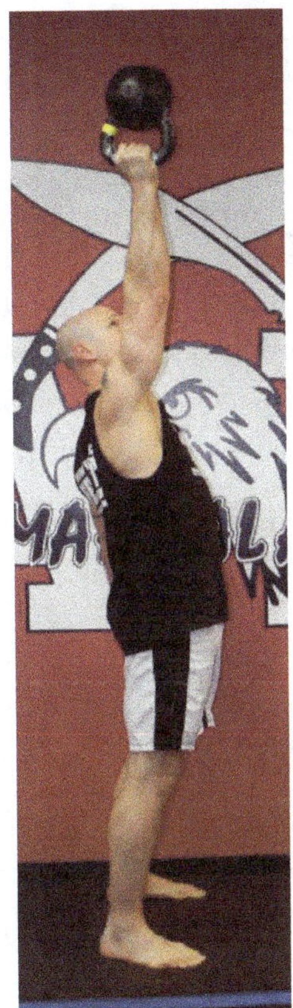

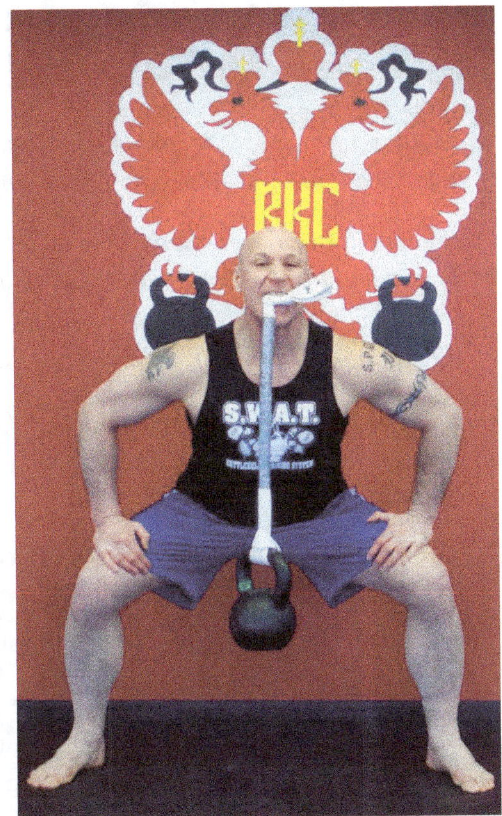

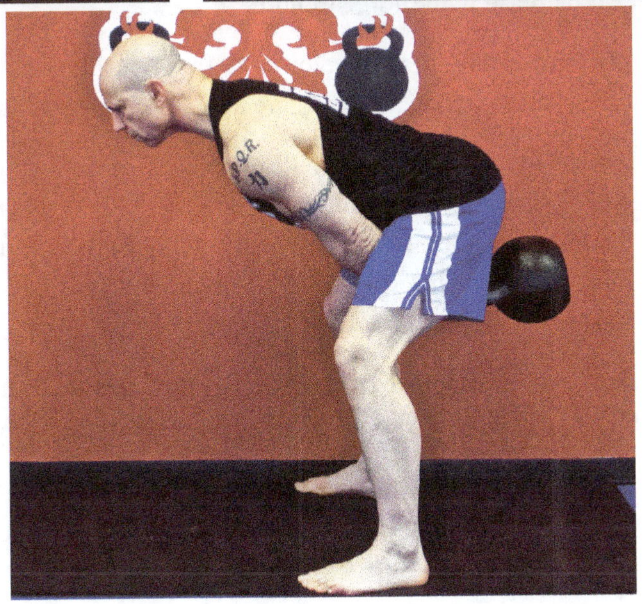

BASIC STRENGTH

In this section, our primary focus will be on bodyweight, simple suspension and man-to-man strength-developing drills.

There are other fantastic methods of strength development available: kettlebells, free weights, sandbags, etc. But there are a multitude of resources available regarding these methods of strength development. The advice contained in this book is catered toward the minimalist.

The calisthenics listed below are some of my favorites for power development and conditioning. There are many others that you may incorporate into your training regimen.

Upper Body Strength is developed through pushing and pulling. By employing a wide variety of Push-Ups, Pull-Ups, Dips, and Handstands, we can develop great strength and durable tendons.

Why You Need It: Someone may try to twist or control your limbs. If they are soft and deconditioned, you will most likely sustain an injury and not be able to free yourself from their grip. Your striking effectiveness will also increase with more strength.

Lower Body Strength is also developed through pushing and pulling. We use various squats and deadlifts to create lower body strength.

Why You Need It: This strength will enable us to deliver powerful kicks more explosively. Our driving power comes from our lower body as well. Pushing someone off of you and standing back up after being knocked down depends on leg strength. Leg strength and conditioning will lessen the effects of leg attacks.

Rotational, Core, and Abdominal Strength is gained through a variety of planks, bridges and abdominal strengthening movements. These are the most important, yet frequently ignored set of exercises.

Why You Need It: The development of a strong core will enable you to sustain a blow and minimize or even eliminate the damage to internal organs.

Neck Strength will increase through the use of the Wrestlers' bridge, 4-way neck dynamic tension and static wall tension. It is essential to have a strong neck. Most people do not work their neck muscles, in fact it never occurs to them.

Why You Need It: You never know when someone is going to grab you by the neck or when something will fall on you. You need to be able to withstand a beat down. A strong neck will also minimize the effect of any shock to your brain.

ROTATIONAL AND CORE STRENGTH

PLANKS

The plank is an exercise that virtually anyone can do, even if you are de-conditioned or suffer from some type of physical handicap. This exercise also serves as a means for you to understand the concept of full-body tension, which will help you in both delivering and absorbing blows.

In all planks, tuck your hips, tighten your butt and adopt a slightly "concave" position as opposed to maintaining a neutral spine.

RKC PLANK

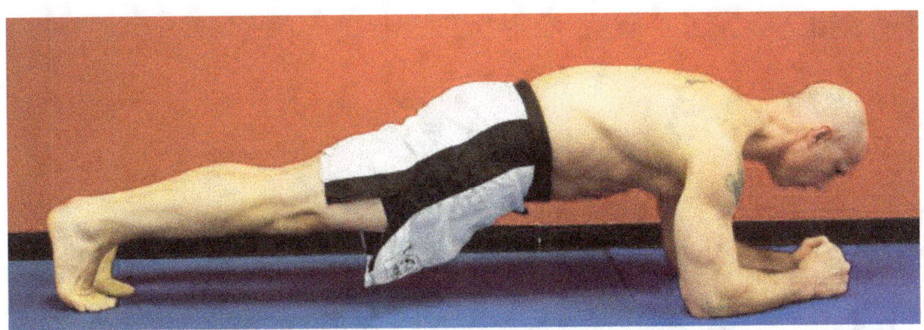

Place your elbows and toes on the floor with your body straight. Start by tightening your abs, butt, and lats, and then move to apply full tension throughout the rest of your body. Your fists should be clenched and located under your face. Practice "breathing behind the shield" by bringing your breath in through your nose, down to the bottom of your lungs, and exhaling through your mouth while keeping your abdominals taut. You should vary your times holding this position, but a 30 second full tension hold is a good place to begin your planking.

OUT AND BACK PLANK

Start in the RKC Plank position. Walk your elbows out as far as you can while maintaining the integrity of your core. Hold for ten seconds, and then bring your elbows back to their original position for another ten seconds. Repeat this sequence for three reps in each position as a starting point.

POWER PLANK

How many of you like to hold a plank for three minutes? Yeah, neither do I. Fortunately the Power Plank allows you to maximize your effort for a condensed amount of time. Assume the RKC Plank position, and then visualize bringing your elbows to your toes and having them meet two feet underground. Apply full-body tension, which is no easy task, for fifteen seconds. Applying full-body tension for fifteen seconds takes a great deal of focus, concentration and practice. The results are fantastic though!

TALL PLANK

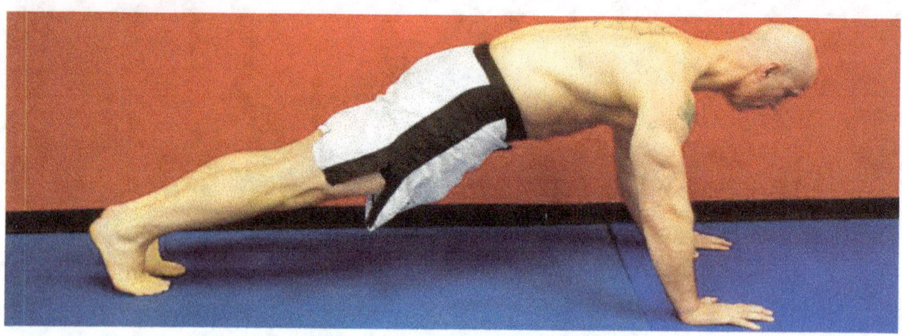

This is essentially the top of your Push-Up. Drive the heels of your palms into the ground as you grip the floor. Tighten your abs and assume the concave position, then draw your knees up and into your quads as your toes are planted into the floor. Start with sets of 30 seconds.

SIDE PLANK (AND TALL SIDE PLANK)

Begin this movement on your side with your elbow on the ground lined up with your shoulder and your feet either one over the other or slightly crossed. Your hips should be perpendicular to the floor and the ceiling. Maintain this position throughout the movement. The slight crossing of your feet is a good starting position for beginners. As with all planks, apply tension to your body. From this position, drop your hip to the floor and then raise it up as high as you are able. For the tall version of the side plank, post your palm on the floor as opposed to your elbow.

ONE-LEG PLANK

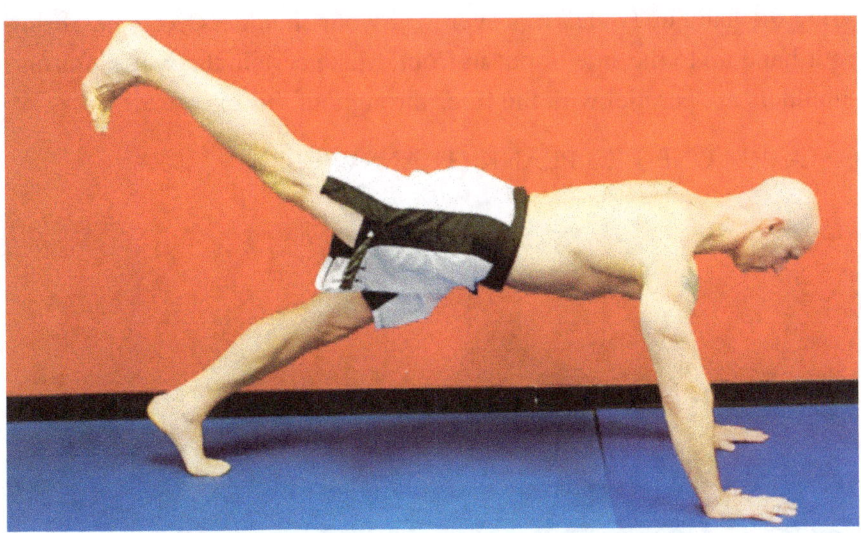

Assume the Tall Plank position and raise one foot off of the ground. Lift your leg as high as you are able while keeping your hips and shoulders in the same plane and parallel with the floor. Repeat the movement on the other side. Hold the position for a duration that allows you to achieve multiple sets. Start with ten seconds on each side and increase both the time and the sets as you become stronger.

ONE-ARM PLANK

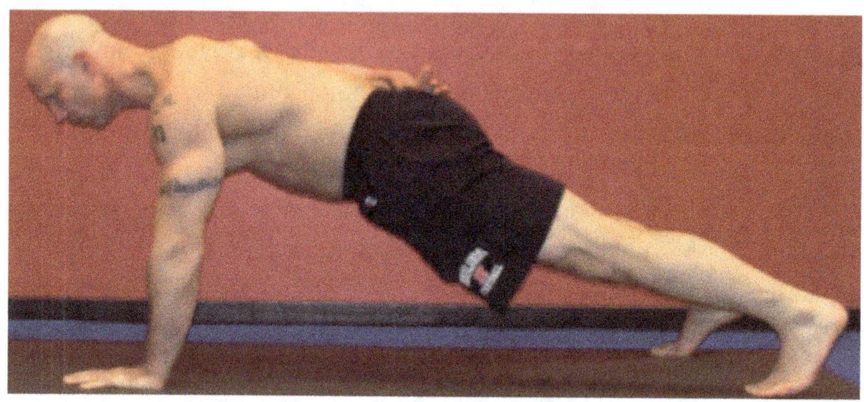

Assume the Tall Plank position and raise one arm off of the ground. Bring the hand up so that it is even with your shoulders. You may bring your hand up to the side or out in front. Make certain that your hips and shoulders are parallel with the floor throughout this exercise.

ONE-ARM/ONE-LEG PLANK (TRANSVERSE)

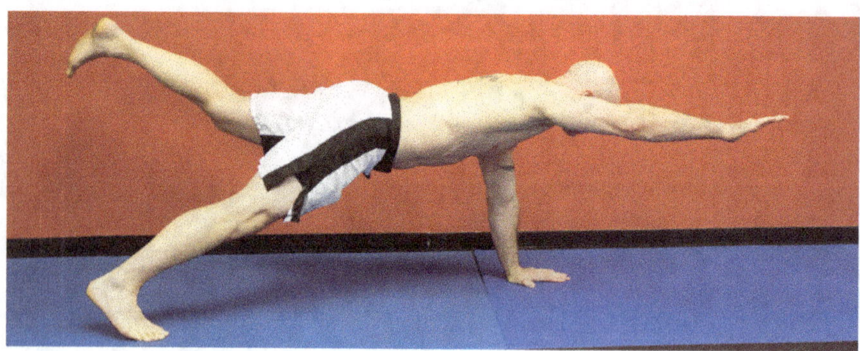

This exercise is to be done in the same way as the One Arm Plank, except that you bring the adjacent leg off of the ground at the same time as your arm. When you raise your right hand, you elevate your left leg and vice versa.

ANGLED PLANK (UP AND DOWN)

If you are just beginning, you may want to start your planks with your hands elevated on a low table, bench, or chair. Once you become more advanced, switch the position so that your feet are raised. This will add difficulty to the technique.

BRIDGES

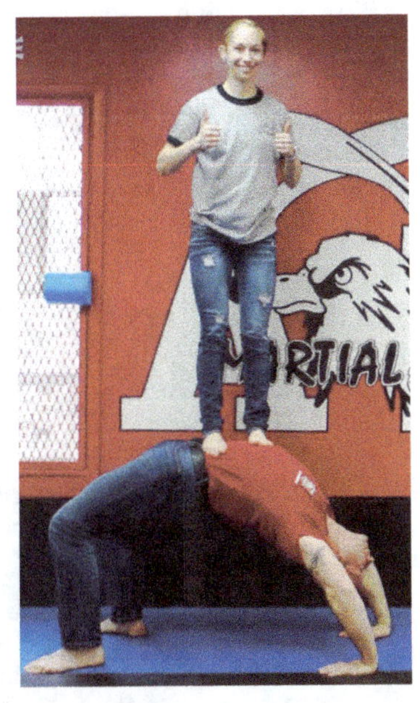

This exercise provides the bridge between your lower and upper body. The spinal erectors are critical to real strength development and core stability. How many times have you seen a huge guy completely incapacitated because he threw out his back? I can almost guarantee that he spends quite a bit more time doing bench presses as opposed to working on his bridge. Don't be that guy. Below are listed some of my favorite variations.

Whatever Bridges you practice, there are several ways to train. One method is to perform a multitude of repetitions. It is important, though, to make certain to pause at the top and the bottom of the movement. This holds true for many other exercises as well.

FLAT (OR GLUTE) BRIDGE

Lie flat on your back and place your arms out to the side at an approximately 45-degree angle. Have your knees bent and as close together as possible with your feet flat on the floor. If need be, place a foam roller, small or large ball, or other object between your knees to help you create tension. Perform ten repetitions. Time under tension is essential. Five to thirty second holds at the peak of the movement are recommended. When you become more flexible, "walk" your shoulders toward your heels and grab your ankles with your hands to help elevate your bridge even more.

RUNNERS BRIDGE

Lie flat on your back in the same initial position as in the Flat Bridge. Dorsiflex both feet, not just the one on the leg that you are raising, but both feet. Contract your glutes and push your hips high toward the ceiling and drive your knee toward your chest while pushing through the floor with the adjacent heel. Maintain this position for two to five seconds. Repeat the movement for five to ten repetitions and then change sides.

STRAIGHT-LEG BRIDGE

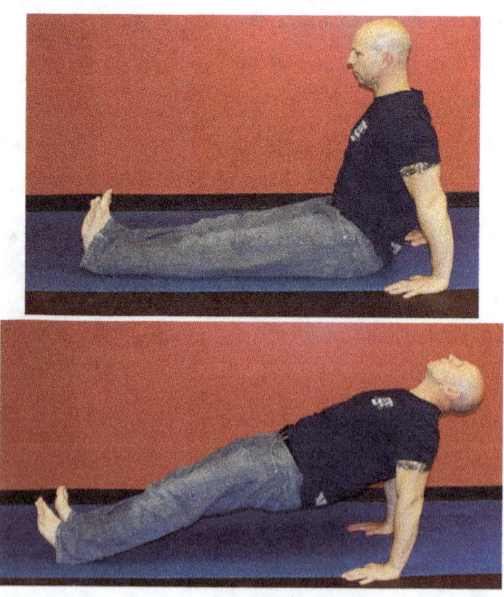

Sit on the floor with your legs straight out in front of you. Sit up tall and have your hands on the floor next to your hips with your fingers facing forward. Squeeze your legs together; they will want to come apart. So, you'll need to contract your inner thighs and control the motion from your hips, all the way down to your metatarsals. Maintain a neutral spine as you drive your hips toward the ceiling. Your head, shoulders, hips and legs should be in a straight line at the top of the movement. Perform 20 to 40 repetitions. Vary the duration of the hold time. This bridge will tax your triceps muscles quite a bit as well.

TABLE-TOP BRIDGE

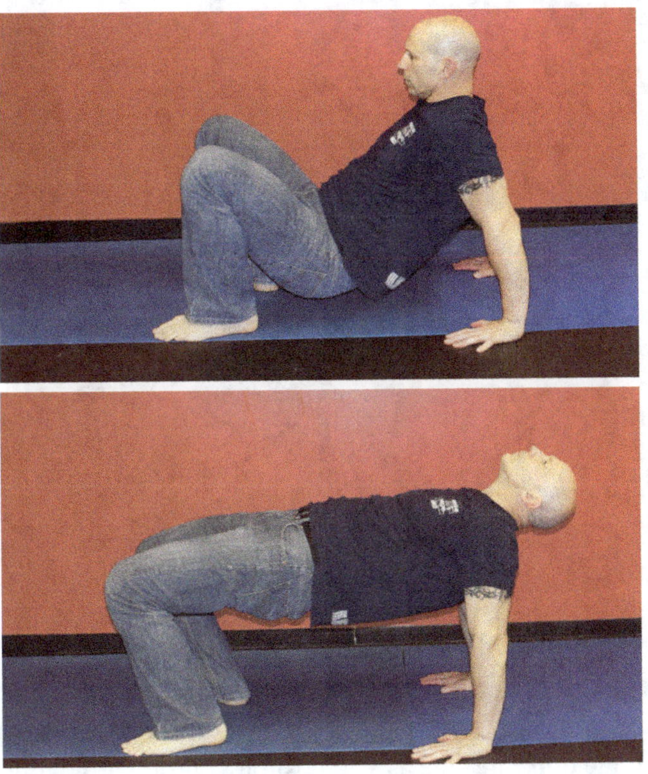

Lie flat on your back and bring your feet close to your buttocks. Keep your knees bent and sit up. Place your hands a little behind your hips with your fingers facing your toes. Maintaining a neutral spine, bring your hips up as high as you are able by contracting your buttocks and tightening your core. Done properly, your body will form a table with your legs and arms at 90-degree angles. Hold for two, five, or ten seconds and then drop your bottom to the ground, touch quickly and come back up. Repeat this movement for five to ten repetitions.

THORACIC BRIDGES

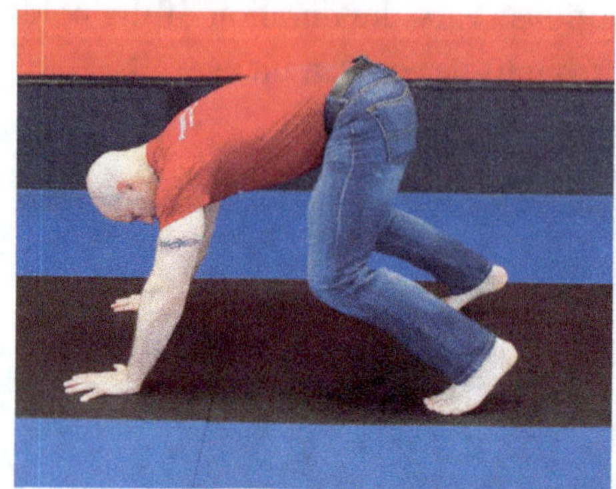
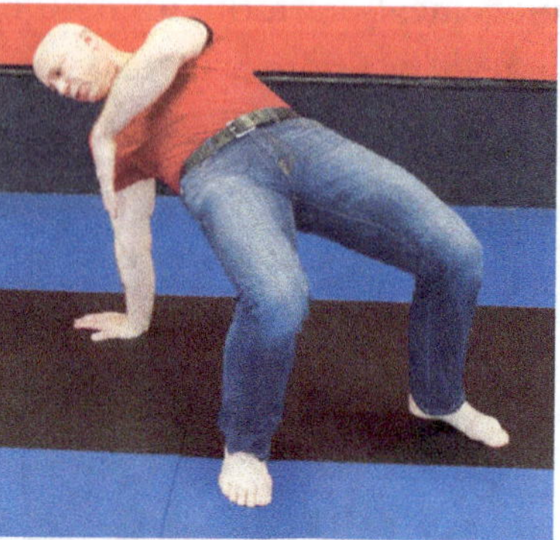

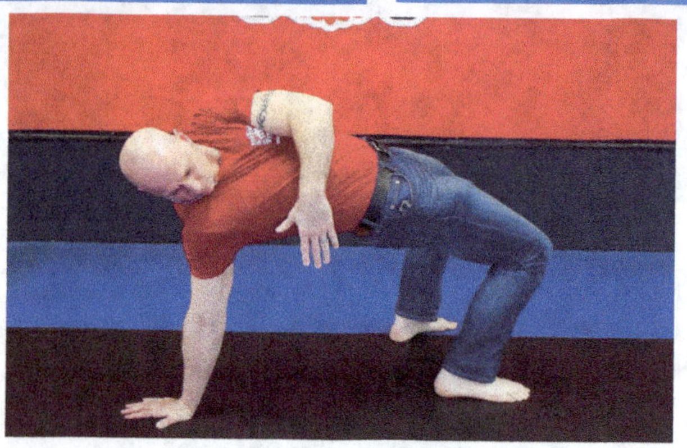

Begin with your hands and feet on the ground, knees flexed so that your feet are almost in line with your hips but slightly behind. If you are going to the right, post on your left hand, then swing your left leg through to the opposite side as you post on your left arm while keeping your shoulder packed (shoulder packing is often described as the act of engaging your lats while pulling the shoulder joints back and down, thus elongating the neck and "packing the shoulder." This movement is the antithesis of "shrugging" your shoulders.)

Reach across your body with your right arm and drive your hips toward the ceiling. Your hips should be in a horizontal position to the floor as you drive them toward the ceiling and your shoulders should be vertical. Repeat this process on the other side for three to five repetitions in both directions.

FULL BACK BRIDGE

Lie flat on your back and bend your knees so that your heels are as close to your buttocks as possible. Invert your hands so that your palms are on the ground with your fingers pointing toward you and on either side of your neck. Your elbows should be pointed directly at the ceiling. Feel free to make any adjustments you may need and creep your hands and feet closer together as you drive your hips upwards. To maximize the effectiveness of this bridge, as well as the others, contract your posterior chain and squeeze your rhomboids together as your hips are raised. Perform ten to twenty repetitions with two to ten second holds.

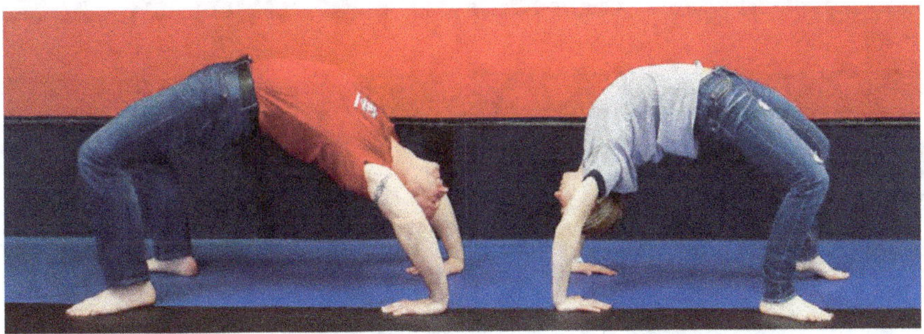

BRIDGE POPS

Lie on the ground and bend your knees enough to allow your feet to be flat on the ground. Drive your hips upward very quickly as you punch across your body and upward. For example, as you thrust your hips upward, punch your right hand up and across to the left side of your body and past your head. Arch your body and turn your head to the same side (left in this case) that your arm is going to. Drop your hips and violently pop them up again. Alternate sides while training.

This movement is crucial when someone is on top of you and you are trying to create space to move. Here's a basic premise to remem-ber:

when you are on top of someone, you want to minimize space to increase your control and pressure. When you are on the bottom, you need to create space to enable you to escape. When practicing bridges for strength, keep your heels planted firmly on the floor. When practicing for application and height, go up onto the balls of your feet.

NECK BRIDGES

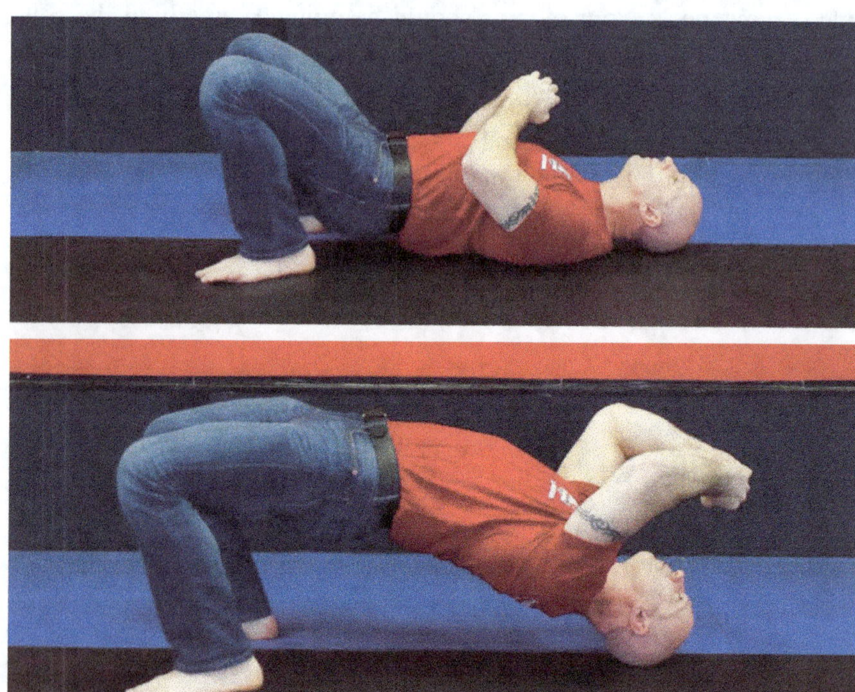

This is a favorite of wrestlers, football players and other athletes in collision and combat sports, since neck strength is essential in these activities. If your neck is weak, you will not last long. Lie on your back as if you were going to do a Bridge Pop or a Flat Bridge except drive up to your head so that your heels and head are on the ground. Once you have developed significant strength with this movement, venture onto the balls of your feet. Next, roll from the crown of your head to your forehead in a back-and-forth motion. You should also incorporate lateral movement and "rolling" motions. Place your hands together and in line with your shoulders as you rock back and forth, side to side and in small circles.

Even though your neck is part of your upper body, I consider this exercise a complete, posterior body movement linking both upper and lower sections of the body together.

PHYSIO-BALL ROLLING

"Sit" on a physioball with your low back on the ball and your feet on the ground. Place your hands out front with your arms slightly bent. Begin to roll yourself around on the ball while trying to maintain contact and not fall off. Roll around on the ball, back and forth, up and down. This is a free-form exercise. This drill is a great deal of fun and helps to develop balance. I include this movement after my bridge work. I generally do this one for 30 seconds to a minute at a time.

ABDOMINALS

The outward visibility of "the abs" are often used as the barometer of fitness, conditioning, and strength. The appearance of abdominals is not nearly as important as their strength, however. The fact that they can be seen is more of a function of diet. Whether your abs are visible or not, they need to be strong.

LEG THRUSTS

Lie flat on your back so that your lumbar (low) and thoracic (mid) back remain pinned to the ground. It's important to keep your cervical spine (neck) off of the floor for most all abdominal exercises. You accomplish this by contracting your abs, not simply lifting your neck and keeping your hips "bolted" to the ground. There should be no space between your low back and the floor. NEVER put your hands underneath your lower back to fill the gap with the floor. Your hands should either be on your stomach, or your fingers should be interlocked and behind your head. Bring your knees up as high as you are able toward your chest, then "thrust" your feet forward with your toes dorsi-flexed (this means the toes are curled back toward the shins). Your feet should be approximately six to eight inches from the ground. Perform 20 to 50 repetitions per set.

CONCAVE ABS (THREE POSITIONS)

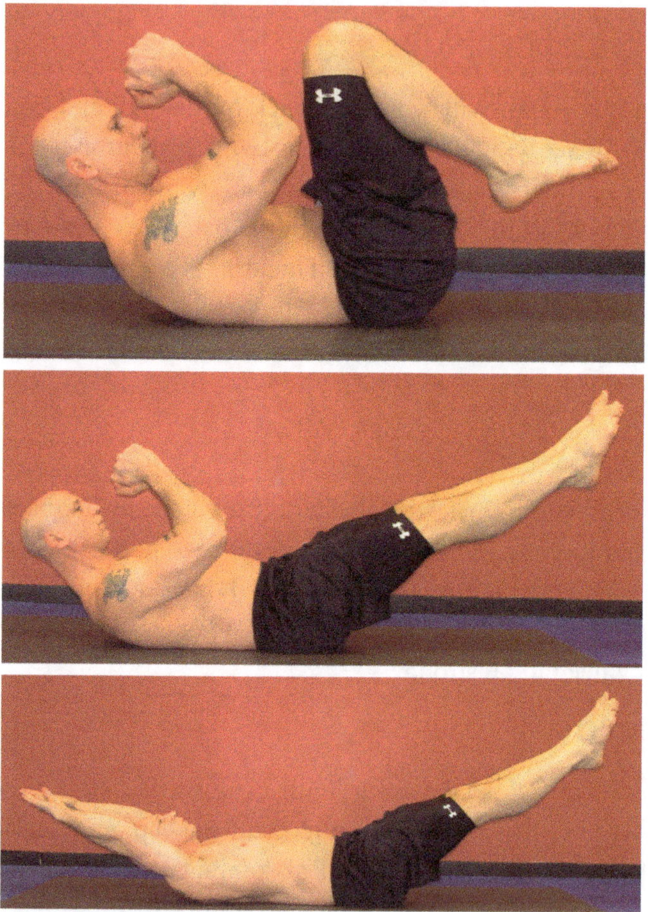

Secure your lumbar region (lower back) against the floor. For the beginner's version, apply full tension as you force your knees into your elbows. When performing the intermediate level, extend your legs all the way out while keeping the tension in your upper body and driving your elbows toward your feet. For the advanced position, extend both your feet and hands all the way out. Be certain to keep your hips down and have no space between the floor and your back. You may have to raise the level of your feet and hands to maintain this position.

There are many ways to use this method to train your abs. You can hold a specific position for 10 to 30 seconds. You may move from one position to another, holding the positions for 10 to 30 seconds before moving on. More advanced students may hold the positions for 60 seconds or longer.

BUTTERFLY CRUNCHES

Start in the Butterfly Stretch position with the bottoms of your feet together and tucked in as close as possible to your butt. Then assume the supine position as with the prior movement, except keep the bottoms of your feet together and as close to your butt as possible. Interlock your fingers and place your hands behind your head with your elbows out to the side and pressed backward as far as is comfortable. Contract your abs and pull your upper body off of the ground so that only your lumbar spine (lower back) is on the mat while keeping your knees as far apart as possible.

On the way down, your head should not touch the floor. There should be tension in your abs for the duration of per set. Perform 20 to 30 repetitions per set, increasing the reps as you become stronger.

BUTT-UPS AND BUTTINATORS

As with most abdominal exercises, start with your cervical spine off of the mat as previously explained. Hold that position and bring your knees up to your chest and then lift your butt upward. For the Buttinator, bring your knees side to and up as opposed to simply raising your hips toward the ceiling. Try to keep your heels as close to your butt as possible throughout the movement. Your knees should be bent the whole time.

WOD (WHEEL OF DEATH)

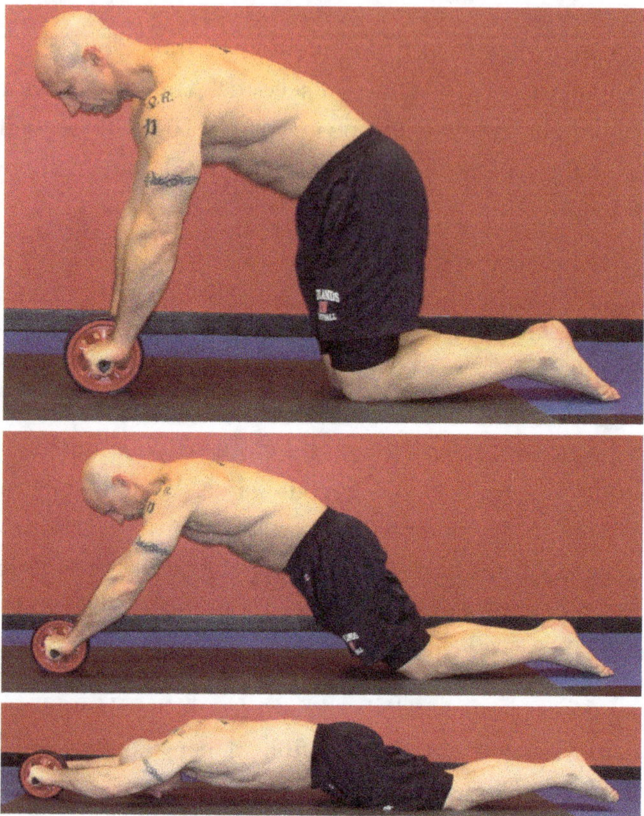

This apparatus has been a mainstay in gyms for eons: the Ab Wheel. This great little tool can be picked up for $10 to $15. We are going to review how to use this equipment properly. Start with your knees together and the wheel in both hands and directly in front of you. Grasp the handles of the wheel and try to "snap" the handle as you fire your lats, abs, shoulders and arms. Maintain the concave or "hollow" position (tucking your hips and head) as you roll the wheel out in front. Only go out as far as you are able while being able to return to the starting position with a smooth motion while maintaining the hollow position.

It is recommended that you place a pencil or weight at the far end of your reach to ensure that you don't overextend yourself. Each forward and backward motion needs to be done under tension and should take anywhere from five to 10 seconds to complete. Start with five to reps each set. When you become more advanced, you can start on your feet.

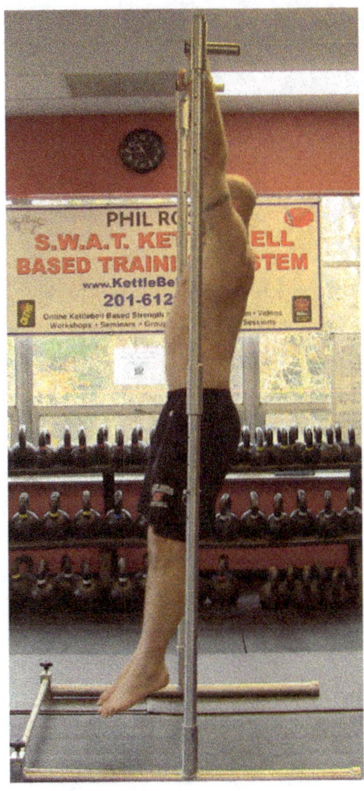

HANGING ABS

The Hanging Abdominal exercise will deliver the most "bang for your buck." There are many variations with various difficulty ratings, but they all begin the same way.

Grasp the bar firmly, with either a thumbless hook grip or full grip (To complete the latter you should grasp the bar with your fingers on one side and your thumb on the other, to create a circle with your hand. To use the former your thumbs and fingers should be located on the same side of the object you are gripping. This grip is used to reduce elbow strain and to grasp something that you can't get your hands around). Pack your shoulders, engage your lats, and shorten your abs by lowering your ribs and drawing your hips up. Do this while maintaining a straight spine. Point your toes and straighten your knees. Apply tension throughout your body and keep your elbows locked. Now you are ready to train! Here are a few of my favorites.

KNEE-UPS AND L-SIT

Hanging from a bar that doesn't allow your feet to touch the ground, assume the Hanging Ab starting position and bring your knees up as high as you are able. I like to raise them to at least mid-chest level. For the L-Sit version, simply extend your legs so that your profile will exhibit an "L". Lower your legs slowly and repeat for ten to twenty repetitions per set.

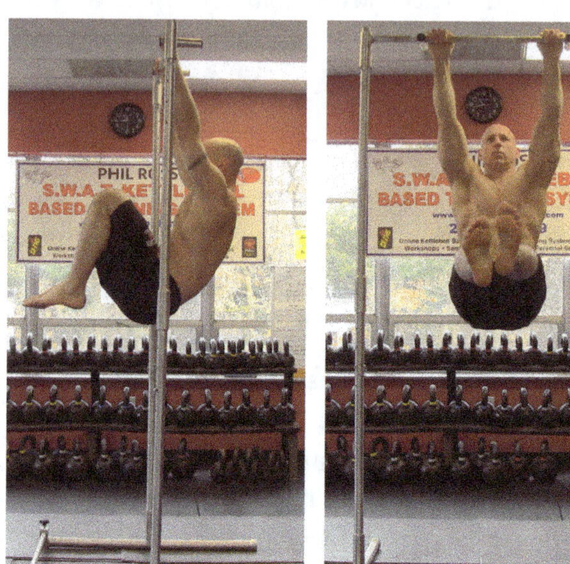

JACK-KNIFES

From the starting position, raise your feet up to the bar. Be sure to keep your knees and elbows locked. Minimize the sway by maintaining full body tension. Sets of five to 10 repetitions are recommended.

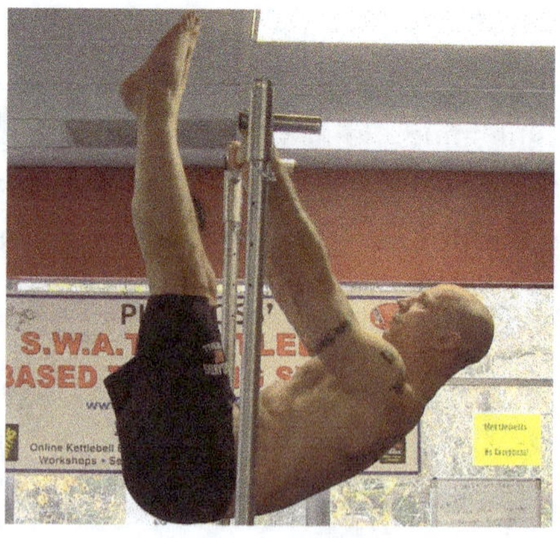

SIDE CRUNCH

Focusing on the obliques and serratus, lie flat on your back and slide your upper body to one side. Have the hand of the side that you slide to behind your head and your legs folded over, so your knees are facing the opposite direction. Place the free hand on your knees. Keeping your shoulders in the same plane as the ceiling, contract your side abdominals and raise your upper body to the ceiling being certain not to twist. This is a very small but effective movement. Generally, 25 repetitions on each side for each set are recommended.

AB CRAWL

This movement is a great deal of fun, but requires some rhythm and coordination. Lie flat on your back, keeping your feet, hands and elbows off of the ground. Your elbows and knees will be close to each other, and your hands will be in line with your face. You will now pick a direction and progress laterally by shifting from having your low back on the ground to having your upper back on the ground. Utilizing a rocking motion as you toggle between your upper and lower body. Make sure that you go in the opposite direction as well and do not let your feet or elbows touch the ground. Start with ten repetitions in each direction.

LEG DROPS

Lie flat on your back with your upper body (cervical spine) off of the mat. Accomplish this by contracting your abs. Position your arms either behind your head or on your stomach. Start with your legs at a 90-degree angle from the floor, squeeze them together, keep your knees straight and toes pointed. Drop your feet down as far as you can while keeping your lumbar spine pinned to the ground. Bring your feet up to 70 to 75 degrees and drop them down to the aforementioned level again. Repeat this movement for 15 to 25 repetitions in each set.

ALPHABET ABS

Begin as you were in the Leg Drop exercise. With your feet, "draw" in the air the letters of the alphabet. Capital letters, no cheating with lower case or script! Needless to say, there are 26 repetitions. You can sing the "Alphabet Song" if you would like.

SQUATS

There is no single lower body exercise more important than squats. Strength, cardio and balance can all be developed and enhanced with this exercise and its variations.

STANDARD SQUAT

Stand with your feet approximately shoulder width apart, and place your hands out in front of you to act as a counterbalance. Actively pull yourself down into the squat. Your feet should be at an angle of no more than 15 degrees, and your shins, knees and hips should all be aligned. Do not allow your knees to protrude beyond your toes. Your spine should be neutral, ribs down and abdominal region taut. Grip the floor with your toes and keep your heels planted, and your eyes should be level with the horizon.

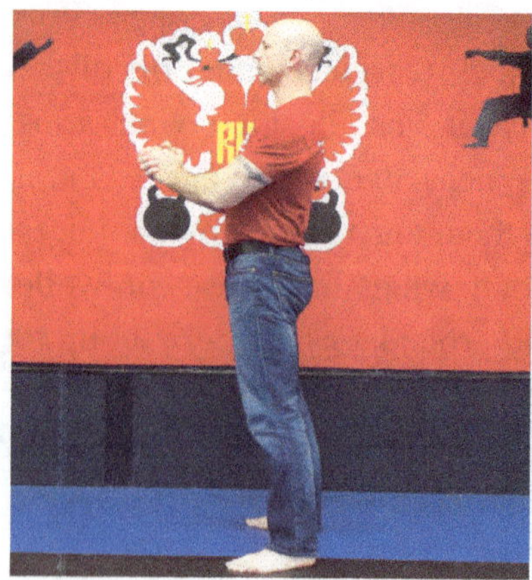
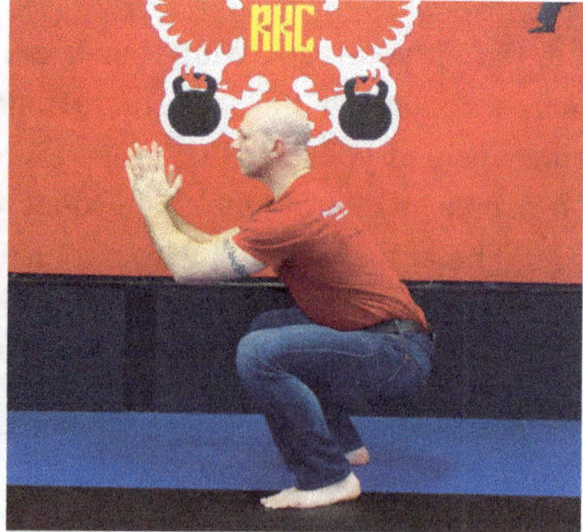

SKEWED SQUATS

This is an incredible squat to help you develop the strength and balance necessary for performing the Pistol or One-Legged Squat. Adopt as narrow of a stance as you can to maintain while still keeping your balance. Plant one foot firmly on the floor and position the other foot next to the base foot so that the ball of the foot is on the ground and in line with the base foot's heel. Most of your weight should be on the base foot. The more weight you can place on it, the better. The stabilizing foot should almost appear as if you are wearing an imaginary high heel with your calf flexed.

Actively pull yourself down below parallel. With practice, you will be able to get substantially below parallel and significantly improve your strength throughout the full range of motion. Sets of 10 repetitions on each side is a good starting point.

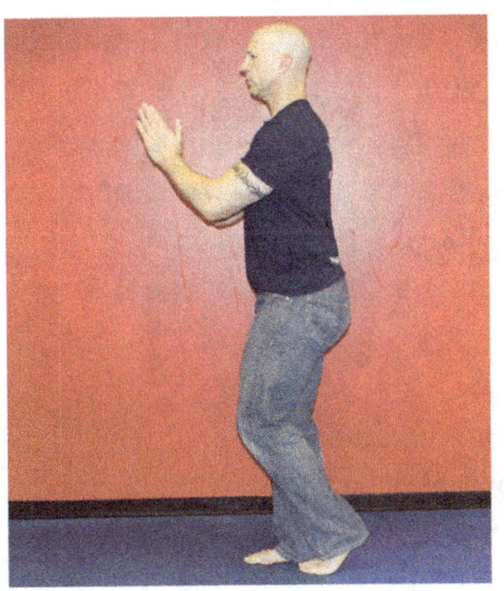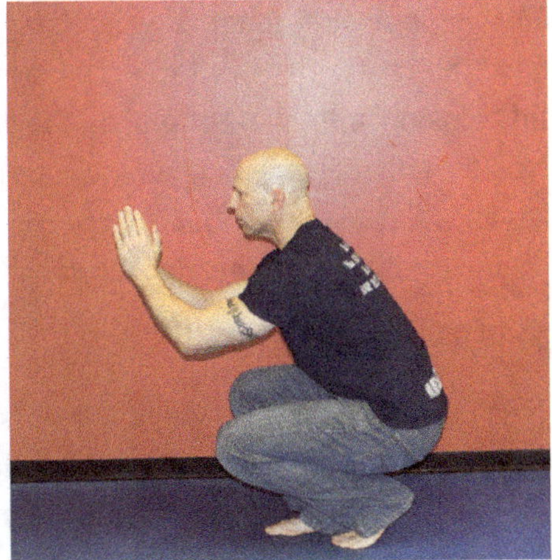

PISTOLS (SINGLE-LEG SQUATS)

This is the most difficult but also the most beneficial leg exercise, period. The training en route to a butt-to-heel Pistol develops balance, trunk stability and incredible leg strength. There are weightlifters that can fully squat 600 pounds, yet they collapse and fall over when attempting the Pistol.

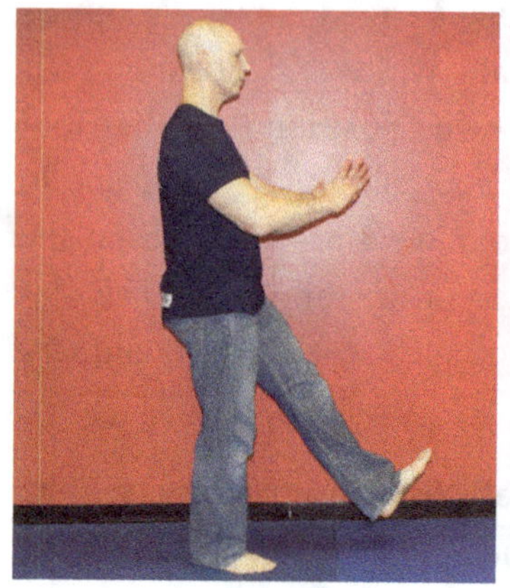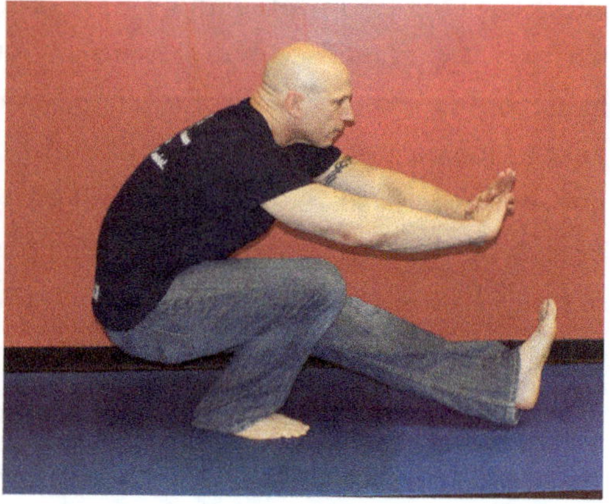

Start by rooting your foot to the floor and extending the other leg with your foot dorsi-flexed. Pull yourself downward as you tighten your abs and put power through the heel of the extended leg. You'll want to have the crease of your hip pass below your knee joint as you maintain full tension into the bottom of the movement. It also helps to create tension and balance when you extend your arms forward. For more advanced versions, raise your arms above your head. Begin your training with one to three repetitions (this is a difficult exercise!).

HINDU SQUATS

This is a fantastic movement for muscular endurance. Begin with your feet relatively close together. The closer the better, provided you are able to keep your feet, knees and hips collinear.

We want to use motion and get into a rhythm for this exercise. Dip down as low as you can, bringing your arms down and to the sides. Explode up and move your arms in a swooping motion in front of your body so that your hands are above your head when you are at the top of the movement and in line with your feet at the bottom. Exhale on the way up and inhale on the way down.

This is a great endurance builder, and 25-50 repetitions per set is recommended.

LUNGES

Stand tall with your feet together and hands at your sides and on your hips. Bring one leg up and step forward, placing your foot out in front only as far as you are able without losing balance. Go deep enough so that the knee of your back leg almost touches the floor. Now return to your original stance by pushing off the foot of the extended leg.

You may do your repetitions on one leg and then the other, or alternate. You may also do a backward lunge by stepping backward instead of forward. You may also Lunge backward and forward on the same leg to mix things up a bit. Do 15 to 25 repetitions with each leg per set.

SPLIT SQUATS

These are great for developing the leg power and coordination needed for lunging inward with a strike or for shooting a takedown.

Stand completely upright with your hands on your hips. Step one foot forward. planting that foot firmly on the ground. Drop the knee of your other leg almost to the floor and be on the ball of your foot on the back leg. Be certain to keep your back straight, spine neutral, and abdominals and trunk tight, while applying tension and stability to your movement. Perform 20 to 25 repetitions with each leg per set.

AIRBORNE LUNGES

This may be the best single-leg movement to perform. If not, it's a close second to the Pistol and much easier on the knees.

Begin standing tall with your feet together. Drop one leg back and guide your knee down to touch the floor slightly behind and next to the heel of your planted foot. Do not allow the top of the back foot to touch the ground as you go up and down.

If you are unable to perform these right out of the box, put your back foot up onto a raised platform like a step or even a large book. Start with sets of three to five repetitions.

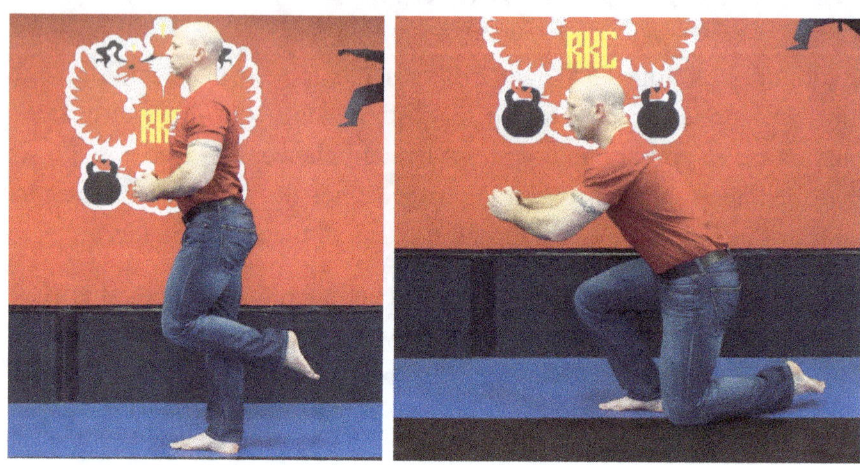

SINGLE-LEG DEADLIFTS (OR ROMANIAN DEADLIFTS), UNWEIGHTED

This movement is great for developing balance, flexibility and the posterior chain. As with most of the lower body exercises, start with your feet together. Maintain a neutral spine and bend forward at the hip while lifting one foot off of the floor and letting it go behind you. Slightly bend the knee of the base leg, adopting a "soft" knee. Keep your shoulders and hips square to each other and the floor as you bring your upper body closer to the floor.

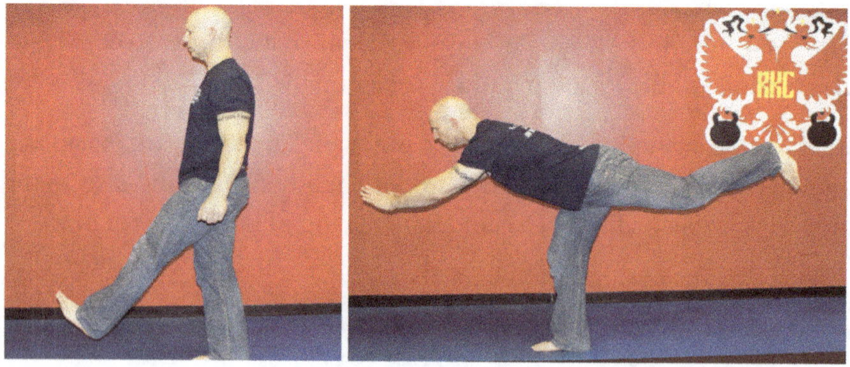

If you can achieve parallel, congratulations! If not, get as close as you can to that position while maintaining the integrity of the technique. To make the movement more challenging, extend one or both arms forward as you hip-hinge into the parallel position.

CALF RAISES

This is not a simple "bodybuilding" exercise. Strong calves will add to your explosive and pushing power. Your calves are also instrumental in your ankle mobility and strength. I practice the Three-Position Calf Raise variation more than the others.

You may either use a step (stair) or any raised platform that enables the full range of motion of your ankle. When you begin this exercise, it is recommended that you use two feet at the same time. Once you have developed greater strength, switch to one foot at a time.

Start on the ball of your foot with your heels in line with your toes and shins. Rise up as high as you can and stretch as far as you can to the bottom by drawing your heels toward the floor. Hold each position for one or two counts. Repeat for ten to twenty repetitions or until you experience the "burn" in your calves. Stretch the calves out by pressing your toes against the step and rocking your knee forward. Repeat the same movement with your heels out and toes together for position two and with your heels in and your toes out for position three.

Start with one set and build up to three of each position. To make the movement more challenging, do one leg at a time by hooking the non-weighted foot behind the knee of the weighted foot. The knee of the weighted foot needs to be locked. You may also hold a kettlebell in one hand or simply slow the movement down and/or hold the top and bottom positions longer for added difficulty.

JUMPS

So how do we address the explosive power required to knock an opponent silly with your kicks? That's where your jumping and bounding training comes in, as they will help you develop greater hip and leg strength.

VERTICAL LEAPS

Set your feet shoulder-width apart. Bend your knees until you reach parallel (or as close to it as you can) and bring your arms back, then rock slightly onto the balls of your feet and explosively drive your feet into the ground as you thrust your fists upward. On the descent, be sure to bend your knees and return to the original starting position. Once there, immediately begin the next repetition. Start with sets of 10 reps and build to 25.

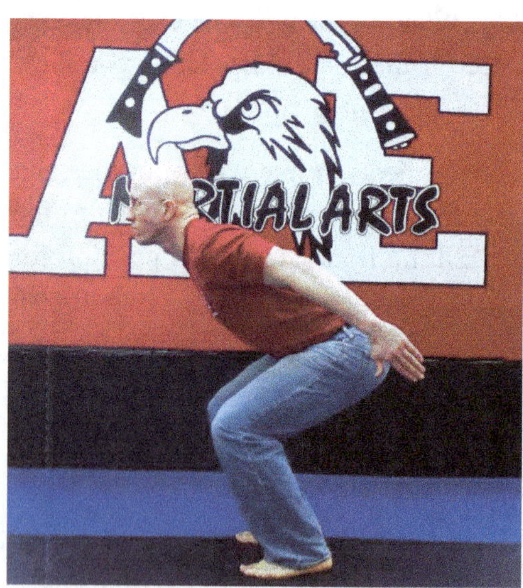
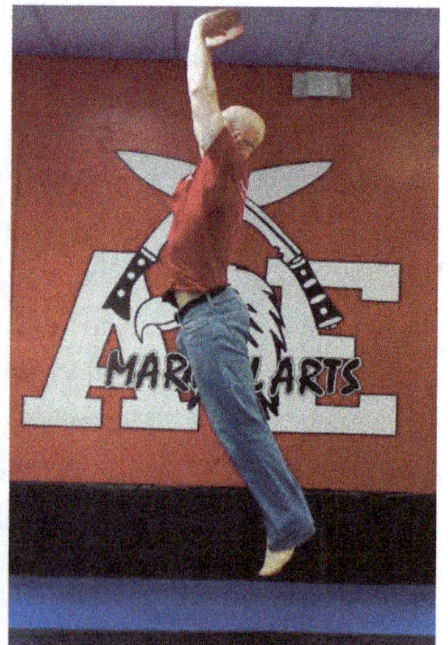

SINGLE LEG HOPS

Stand tall and raise one knee up as high as you can and hop forward by pushing off of the base foot. Land on the same foot and repeat this movement. Start with 10 to 15 repetitions on one foot and then repeat on the other. Try three to five sets for each leg and then increase as you build your strength and endurance. You can also do this for time or distance as well.

LUNAR LEAPS

No, we are not doing impersonations of the legendary pop star Michael Jackson, but we will be performing an extremely beneficial movement nonetheless. We will be practicing lateral bounding.

Imagine you are on the surface of the moon. Shift your weight onto one foot and leap forward and slightly to the side at approximately a 45-degree angle. Pause on the foot that you land on, and without putting the other foot down, drive off of that same foot and repeat the 45-degree angle leap to the other side, once again landing on the foot previously in the air. You will be both landing and pushing off of the same foot, alternating with every other step.

Your pause on each foot between your landing and take-off should be at least one full count. Keep the image of "bounding on the moon" in your mind while performing this exercise. Start with 10 to 20 repetitions on each leg for two to three sets.

POWER SKIPS

When you were a child, you may have skipped around during play. Kids tend to do this naturally. In this exercise you will drive one leg off of the floor as you thrust the opposite knee and elbow into the air. As you land, switch sides. The "Power" part comes when you thrust off of the floor and upward with as much power as you can muster. Do this for 30 to 60 seconds.

LEAP-UPS

Start with your knees slightly bent, and then quickly bring your knees up to your chest (or as high as possible). Land with your knees slightly bent and repeat this movement for 10 to 20 repetitions for three sets. It is important to land on the balls of your feet and not on your heels, and to minimize the time your feet are on the floor between reps.

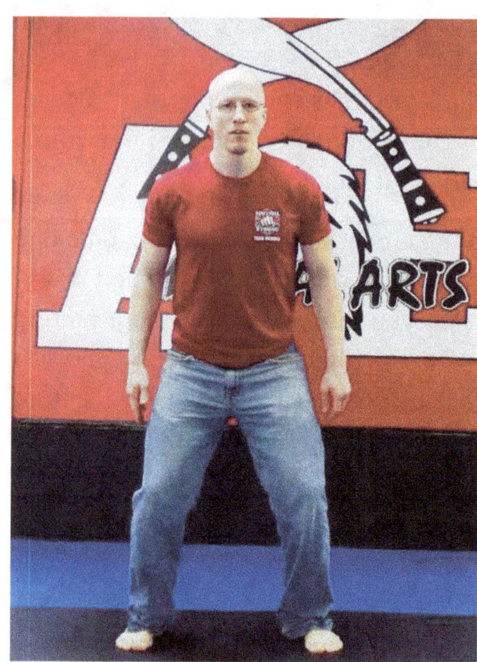 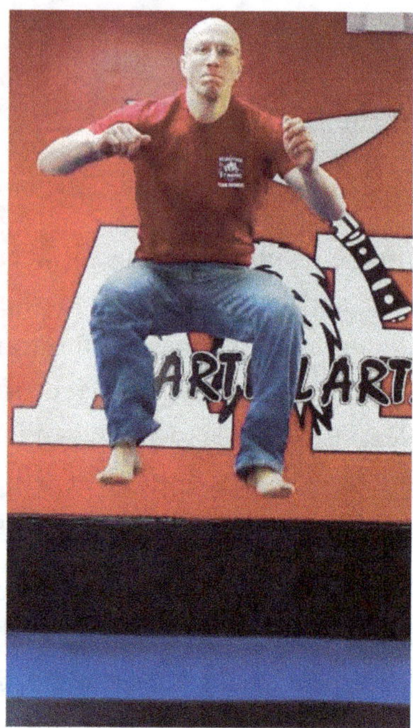

BOX JUMPS

There are a variety of boxes and heights that you may use. Whether you choose metal, wood, plastic or foam mats, be sure that they provide a stable base and will not topple over. If you do not have the means to secure any of these, bleachers or a bench bolted to the ground are excellent substitutes.

Bend your knees and set your arms back as you shift onto the balls of your feet. Explode upward and shoot your hands forward as you launch yourself onto the raised surface. Land with bent knees and then jump backward off of the platform. Keep your knees bent as you land to absorb the shock and prepare for the next repetition.

Some of these workouts go for speed, and for others you will want to slow the pace a bit, especially when you are jumping on to a higher platform. When training for power, do sets of 10. When emphasizing speed, do your sets in 30-to 60-second increments.

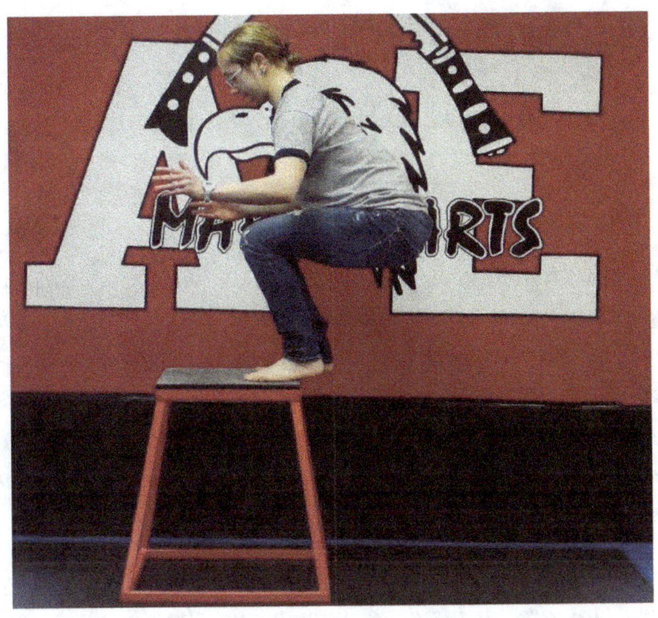

With respect to the latter scenario, you will begin with your hands out to the side, palms out and your feet approximately shoulder-width apart. Bring your knees up to your chest quickly as possible as you raise your palms to the ceiling. As you land on the balls of your feet, immediately repeat the motion. You want to minimize the amount of time that your feet are in contact with the ground. Perform sets of 10 to 20 repetitions.

CALF THRUSTERS

Place your hands on your hips and quickly rise onto the balls of your feet. Keep your head level and your back straight as you go up and down. When you do this for speed, execute a hundred reps per set. When you are going slowly, do 25 to 50 repetitions per set.

UPPER BODY STRENGTH: PUSHING, PULLING AND NECK

(ISOMETRIC AND DYNAMIC TENSION)

PUSHING

Push-Ups and Handstands are essential to building a strong frame. Please be certain you can execute a strong Plank prior to attempting Push-Ups. I see far too many people trying to perform a Push-Up and their elbows are flaring, their backs are sagging like horses ready for the glue factory, and they are dropping to their knees and moving their heads around as if they were bobbing for apples. Simply stop and work on your planks.

The knees on the floor Push-Ups will NOT make your Push-Up better. These Push-Ups are an insult to women and should not be employed. Master your Plank and then start with Wall Push-Ups and gradually decrease the angle with various levels of Incline Push-Ups until you have your hands on the floor and are cranking out solid Push-Ups!

There are some fantastic progressions for Push-Ups and other body-weight exercises in the *Convict Conditioning* Series. I would strongly recommend employing these progressions for maximum Bodyweight strength development.

PUSH-UPS

Push-Ups are my favorite of all bodyweight exercises. If there is a floor available, you can train. You want to achieve full-body tension in all variations. Tighten your core, buttocks, etc. You also do not want to flare your elbows. On most Push-Ups, you should have your elbow pits facing forward as you grip the floor with your fingers and drive the lower outside of the heel of your palm. Actively pull yourself down to the floor or at least to a fist's distance above. Maintain a neutral spine, and do not lift your head up too high or allow it to droop downward.

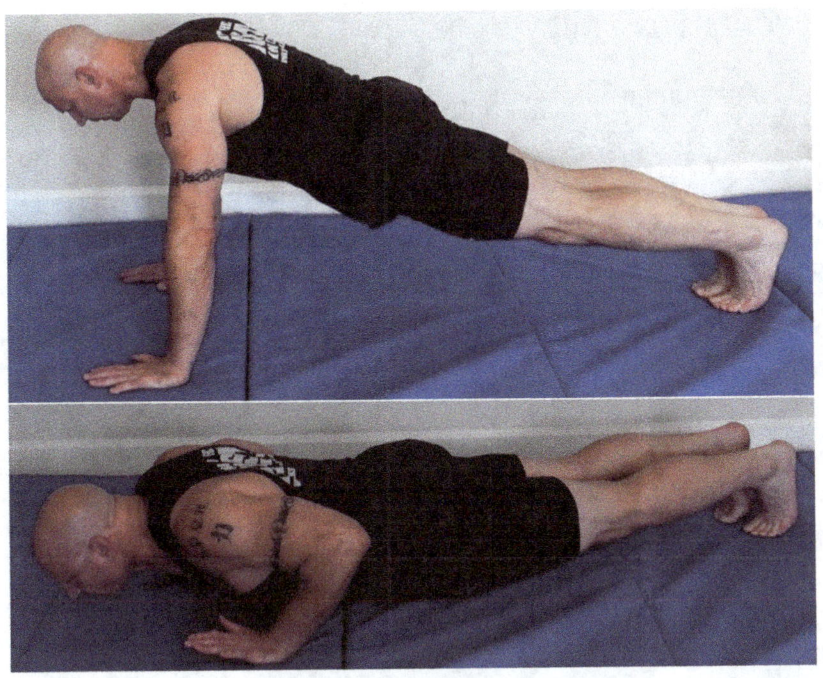

STANDARD (RKC) PUSH-UP

With palms flat on the ground, spread your fingers wide and grip the floor. Corkscrew your palms into the floor so that your elbow pits are facing forward. Actively pull yourself down to the floor and exhale as you push yourself up. Inhale at the top and repeat. Each direction of the repetition should consume one full count.

10-SECOND PUSH-UP

Begin as you would for the RKC or Standard Push-Up. Using a timer, or a clock or simply counting, take 10 seconds to lower yourself to the ground, then touch and count for 10 seconds on the way up. Full-body tension is employed, as well as your full range of motion. The goal here is to be moving for the duration of the exercise, only pausing momentarily at the bottom and the top. Start by doing two to three repetitions and work your way up to sets of five. There is also a five-second version of this movement.

KNUCKLE PUSH-UP

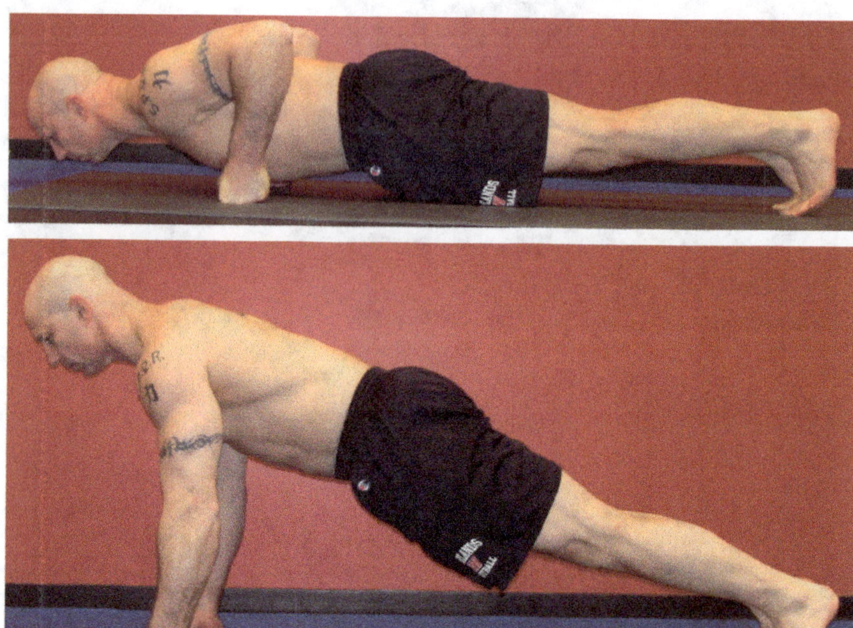

Place your front two knuckles on the ground. Make certain that you don't rock backward or have the last three on the ground. Your front two knuckles (index and middle finger knuckles) need to be aligned with the radial and ulna bones of your forearm. You should perform these Push-ups on a hardwood floor or on bricks to condition and develop calluses on your knuckles.

WIDE-GRIP PUSH-UP

Place your hands wide apart, beyond shoulder width and keep your fingers pointed forward. Be sure to keep your elbow pits facing forward, it's a little more difficult to do with your hands set wide apart.

TRIANGLE (OR DIAMOND) PUSH-UP

Set your hands directly below your chest with the thumbs and forefingers touching to form a "triangle" or "diamond" on the floor.

FINGERTIP PUSH-UP

Position your fingers on the floor so that only the tips are in direct contact. As you become stronger, subtract fingers from the floor one by one. There are many people who can perform one-and two-finger Push-Ups.

ARCHER PUSH-UP

Begin as if you are going to perform your standard Push-Up. Shift side to side as you extend the one arm and place most of the weight on the other as you straighten it out. You are swooping your chest to the floor as you complete the exercise.

WALK-THE-PLANK PUSH-UP

Perform a Push-Up and then move one hand (right) to the other (left), shift that hand out (left), and repeat the "walk" and Push-Up sequence. Once done, repeat the movement in the opposite direction.

MEDICINE BALL PUSH-UP

There are several variations of Push-Ups that one can perform with a medicine ball. You may place your hands in the middle of the ball and do Close-Grip or Triangle Push-Ups. You may also have one hand on the ball and the other on the floor as you execute your Push-Ups. You may also slide the ball in and out with one arm or roll the ball from hand to hand as you do your Push-Ups. Have some fun with it. When doing the stationary types start with sets of 20 to 30 repetitions; with the moving Push-Ups, begin with 10 reps on each side.

FURNITURE-SLIDER PUSH-UP

Purchase a couple of furniture sliders from the hardware store, or you can use plastic knee pads as a substitute, which is what I did after carpet installers left a pair behind in my garage. I started playing around with them and got a great workout by taking turns sliding one hand either out to the side or straight out in front. You should begin with five repetitions in either direction.

BACK-OF-THE-WRIST PUSH-UP

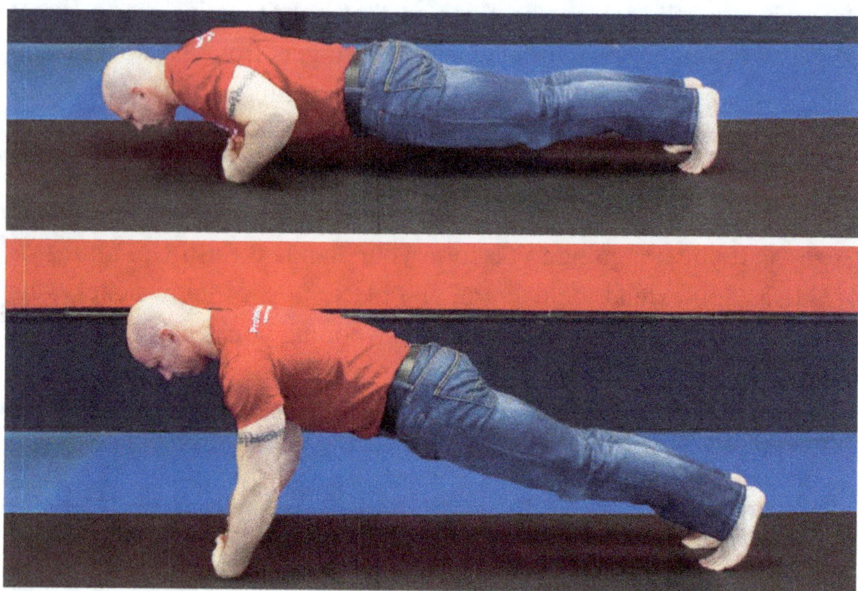

Bend your wrists toward your inner forearms and put your fingers together as if you were trying to pick a cherry. Place the back of your wrists on the floor and assume the Push-Up position. Keeping the back of your wrists planted, begin your movement.

These may be painful for beginners, but they are a great conditioning method for your wrists and forearms. Start with five to 10 repetitions.

ONE-ARM PUSH-UP

If you have been practicing your Push-Ups without your elbow pits forward or if your lats have not been engaged, you will not be able to perform a One-Arm Push-Up. If this has been the case, revisit your push up technique.

We do our One-Arm Push-Ups on either our palms or knuckles. The knuckle version is more difficult. Stabilize yourself on one hand, then place the other behind your back or on your hip. Actively pull yourself down so that the shoulder of your suspended hand touches the floor. Full-body tension is imperative.

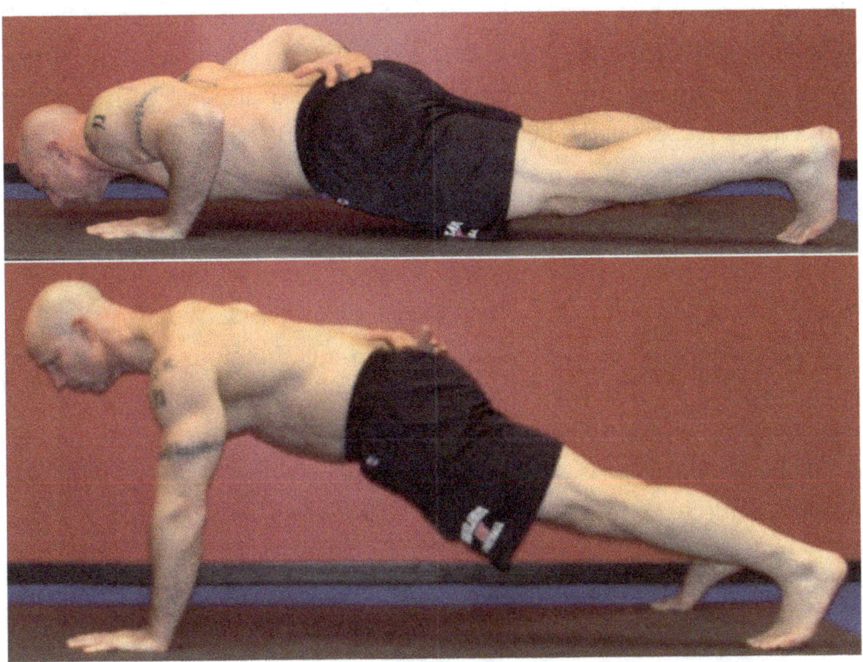

Single-arm pumps are a good way to prep you for the one arm push up. You may only do partials while you are working on getting the full Push-Up in. The closer your feet are together, the more difficult the Push-Up is to perform. This goes for most variations.

ONE-ARM/ONE-LEG PUSH-UP

This is one of the most difficult Push-Ups to perform from the supine position. A great deal of core and contralateral strength is required.

Start in the Push-Up position, migrate to one arm, and then lift the adjacent foot off of the ground. Actively pull yourself down so that the shoulder of the suspended hand touches the floor. Once this has occurred, drive your body upward by employing full tension in your body and contracting your muscles as you return to the top position. Do one to five repetitions on each side.

PLYOMETRIC PUSH-UPS

There are several variations of the Plyometric Push-Up for you to choose from. While performing any of them, it is important to "pop" your body off of the ground and to maintain the plank position. Drop down and explode up. On these Push-Ups we are not utilizing the active negative, so make certain that you are proficient at the standard Push-Ups before attempting any of the Plyometric versions.

The variations are determined by your hand position. Here are a few of my favorites: Standard-Width and on your palms, Close or Triangle, Wide, Knuckle, Single-Arm, and Back of the Wrist. We also practice changing the position of the hands in mid-air. Example: Start on your palms, switch to knuckles, and then to wrists every repetition. Begin your training with 10 repetitions. The higher you "pop up", the more difficult the Push-Up is. There are some people that can pop from the floor to a fully standing position.

HANDSTANDS

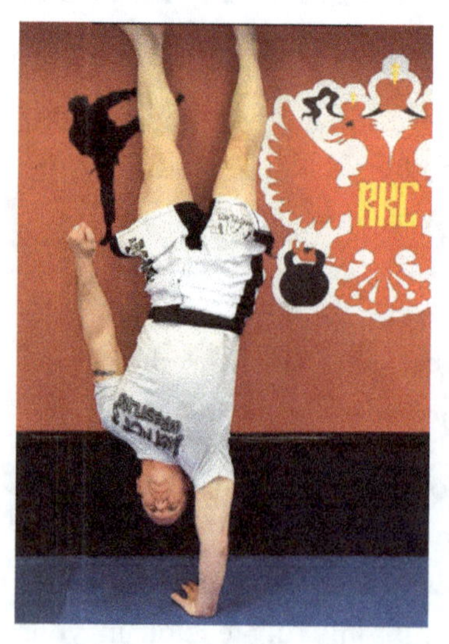

Handstands are an incredible strength-developing exercise. I do Handstands virtually every day. There are many, many Handstand variations. We're going to address three, although I advise you to practice Crow Stands prior to your Handstand training. They will help you build the strength and balance required for Handstands.

CROW STAND

Kneel on the floor and spread your fingers out as wide as you are able while still allowing you to "grip" the floor. Set the inside of your knees on the outside of your elbows and administer enough tension for you to maintain this position with only your hands on the ground. In the beginning, you may have to put your toes on the floor to balance yourself. Start with 10-second holds and build your way up to one minute. Once you are able to do a full minute, you have developed sufficient strength, balance and tension to embark on the vertical position.

FACE-THE-WALL HANDSTAND

Start with your hands on the ground and your feet toward the wall. Now, "walk" your feet up the wall and assume as vertical a position as is comfortable for you. Try to hold this position for five to 10 seconds before crawling back down. Once you are able to have an almost completely vertical position with your face very close to the wall and can hold it for 30 to 60 seconds, you are ready to attempt the next progression.

WALL HANDSTAND

Place your hands on the floor approximately 6-10 inches away from the wall. Grip the ground firmly, straighten one leg and use the other to kick up to the vertical position. Use the non-kicking leg to steady yourself against the wall. Lock out your elbows and pack your shoulders, making your neck long. Focus your eyes on the wall on the other side of the room rather than the floor. Dorsiflex your feet to aid in the creation of tension. Gradually begin to pull one foot away from the wall, and once you are confident doing this pull the other one off as well until you are free-standing in your Handstand.

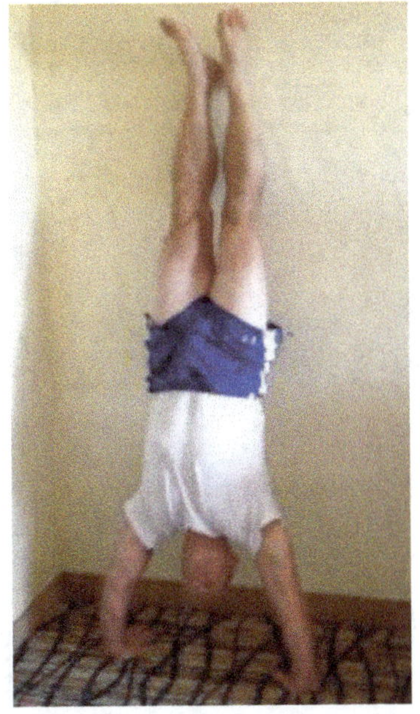

This is also a great time to practice Wall Push-Ups. These will help you develop additional strength, tension and balance in this position. Try to bring your head to the ground before you go back up. If you want more of a challenge, do these Push-Ups from a raised platform(s), parallel floor bars or even on kettlebells. This will enable you to get your head down lower.

FREESTANDING HANDSTAND

There are several methods that will work here, but this is my favorite: spread your fingers out and grip the floor with your hands. Bend your elbows and extend one leg out behind you. Attempt to get your face as close to the floor as possible and press yourself up as you perform a gentle kick upward with the leg that is on the ground.

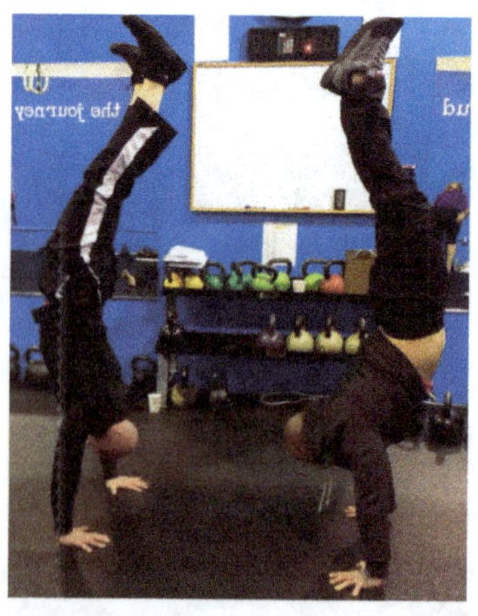

While performing the maneuver, fix your eyes on an object (usually a wall) across from you as opposed to looking at the floor. Drive your palms into the floor and create tension all the way through your heels while adopting a straight body. When it feels as though you are going to topple over, it means you've reached the position that you will steady yourself from. Bear these words in mind when practicing.

You will also experience this feeling when you are practicing your Wall Handstands as you take your feet off of the wall. Try to hold yourself up as long as you are possibly capable. Generally, when first performing the Freestanding version, one can only hold this position for a few seconds before losing their balance. You will eventually build your strength and balance in this position.

You will lose your balance and fall, this is inevitable. The two methods of failure recovery that I have used are the roll out and the pirouette. The pirouette is the preferred method. It requires less space than the roll-out, and if the landing surface is not soft or has obstructions, injury may result from a roll-out. Additionally, practicing the pirouette helps you develop better balance. The roll-out will require you to tuck your head, bend your elbows and roll across your back while bringing your knees up to your chest. When practicing pirouette, shift your weight from one hand to the hand of the side that you are falling to. As you bring one hand off of the floor, keeping your feet together, bend at the hips and rotate 90 degrees as you set your feet on the floor.

When your Handstands become solid and you are able to determine when you'd like to come down, you should try to "pop" out of the position. I start by bending my elbows and quickly pushing off of the ground and then snapping my hips as I drive my feet into the floor and come to a full, upright position. This ending is very akin to how a gymnast finishes their floor exercises, and you'll feel like you've really accomplished something when you can do it.

PULLING

Pull-Ups, Rowing Motions, and Partner Lifts are the most effective means to develop pulling strength without equipment. Pulling is essential to fighting and lifting or carrying. Our pulling strength determines if we are able to move an opponent around and grab, hold and lift them.

During these exercises pay particular attention to your elbow health. Make certain that you warm up your elbows and arms prior to any heavy pulling exercises. If you overdo your pulling training, your elbows will be the first to let you know. Gradually build to, do not rush to, advanced movements and large rep sets until you have properly prepared your joints and tendons. Soft tissue injuries can result if you push too hard too soon.

PULL-UPS

There are endless Pull-Up variations with different difficulty levels, but what follows are my favorites. I chose these variations because, with proper training, most people will be able to perform some version of them. Additionally, by increasing the rep count or by performing the movements slowly, even the advanced practitioner will be challenged. Most of the movements lend themselves to grip width adjustment, yielding further variation to your training.

Pull Ups are an incredible barometer of strength, especially when calculating strength-to-bodyweight ratios. If you cannot lift yourself off of the ground you are either too heavy or not strong enough for your weight. When considering abdominal strength, Pull-Ups are a fantastic indicator. Have you ever seen anyone who can perform twenty Pull-Ups and has weak abs? I haven't.

PLANK PULL-UP

Position yourself under a bar and utilize a thumbless grip. Have your arms fully extended at the bottom and assume an upside-down plank. Your toes should be dorsiflexed, and your body should have full tension. Pull yourself up so that your chest touches the bar. That complete motion constitutes a full rep. If you cannot complete a full rep, either change the angle of the bar to make it easier and/or hold the top position at full muscular contraction to develop more strength. Holding the top and bottom positions of your Pull-Ups is a great way to both develop and enhance your strength.

TACTICAL PULL-UP

Completing a Pull-Up generally means pulling your body up so that your chin significantly clears the bar. Your palms face forward so that the backs of your hands are facing you. In the Tactical version, you adopt a thumbless grip, pack your shoulders, tighten your abs and pull yourself up. There is no, nor should there ever be, any "kipping" of the body when performing Pull-Ups. Kipping, which means swinging your body around to gain pulling leverage, does not promote strength development; nevertheless it is useful when performing a Muscle-Up.

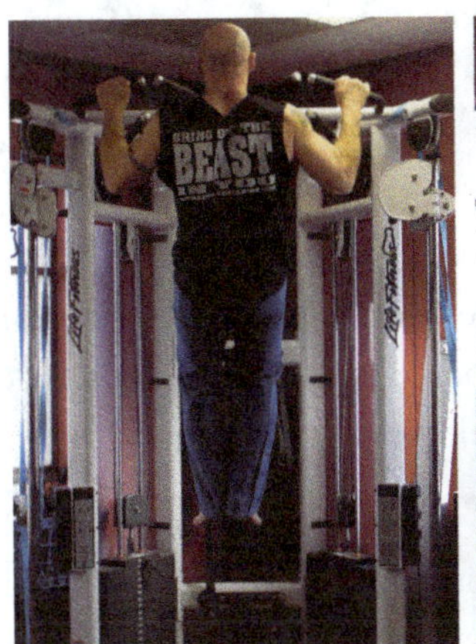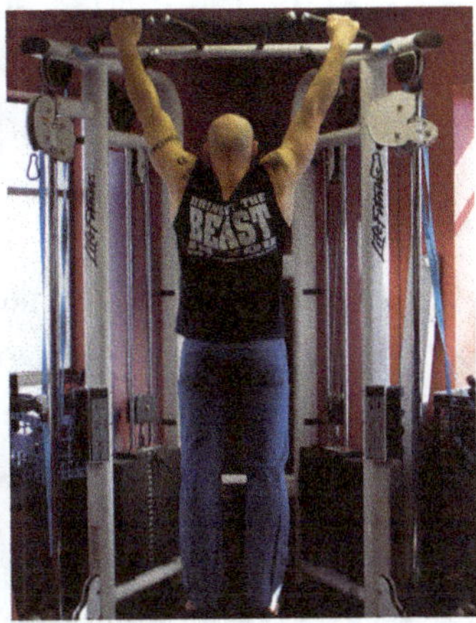

CHIN-UP

The Chin-Up is simply a Pull-Up with your palms facing you. I find these a little easier to perform due to the increased incorporation of the bicep muscles. This motion is also a little friendlier to the elbows and shoulders. As you become older, performing Chin-Ups as opposed to Pull-Ups is recommended to help avoid injuries. All other aspects of the Pull-Up remain consistent.

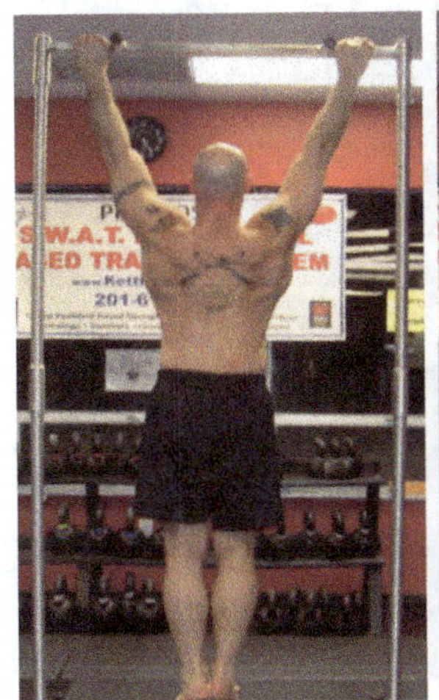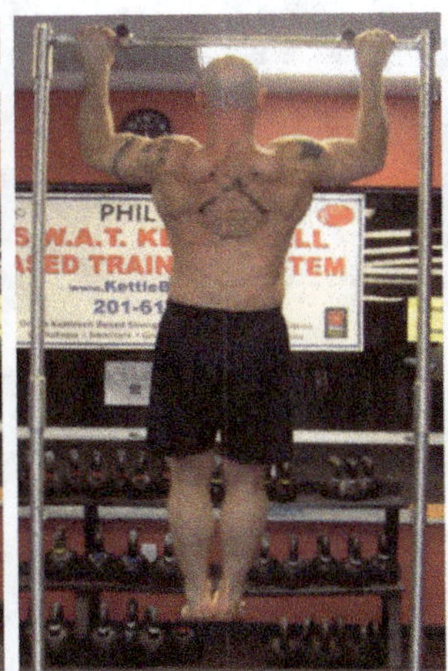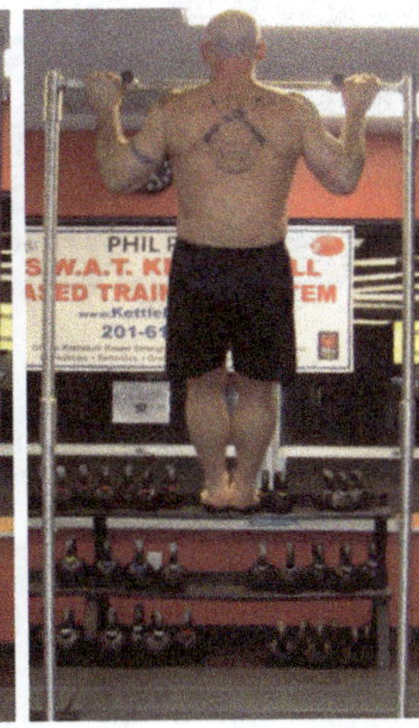

WIDE PULL-UPS

I like to utilize the thumbless grip on the Wide Pull-Ups, just as I do with the Tactical Pull-ups. This exercise is more difficult than the aforementioned versions due to the widened grip. The outer lats are taxed quite a bit with this movement, and it helps to broaden the back.

TOWEL PULL-UPS

Take a towel and fold it so that it takes on the shape of a rope and drape it over a bar. Grip tightly and pull yourself up. This adds an element of instability to the movement and develops your grip strength.

You may also use a towel in a hotel room to practice. Place the towel on the top edge of the bathroom door (it's usually a very sturdy door), take a thumbless overgrip, bend your knees so that your feet are off of the floor, and pull yourself up.

KARATE-BELT ROWS

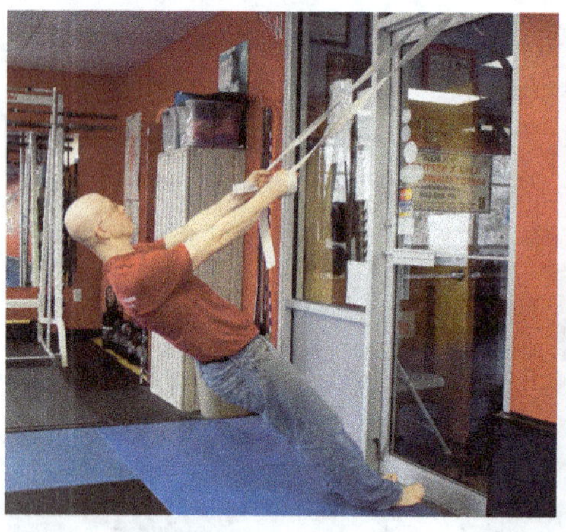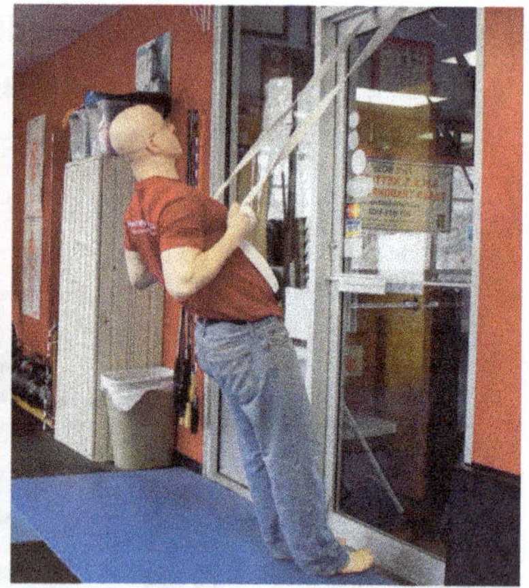

These may be done with a door or tied to a bar and with one or two arms. If you are practicing the door version, tie a knot in one end of one or two belts. Put it, or them, over the top of the door and then close the door tightly. Lean back and pull yourself upward. You may loop handles in the belt on the gripping side if necessary. I tend not to do so, since the loops make it easier to grip and thus rob you of additional grip strength training.

When using a bar, as on a Smith machine, for example, make a slip-knot with the belt. Loop it over the bar, tighten it and lean back. The bar version allows you to train with a variety of levels.

Always use a full range of motion while training in these (and most) movements. When performing the one-arm version, keep your shoulders square. This will aid you in developing greater core strength and allow you to take full advantage of the unilateral movement, thus making your body work harder by recruiting more muscle stabilizers.

LAT PULLS

Lie flat on your stomach and reach forward as far as you can while keeping your hands in line with your shoulders. Bend your knees so that your lower body looks like a frog swimming and bring your legs together as you pull yourself up to your hands. Then rinse and repeat.

This movement is best performed on a mat or smooth floor as opposed to a carpet. Start with 10-15 pulls in accordance with your fitness and strength levels.

NECK STRENGTH

The development of a strong neck is essential to survival, as you'll see when looking at the size of the necks of collision- or combat-sport athletes. They are huge. Why is this?

It's because the neck is the shock absorber for your brain. The stronger your neck is, the less shock your brain will suffer and the fewer traumas your body will have to endure. This holds true not only in combat, but in case of a fall or a car accident.

DYNAMIC RESISTANCE FOUR-WAY NECK

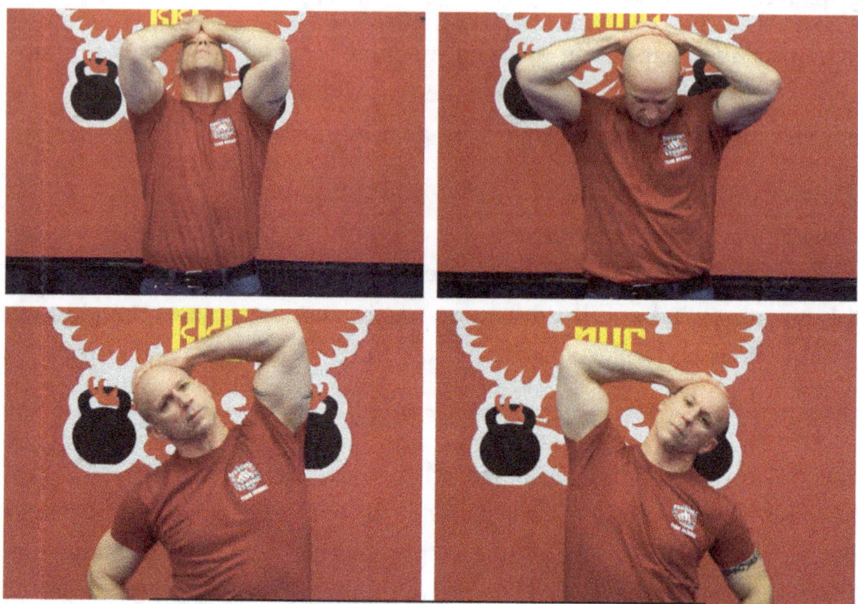

Tilt your head all the way back and place your palms on your forehead. Providing counter-pressure with your hands, move your head all the way forward for a count of 10. Now place your hands on the back of your head and repeat the movement in the opposite direction. After you have done back and forth, tilt your head all the way to the left and place your right hand on the right side of your head and move your head all the way to the right, counting to 10 once again. Repeat the movement to the left side. It's important to note that you should use a full range of motion and keep steady pressure for the full count of 10 in each direction.

BACK-PRESSURE NECK

Stand with your heels close to the wall and place a folded towel on the wall and behind your head. Apply pressure backward into the wall for a count of 10. Relax for two seconds and repeat for 10 repetitions. Perform three sets of this movement.

PARTNER TRAINING

If you do not participate in external resistance training with kettlebells, sandbags, barbells and the like, to maximize your lower body strength in particular you should work with a partner. External Resistance, defined as any other weight than that of your own body, is needed to develop your highest level of strength, so if you don't have equipment a training partner will come in most handy.

It is good practice to have a partner close to your size and weight, especially when you first embark on partner training. This is not always available, however, so you'll need to work with what you have.

PARTNER SQUATS

Direct your partner to climb onto your back, as if you were going to play "Chicken Fight." Loop your arms around their legs at knee level and actively pull yourself down. Only pull yourself deep enough so that you are able to get up! If you bottom out, simply have your partner get off.

The number of repetitions that you do depends on the strength that you have developed during your solo squat training. However, starting with five to 10 repetitions is a good place to begin. If you can only do two or three reps per set, you will want to improve your strength in your solo squat work and/or incorporate Trust Squats.

TRUST SQUATS

This exercise does not add additional weight, but it enables both parties to safely achieve a deep squat, thus expanding their range of motion by going well beyond parallel. Start by facing your partner and grasping their hands, right to right and left to left. Straighten your arms and lean back as far as possible with your feet approximately one foot from your partners' and shoulder width apart. Actively pull yourself down in unison with your partner. Keep tension in your body as you drive your feet into the ground and propel yourself upward.

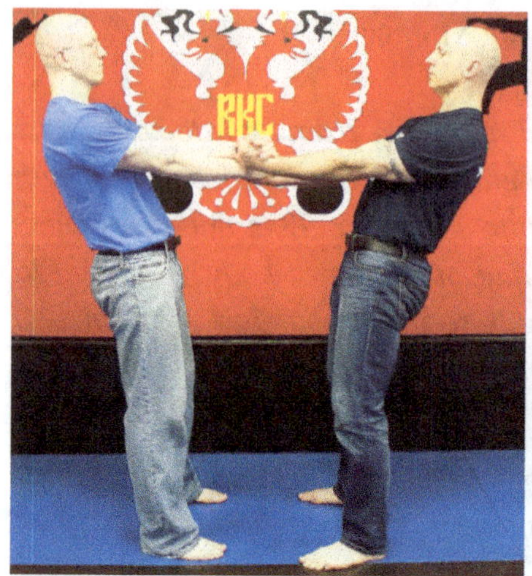

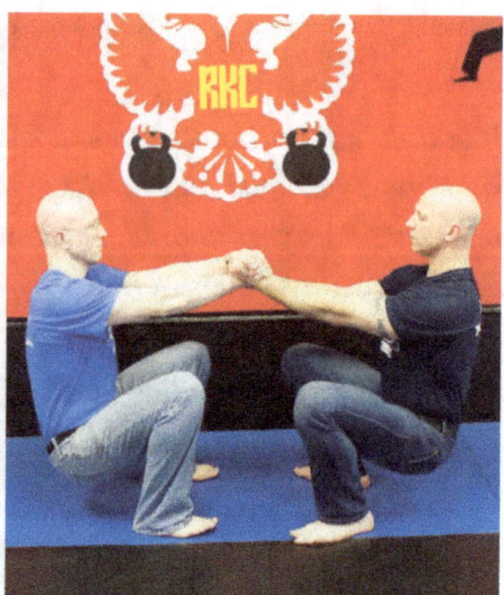

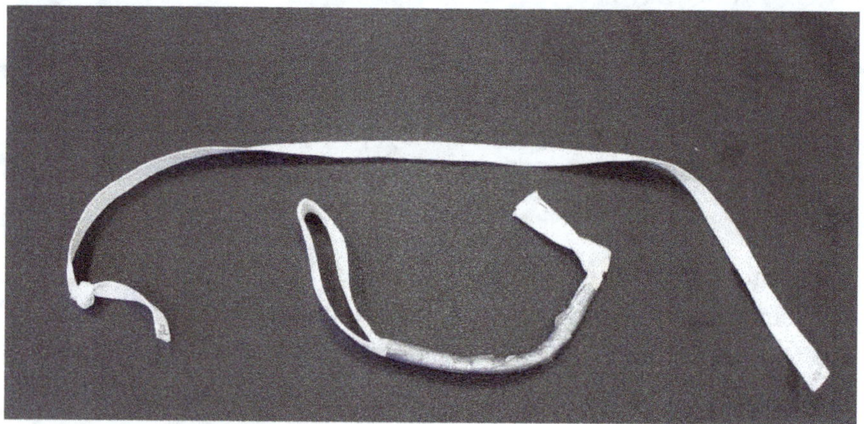

Knotted karate belt & bite belt.

You do not have to be close in weight to your partner to do this exercise. If you don't have a partner, use a karate belt in a doorway. Repeat this for 20 repetitions in each set.

PIGGY-BACKS

Assume the position that you did in the Partner Squats and run with your partner on your back. Perform laps alternating with your partner. It is recommended that you run in a straight line, since making cuts and turns with someone on your back may result in injury.

STANDING LIFTS

There are a variety of standing lifts that you may perform. These are fantastic for developing coordination and real, functional strength from having to adjust to the shifting weight of your partner. These lifts also develop the explosive power and hip pop necessary to rip an opponent off of the ground.

BODY-SLAM LIFT

Facing your partner, thread your left arm through their legs and situate your right arm over the left side of their neck. Lift and tilt them toward the right side so that they become parallel to the floor and perpendicular to you. If you were to finish the slam, you would continue the movement until the opponent's feet were above your head. You would then pile-drive their head into the ground. However, we are simply using this lift to create

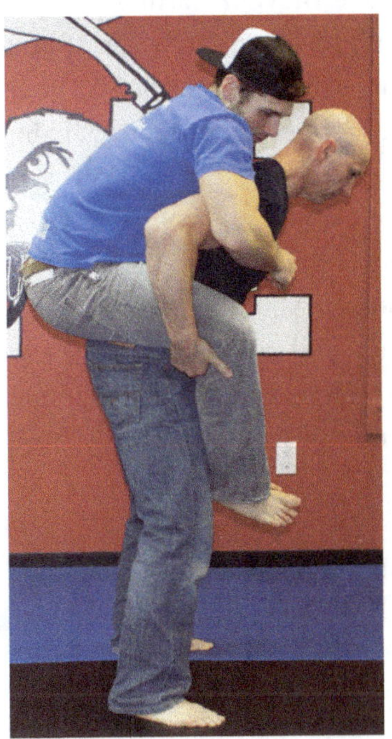
Piggy back.

strength at this point. Repeat this for five repetitions on each side for each set. Add more reps as you become stronger.

DOUBLE LEG LIFT

Face your partner and put your head to one side as you shoot in for a takedown (shoot means going low, stepping forward and grabbing one or both of your opponent's legs to set them up for a takedown). Pin your inside ear to your partner's body, arch your back, look upward, and lift them off of the ground. Repeat this process on alternating sides. Practice this drill with the clock set to 30 seconds and alternate with your partner. Increase the time to a minute when you become more conditioned.

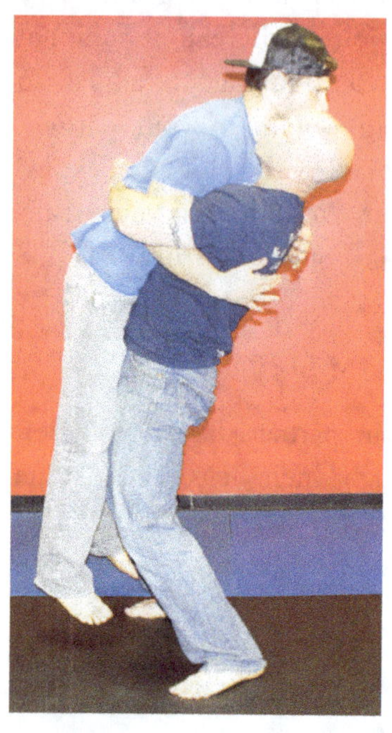

ONE-ARM BEAR-HUG LIFT

Trapping one of your partner's arms, grasp them low about the waist. If you have their right arm trapped, your right hand should be facing palm down on your Gable Grip. As you sure up the Gable Grip, roll your wrist toward you and into their floating ribs, step in and lift. You don't have to hurt your partner; just use enough power to make sure you have the technique down solid.

DONKEY CALVES

Start by hinging your hips so that your upper body is at a 90- degree angle. Support yourself with your extended arms on a bench or another sturdy surface. Have your training partner sit on your lower back, facing toward your head. Perform calf raises from this position. There are three basic positions to use for these exercises: toes pointed in, toes pointed out and toes pointed straight ahead.

PARTNER DEAD-LIFT CARRIES

Have your partner get on their hands and knees on a matted surface. Approach them from the back, straddle them and wrap your arms around their waist and use the Gable (or thumbless) Grip. Lift your partner up and move them forward. If they are too heavy for you to move them on your own, have them assist you by pushing off of the ground with their hands and feet.

TOWEL TUG-O-WAR (LAT PULLS)

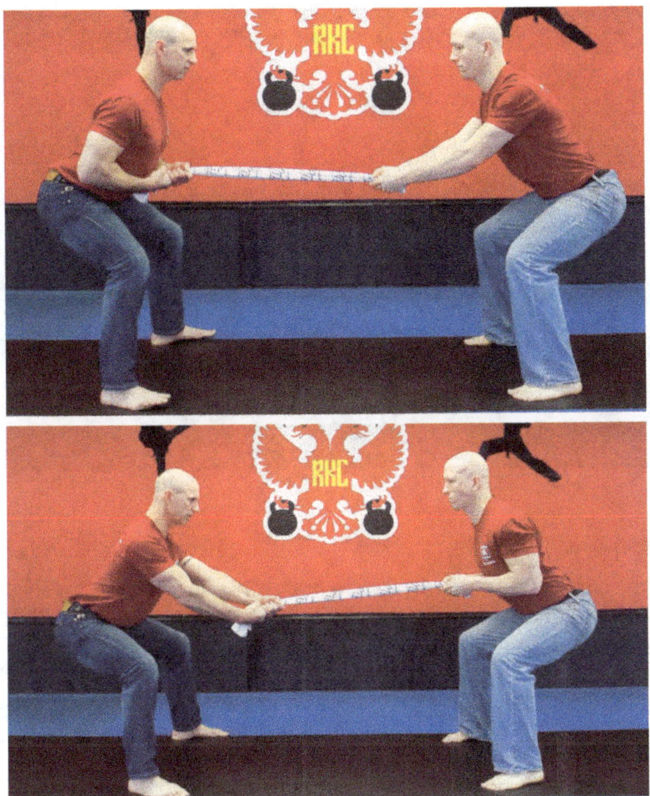

Take a standard-sized bath towel and fold it the long way until you cannot create any more folds. Standing face-to-face, each person bends their knees, bends at the hip and maintains a neutral spine as they grasp the towel. One person has their arms bent and the towel close to their body. The other has their arms fully extended.

Next, you apply tension as both people pull on the towel. Even though both parties are pulling, just enough tension is applied to allow for a five-second pull in each direction. Repeat five to 10 repetitions in each direction. Maintain a neutral spine and "athletic stance" for the duration of the movement.

TOWEL TRICEPS

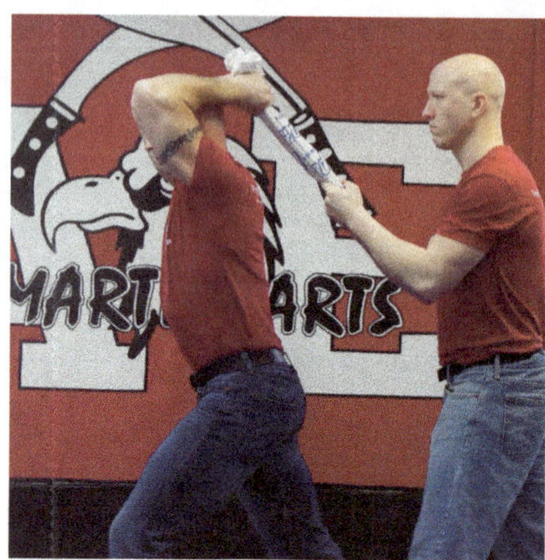 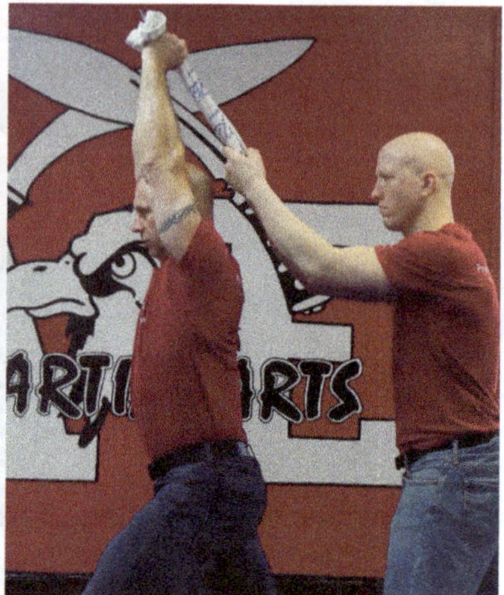

You'll need one towel between you and your partner. Configure it as did for the Tug-o-War. The person working the triceps will grasp the two ends of the towel, elbows bent so that their hands are behind their head and their elbows are pointed upward. A "U" will be formed by the towel and will be positioned in the middle of their back. They will adopt a staggered stance with one foot back for added balance. The partner will be behind and grab the towel at the bend. They will apply tension so that it takes effort for the person with the two ends to completely lock out their elbows. On the descent, the elbows must be unlocked, and then the person pulls the towel down as resistance is being applied. Repeat this movement for three to seven repetitions per set. There should be minimal body movement during this exercise.

PARTNER DRAGS

Have your partner lie flat on their back. Have them grasp a martial arts belt firmly in their hands, elbows flexed. Face your partner so that your feet are about one foot away from their head. Using two hands (or one if you are very strong), grab the belt and pull your partner backward. Repeat this movement for as long as you are able.

PLOW-HORSE

Have your partner wear a martial arts belt. Position yourself directly behind them. Grab their belt with one or two hands while you are behind them. They will adopt a Front Stance (70 percent of their weight on the front leg and 30 percent on the rear one) and step forward as you are applying tension in the opposite direction. You want to apply only enough to make it difficult for them to walk forward.

If the person holding the belt is very strong, use one arm to hold it. If you need to use two hands to apply more backward tension, do so.

LEG-THROWS

One of the old-time gym favorites! Be certain to keep your lumbar spine "bolted" to the ground. You can accomplish this by contracting your upper abdominals and forcing your hips to the ground simultaneously, as you assume the supine position. Next, your partner will stand with their feet at your head, and they will be facing the same direction as you. Reach your arms upward and behind you and grab their ankles. Now raise your feet up quickly and once your legs reach 65 to 75 degrees, your partner will push them downward so that your feet wind up approximately six inches off of the ground, after which you bring them up quickly again. You may also have your partner throw your feet to either side.

Start with 10 repetitions and direct your partner to only apply enough downward thrust to push your feet to within six inches of the ground before you bring them back up. To make this more difficult, you can have your partner push down on your thighs directly above your knees as opposed to pushing your feet. Once you become stronger, work your way up to 30 repetitions per set.

DOG STANCE

One partner assumes the Dog Stance, positioning on all fours. The other sits on their back while facing the opposite direction and hooking their feet inside the thighs of their partner. The top person leans backward as far as they can go. Simultaneously, the bottom person (in the dog stance or "referee's position") uses their head to push against the low back of their partner, both as the top person goes up and down. Repeat for 10 repetitions and then switch positions.

PARTNER PLUMB

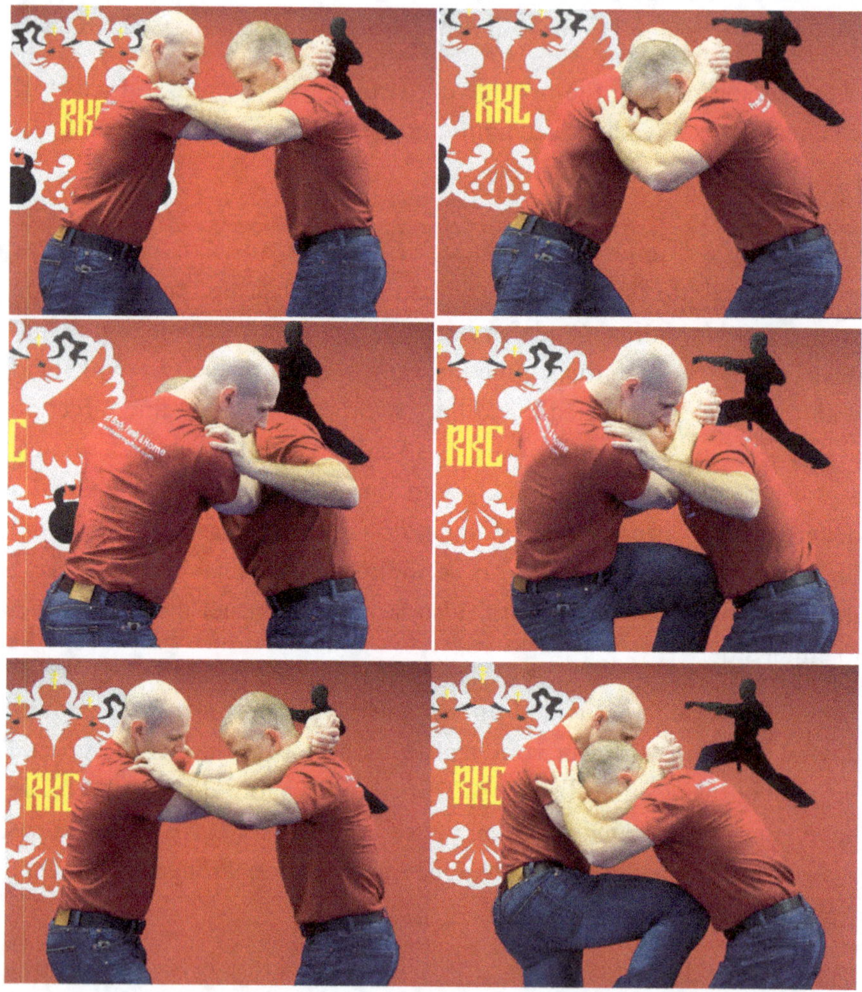

Face your partner, and start by having one of you apply a Gable Grip around their partner's neck and pinching their elbows close together. Start slowly and then build speed and tension as you shake and move your partner about. Do this for 15 seconds, and then switch roles. Repeat this movement three times each. Once you become adept at this movement, you can add time and increase the sets.

ISOMETRICS AND DYNAMIC TENSION

SAMPSON PRESS

Stand in a sturdy doorway. Place your arms from your palms to your elbows on the inside of the door jam and press outward. It is important to tighten the whole body as you push outward. Hold the full tension position for 10-15 seconds. Repeat three to five times.

REVERSE SAMPSON PRESS

Begin as you would in the Sampson Press, except place your arms at your sides with your palms facing you. Place the back of your hands against the door jam and tense your body as you press outward with the back of your hands. Hold this position for 30-60 seconds with full-body tension. Repeat this for two to three times per workout session. Upon completion, it's fun to step out of the doorway and allow your arms to go upward on their own!

BICEPS AND TRICEPS

Stand tall with your feet shoulder-width or a little less apart. Pack your shoulders and engage your lats. Put your hands together with one hand palm down and the other palm up. Keep them fairly close to your body. Push down with the top hand as you are providing resistance with the palm up bottom hand.

Perform the same movement in the opposite direction, thus working the triceps on one arm and the biceps on the other. Repeat this movement for five repetitions, three seconds up and three seconds down, and then switch arms. Be certain to employ full-body tension while executing this movement.

SQUAT AND HOLD

Stand with your feet shoulder-width apart. Applying full body tension, assume five different positions during the full range of motion. These positions are:

Top - Knees locked out.

One-Third Down - Bend your knees slightly so that you are halfway between standing and mid-squat.

Half-Way Way Down - Bend your knees so that you are halfway between standing and the bottom of your squat.

Two-Thirds Down - Bring yourself below the parallel position (the hip joint dipping below the top of the knee).

Full Bottom - Lower yourself to the utmost bottom of your squat. Be sure to avoid the "tail tuck."

Hold each position for a five-second count. Move from position to position. Mix it up; they don't need to be done in order. Start with 15-20 repetitions per set.

LYING SQUAT

Lie flat on your back and dorsiflex both feet. Place your hands on the floor at your sides and lift your head off of the floor by contracting your lower abs. Bring your knees up toward your chest or as high as you can possibly go. Have your training partner grab your instep with a hook grip and then pull your legs until they are straight. Don't offer a hundred percent resistance; you will get pulled across the floor! Once your legs are straight, repeat the process in the opposite direction. Repeat this for three to five repetitions per set.

ENDURANCE

High-stress situations demand massive anaerobic and aerobic capacity. During a street confrontation, you will experience an incredible adrenaline dump. The better condition you are in, the better your chances will be in managing the onset of weakness, shortness of breath and tunnel vision. Also, you may have just gone through a hard day (or night) of work and may be exhausted. If you are in better condition, you will be able to handle daily fatigue better.

WHAT ARE SOME OF THE BEST TRAINING METHODS TO EMPLOY?

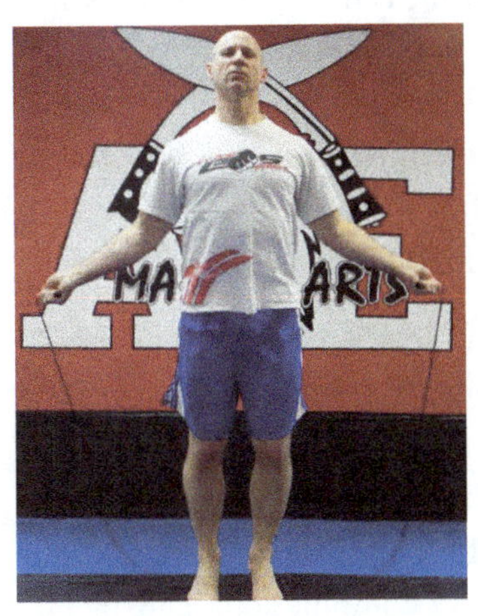

Skipping rope is the single best aerobic activity for a fighter. We begin every training session with three to five minutes of skipping rope. You need not perform double-jumps, crossing the rope or other fancy rope tricks to gain the benefits of jumping rope.

Why is jumping rope so good? For starters, you can do it anywhere. If it's cold or snowing or too hot outside, it doesn't matter. You can jump indoors. The coordination of moving your hands and feet in rhythm with each other, plus the shifting of weight from one foot to the other prepares one for moving and striking.

Burpees facilitate anaerobic conditioning and also help us to train to use the sprawl, which is a maneuver used to defend the legs against a single- or double-leg takedown.

Bag Work offers the best combination of skill-building and endurance training. There are additional bonuses of power development and body hardening. You will find routines listed in Chapter 14.

Grappling is possibly the best man-to-man strength building endeavor you can participate in. Pushing, pulling, balancing and reacting to the movements of another human as you vie for position develops incredible strength and body awareness. Grappling also contributes to the hardening or callusing of the body. Wrestlers and grapplers are notoriously tough due to the grinding nature of their training.

MIRROR OR SHADOW TRAINING

The Sprawl and Brawl drill is a great way to conduct a solo MMA (Mixed Martial Arts) warm-up or endurance-building regimen.

Stand in front of a mirror and practice your movement (footwork, slips, bobs, weaves, parries), kicks, punches and combinations, and every ten to fifteen seconds or so, drop to a sprawl and pop back up. Throw a knee every time you come back to your feet. Most likely, your opponent's head will be at your knee level after your sprawl. It's recommended to perform two-minute rounds with 30 seconds of active rest.

Shadow boxing, kickboxing or defensive tactics may all be practiced in front of a mirror. Practice your movement and strikes in a series of combinations while imagining executing them on an opponent. Set a timer and explode into the techniques. Practice should be pointed and have purpose. Repeat specific maneuvers for a chosen number of repetitions or specific duration. The techniques, combinations and tactics are listed in chapters 9, 10, 12, and 13. Use the same time criterion as used in the above.

The Wall Drill for kicking is the single best exercise for perfecting your kicks and developing the power of your higher kicks. I have to tell you, this drill does NOT get any easier with practice. You simply develop better kicks. Start by placing your right hand on the wall, with your right foot about a foot away from the wall and your left up, level with your head and facing the opposite direction so that you are perpendicular to the wall.

All of these kicks are to be done slowly. A solid two to three seconds (longer to make it more difficult) in each direction is about right. Look toward your left hand and do the 10 repetitions of the following five kicks:

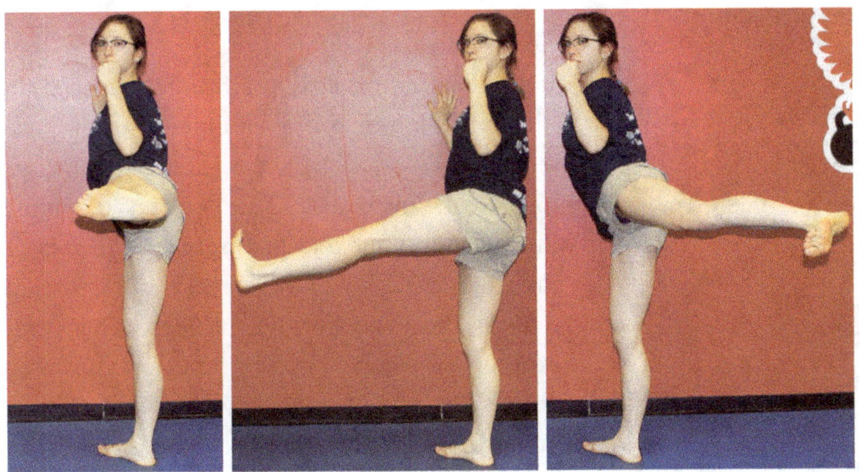

Side-leg raise | Forward crescent circles | Backward crescent kick.

SIDE-LEG RAISE

Dorsiflex your foot, keep the leg that you are lifting in line with the base leg and lift it as high as you are able to *without* bending your back. Don't focus on the height of your kicks; concern yourself with your alignment. After the tenth repetition, hold the leg in the up position for two counts of 10.

FORWARD CRESCENT CIRCLES

Move your foot forward and bring it up as high as you can. Once you have reached the peak start to bring your foot to the back, keeping your leg up as high as you can especially when your foot passes the halfway point of your body and goes behind you. The circles should be slow, deliberate and at the full range of the movement.

BACKWARD CRESCENT CIRCLES

This is the same movement as the previous one, but with one exception :start the movement backward with your heel leading the way as opposed to your toes.

SIDE KICK

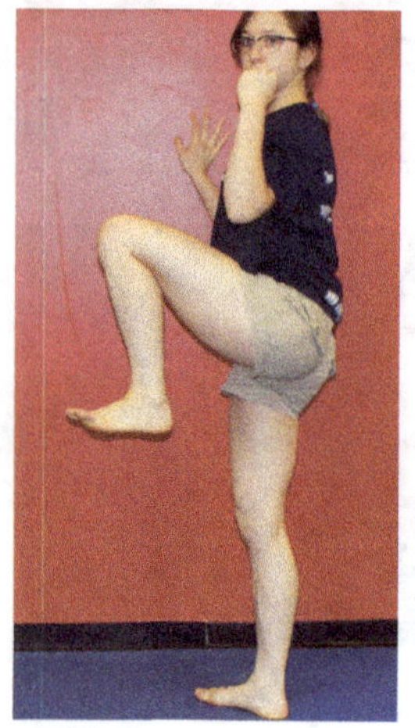

Side kick.

From the starting position, bring your knee up high so that your heel is in line with your base leg. Turn your foot on the floor so that your toes are facing the wall and rotate your hips, thus turning your foot and pointing the toes of the chambered leg to the ground (a chambered leg has the knee up and the leg drawn back poised to kick). Slowly extend your leg outward as if you were driving your heel into your target. Return your kick slowly to the starting position. Repeat for 10 repetitions and hold in the out position on the tenth repetition for two counts of 10.

ROUNDHOUSE KICK

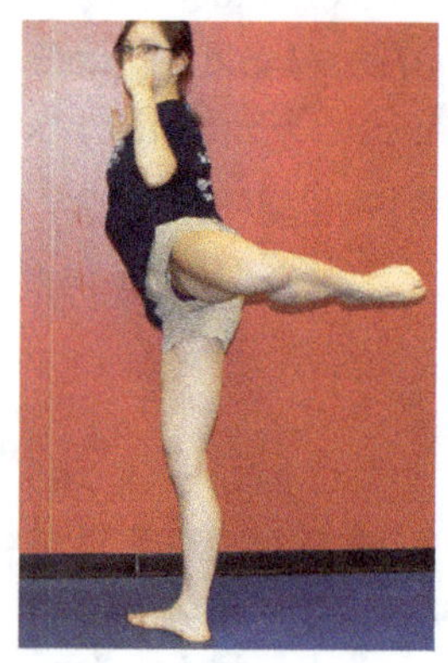

Roundhouse kick.

Pull the kicking knee back until it is aligned with your hip. Plantar-flex your foot so that your toes are pointed. Extend your leg but be sure to keep your knee in exactly the same spot. Bring your foot out and back to full extension and full flexion for 10 repetitions. On repetition #10, hold your foot in the extended position for two counts of 10.

Then you should repeat these movements with the other leg.

BODY CONDITIONING

You need to forge your body into a rock-hard form. Your goal is to create a well-conditioned, durable, calloused and resilient body, which will prepare you to handle any physical emergency.

This should be done to the extent to which you turn your body into a machine that is able to withstand an attack and return an onslaught. To what degree you develop this ability depends entirely on how much effort you are willing to put into it.

One key aspect to achieving a high level of conditioning is to toughen the body to prepare it to withstand trauma. This includes the entire body: hands, arms, shins, thighs, torso, etc. A great deal of this will be accomplished with actual sparring. However, to maximize the toughness of the body, specific hardening drills are necessary. This is called **callusing of the body**.

Conditioning of the shins, knees, elbows, hands, wrists, and fingertips is imperative for having a body that is strong and able to withstand an attack. You need to forge your limbs into "steel implements." The use of sand, rice, pebbles and even crushed glass will toughen your fingers, hands and skin. There is a partner forearm-toughening drill that works wonders as well.

Use of a Makiwara: A Makiwara comes in one of several configurations. For instance, you can wrap wood in cloth or rope. Or it can be a brick wrapped with rope or buckets filled with sand, pebbles or even crushed glass. Strike with your front two knuckles, the edge of your hand, palm, and fingers. Always begin lightly and then increase the power of your strikes gradually as you become more conditioned. If you are using buckets, strike downward into the bucket filled with material. Start with sand, progress to pebbles and then on to crushed glass if so desired. This will toughen the skin and strengthen your hands for striking. This may take several months to years to build the desired callusing and bone density.

Make certain that the surface you strike has some give, and DO NOT mount it on a wall. The energy will get transferred back to your shoulder, elbow and wrist. Be forewarned, if you become overzealous you will injure yourself and prolong your conditioning process unnecessarily.

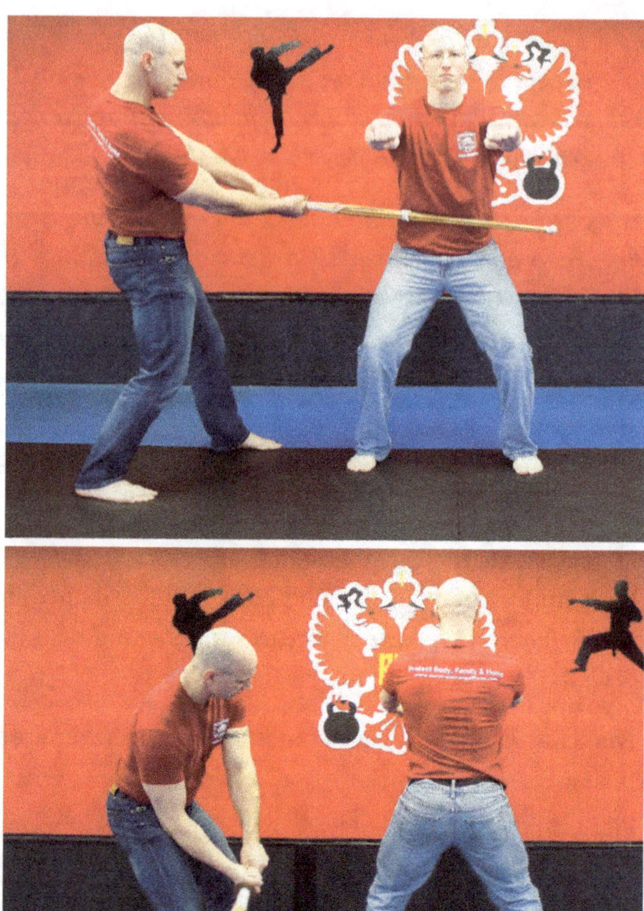

The Wing Chun wooden dummy is also great for toughening the body: forearms, palms, feet and shins. There are a variety of books and videos on the techniques for training with the dummy. The downside of this training is the size of the piece of equipment and mounting it, this is why I haven't used one in 30 years. The other prescribed methods of body conditioning described in this book will be more than sufficient and take up less space. You would be better suited allocating the space and your funds toward a hundred-pound Muay Thai or heavy bag for boxing.

When working with a partner, one of the best conditioning workouts is the Two-Position Forearm- Conditioning Drill. Stand facing your training partner in a fighting stance, and each of you will put your right foot forward. Place the backs of your forearms so that they are against each other. Simultaneously, bring your forearms down so that your fist is at knee level, and bang the backs of your forearms together. Immediately bring them back to the original position and bang them together again. Repeat this process for repetitions or time. The amount of time or number of repetitions depends on the conditioning level of you and your partner. Add in more hip movement and harder strikes as you become stronger and more conditioned. As with all of these body-conditioning exercises, start slowly and increase the speed and power of the callusing technique as your body becomes more accustomed to the trauma.

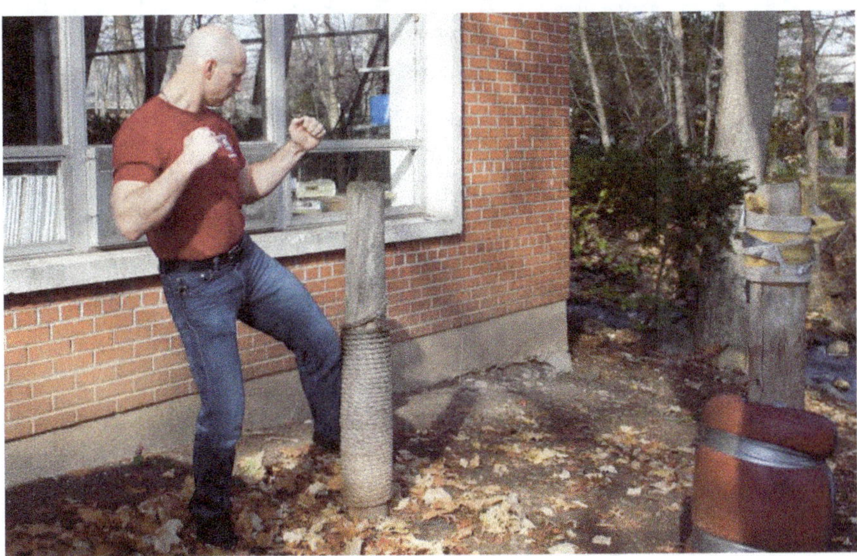

My all-time favorite for shin conditioning is using a fencepost wrapped with foam, carpet, or rope. At our studio, we have two kicking posts outside. One is wrapped in foam, and the other is wrapped in 3/4" rope.

If you only have space for one, then I suggest wrapping it with a thick-pile carpet.

If you do not have access to a kicking post, there are other methods to prepare your shins for combat. You may use a rolling pin and run it up and down your shins. Couple this with light taps from a rattan stick up and down the full length of the shin bone. Additionally, your heavy bag work will contribute to the hardening of your shins, as well as your knees, elbows and hands.

How does this work? You will experience microbreaks in your shins, which sounds bad but is actually important for toughening up that area. They will heal, thus resulting in thicker, denser shin bones.

Many of my training partners have complained about how "hard" my shins are. My Shin Kicks and Cut Kicks have yielded favorable results in competitions and street applications. At one time I experienced a trilateral, spiral fracture, which was a highly unusual injury. Upon reading the X-ray in the emergency room, the physician came to me with a pale look on his face. He had thought that I had some type of "strange disease" or cancer. He went on to explain that he'd never seen anything like this before and was extremely concerned. I told him to relax and then assured him that what he saw was normal for the activity that I take part in. He was relieved. He also became one of my students and has been since 2002!

Do not start your training with hard strikes; this will injure you. Progress slowly after starting out with light, controlled strikes. As with all body conditioning, if you allow yourself to get carried away you may get injured and then you will miss training. Again, build slowly and condition over time. Body conditioning and callusing is a marathon, not a sprint.

GRIP STRENGTH

The development of a strong grip is quite possibly the most important attribute to have as a good fighter. The ability to grab, hold, crush and pull is fundamental to your ability to defend yourself and continue to fight. Your grip will be significantly enhanced through many of the exercises contained in this book, and that is fantastic news for you since grip strength is so essential.

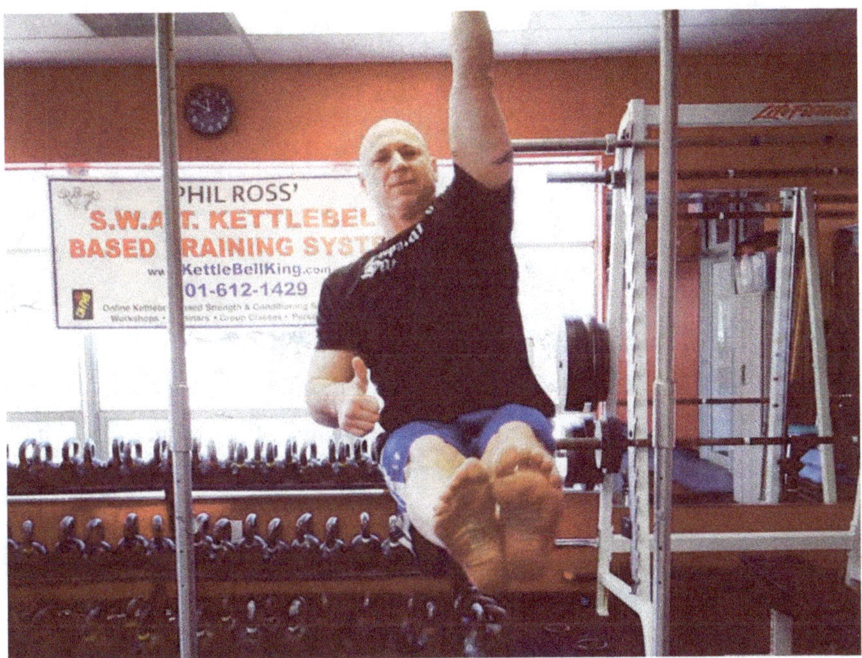

As your grip strength increases, you will need to grab, twist, hold and crush with more and more force. We have a significant number of exercises for grip strength listed earlier in this chapter, specifically exercises using a belt or a towel.

Some additional training methods will include Fingertip Push-Ups, which are great. Squeezing hand grippers or a tennis ball are fantastic as well. Then there is the Spear-Hand Thrust, in which you plunge your hand into a bucket of rice or sand and grip, twist and squeeze. You can crumple a newspaper one sheet at a time. And you should hang, simply jump up, grab onto a bar and hang. Use two hands, or one hand and bring your legs into an L-Sit position. Hang for a time in various configurations. Start with 30 seconds and then increase. If you are able to support your weight for two minutes or more while hanging from a bar, it means you've developed good grip strength. Obviously, the heavier you are, the more difficult the task, but this movement, like many bodyweight movements, is a good indicator of how much you should weigh.

There are many other grip-enhancing exercises. But these are some of my favorites, and they are the most economical and easily accessible.

WRIST STRENGTH

Grappling will do a lot to condition the wrists. But specific exercises can be very beneficial for not only making them strong, but also flexible and resilient.

As mentioned earlier in this chapter, Knuckle Push-Ups and Back-of-the Wrist Push-Ups are great for wrist strength and range of motion. Then there are the various wrist-stretching exercises, palm up with a straight elbow, and palm down as well. We also use a variety of wrist rotations and stretches. Some of the best stretches for the wrists and forearms involve placing your hands palm down, on the floor or against a wall. On the wall, have your fingers facing the ground so that the underside of your wrist is facing upward. While kneeling on the floor, have your fingers facing you. For either of the positions, shift your weight toward your fingers while keeping your palms flat on the surface. Rock back and forth, changing the amount of pressure. Perform the exercise for a minute or so for each hand. While on the floor, do both hands at once.

Another great strength, conditioning and flexibility exercise is the Wrist Lock Drill. Not only do you gain the aforementioned from this training drill, but you also learn how to move while in a Wrist Lock and position yourself properly to respond once you have gotten away.

Start by facing your partner. Reach out and grab their wrist, then respond with a Wrist Lock. They, in turn, will go with the technique by either turning or rolling and re-grabbing you with a Wrist Lock. Repeat this process of locking, grabbing, re-grabbing, and countering for 30 to 60 seconds per round. The specifics on executing several Wrist Locks are listed in Chapter 8, titled "Grips and Locks."

When you become more advanced, you can use tools such as bamboo shinai and, eventually, wooden dowels to toughen and condition these areas. Though not normal to mainstream training, they have proven to be very effective for many practitioners.

Physicality is extremely important for both your body and your mind. You will need strength and endurance to be able to defend yourself at the highest level under the worst circumstances.

Training Sessions

No one has the ability to choose when they will be attacked or faced with a dire situation in the street. Victory favors the prepared. You may have just gotten off of your shift at work and are completely exhausted, and then you get attacked. If you are in good condition, your chances of survival are increased. If you are too weak and fatigued to respond, you will perish.

Listed below are a few examples of training sessions that we use on a regular basis. We address speed, agility, endurance, strength, mobility and flexibility in these sessions. Feel free to design your own based on the information in this book.

TRAINING SESSION EXAMPLES

ENDURANCE CIRCUIT

Jump rope for two to three minutes, perform bo-staff stretching, free-hand stretching or a combination of both for 10-12 minutes to get ready for your circuit. Be certain to include bridges in your warm-up.

The circuit is as follows:

- Jump Rope: 100 Skips
- Push-Ups: 10 to 25 reps (various types and difficulties)
- Jump Rope: 100 skips
- Standard Squats: 25 reps
- Jump Rope: 100 skips
- Pull-Ups: 80% of Max
- Jump Rope: 100 skips
- Split Squats: 15 reps on each side
- Jump Rope: 100 skips
- Dips: 10 to 15
- Jump Rope: 100 skips
- Abdominals: Wheel of Death, = 5 reps; Leg Thrusts, = 30 reps

Repeat this circuit three times.

STRENGTH CIRCUIT

Take your time and make certain that you have 30 to 60 seconds of rest between exercises. Low reps are in order, one to five for beginners and one to 10 for more advanced practitioners. The reps should be based on 70 to 80 percent of your max effort per exercise. Remember, our goal is strength development, not cardiovascular endurance.

Jump Rope for two to three minutes and make certain that you focus on warming up your joints thoroughly to prepare yourself for the task ahead. You will be stressing your joints with these more difficult movements:

- One-Arm Push-Ups
- Single-Leg (Pistol) Squats
- Pull-Ups
- Back Bridge (Full or Table-Top)
- Handstands (to your level)
- Air Lunges
- Hanging Abs
- Plyometric Squats

- Calf Raises
- Four-Way Neck

Repeat this circuit four to five times.

STRENGTH AND ENDURANCE BODYWEIGHT CIRCUIT

Jump Rope for three minutes and loosen up your body from the ground up with ankle rotations, small knee circles, hip rotations, shoulder circles back and forth, wrist rotations and neck stretching. The warm-up should take seven to 10 minutes.

Set your timer for fifty seconds of work and 10 seconds of rest between each movement. Work to your "reasonable max," not to burn out but push yourself. If you can't do the movements for the full 50 seconds, use a regression. Example: Let's suppose that it takes you 30 seconds to do six Pull-Ups and there are twenty seconds left in the set. Perform Plank Pull-Ups for the remaining twenty seconds. Do five rotations of the below-listed exercises for a total of 45 minutes. At the end spend three to five minutes on your cool-down and stretch.

1. Handstands
2. Dips
3. Hanging Abs or other Abs
4. Push-Ups
5. Squats
6. Bridges
7. Lunges
8. Pull-Ups
9. Calves

Cool Down and Stretch.

Chapter 5
Weapons of The Human Body

The human body, with all of its frailty and potential target areas, has some built-in weapons. The key is to condition them and know how to apply them properly. We'll start from the bottom and work our way up, describing the available weapons and how to use them best. The specifics of the execution of the actual techniques will be addressed in Chapter 9.

THE FOOT

The foot has several basic areas and positions suited for attack. First is the heel. I put the heel as number one because the use of the heel as a weapon takes very little skill and is a great loosening-up or distraction technique, as well as a fantastic finisher. It's also a great counterattack to employ when grabbed from behind. To use the heel, it's best to dorsiflex the foot and stomp downward. This position creates the most tension in the foot and focuses more force per square inch on a smaller area. The primary techniques to use are Stomps, Shin Rakes, Mule, and Push-Kicks.

The Ball-of-the-Foot Front Kick is a thrusting technique that can be delivered to virtually any part of the body from the shin to the chin. As opposed to Front-Snap Kick which is only good when used to strike the groin or the chin.

The instep of the foot is a great spot to strike with when delivering a Roundhouse Kick. The instep is located between the toes and the ankle of the foot. It is best to have the area between the arch and the ankle as the focal contact point with the desired target.

THE SHIN

The use of this area for striking was made popular by Muay Thai, but has been in use for many, many years and in a multitude of cultures prior to the recent Thailand-inspired fame.

A well-conditioned shin bone is like a baseball bat. We achieve this advanced state of hardness through a gradual conditioning process. Start slowly and gently at first. You will not condition your shins overnight! Try to avoid causing your shins to bruise, bleed or get severe bumps. Discoloration and soreness are to be expected. However, do not take it to excess; if you injure yourself, you can't train.

Over time, you will create microfractures in your shins. They will heal and result in calcium deposits. As they multiply, the shin becomes harder and denser. Repeat this cycle of healing enough times and you will have forged a formidable pair of weapons! The primary attacks using the shins are the Cut Kick, Shin Kick and Rip Kick.

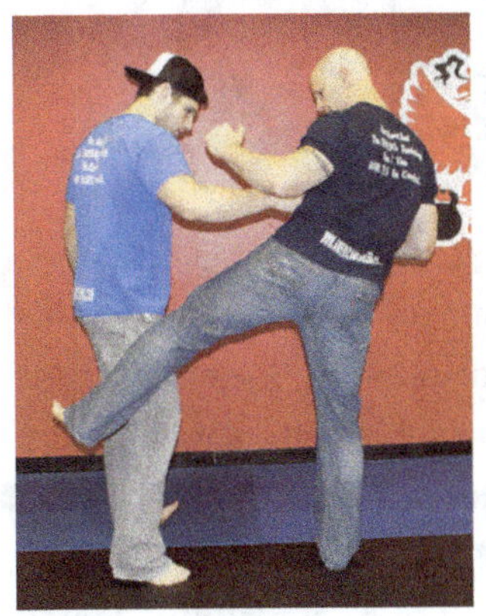
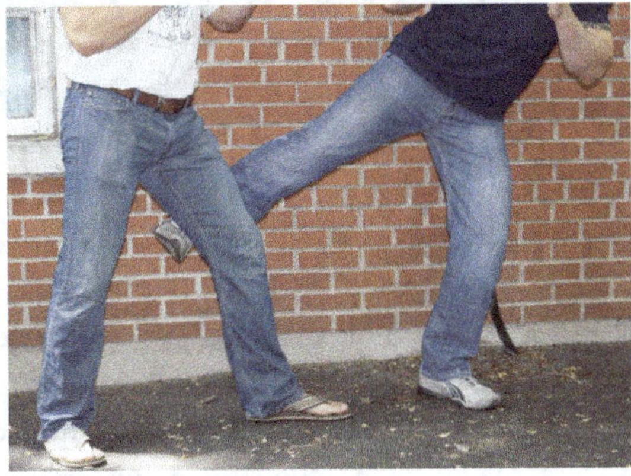

THE KNEE

The most powerful strike that the human body can deliver is the Flying Knee. It can land with a force comparable to being hit by a car traveling 35 mph.

The Flying Knee may not be practical for most people to use. But simple knee strikes are very easily administered to the femoral artery (inner thigh), the perennial nerve (outer thigh), bladder, solar plexus, kidneys, ribs and groin. Once you've doubled your adversary over with a well-placed strike (or strikes) to the aforementioned soft tissue areas, strikes with the knees to the face and head are easily delivered. You won't stop, but keep throwing the knees until your assailant drops to the ground giving you ample time to escape.

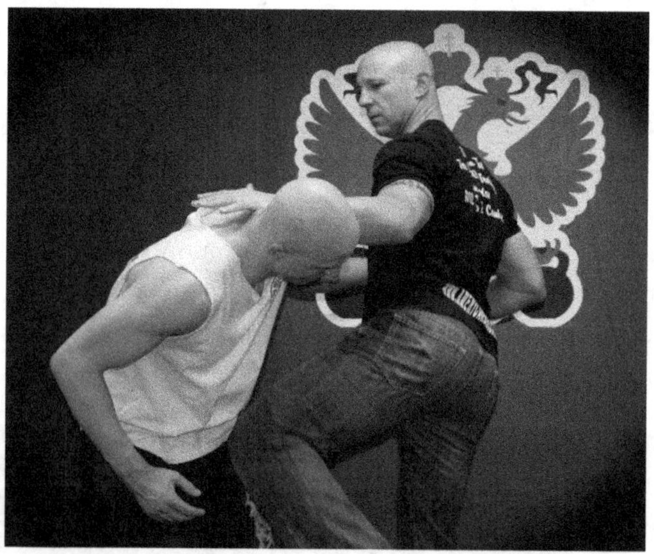

There are several ways to secure a grip on your opponent when administering Knee Strikes. One method is referred to as the Plumb. To use the Plumb, or Thai Clinch, grab your opponent with both hands behind the neck. Do not interlock your fingers. Instead, use a palm-to-palm, also called the Gable grip. This grip is the most effective grip available. Several years ago, the top Division 1 NCAA wrestling teams conducted tests on the various hand grips. The Gable Grip (palm-to-palm) won, hands down (pun fully intended).

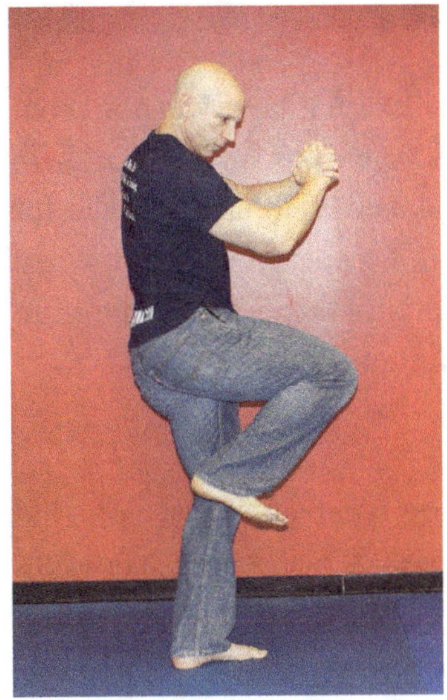

Knee drive and Muay Thai clinch.

Another method comes into play when you are on the side of your opponent and they are doubled over (bent at the waist). Take one arm and place your hand on the back of their neck with your forearm positioned against their jaw. The other arm is threaded under their arm with your hand placed on their back. From this position you are able to levy Knee Strikes to the face, ribs, stomach and the peroneal nerve of the leg closest to you. This position also makes it difficult for your opponent to turn into you to grab you because you are controlling their head. There are two other distinct advantages to this position. You are able to see the surrounding area, and you are positioned to throw your opponent either to the ground or into another assailant.

The Spring-Board Knee is simple and extremely powerful. The strike is delivered at close range. Stomp one foot hard into the ground and then "spring" upward as you drive the other knee into your opponent's body. More power is garnered by this method due to the plyometric nature of delivering this strike.

The Flying Knee is the most powerful, yet the landing percentage is not as high as the other methods for delivering the knee. When you literally "launch" yourself at an intended target, you gain sheer power from the movement and speed generated; plus, you eliminate the friction with the ground. This is a risky move, and you stand a greater chance of missing. I would only recommend this strike if you catch your opponent completely off-guard or as a finishing technique once they have sustained a significant amount of damage and are unable to move quickly.

THE HIPS AND BUTT

On the surface, the hips and buttocks seem like unlikely weapons, but their applications are many. You can use your hips and buttocks to smash into your opponent to break their balance or to create space for you to deliver other strikes or to facilitate an escape. In addition, when grabbed from behind, smashing your butt into the attacker's groin is an effective distraction and space-creating technique.

THE SHOULDER

The shoulder is a great, unorthodox striking weapon. When you find yourself in the Grappling and Trapping Ranges (Covered in Chapter 8), smashing your shoulder into the opponent's face is extremely distracting. The shoulder is also a good lead-in on a takedown. Drive your shoulder into the solar plexus, stomach, or chest as you perform your takedown. Follow this to the ground as you drive your opponent to the floor. When you find yourself slightly crouched and under your opponent's chin, explode upward and drive your shoulder into their chin.

THE ELBOW

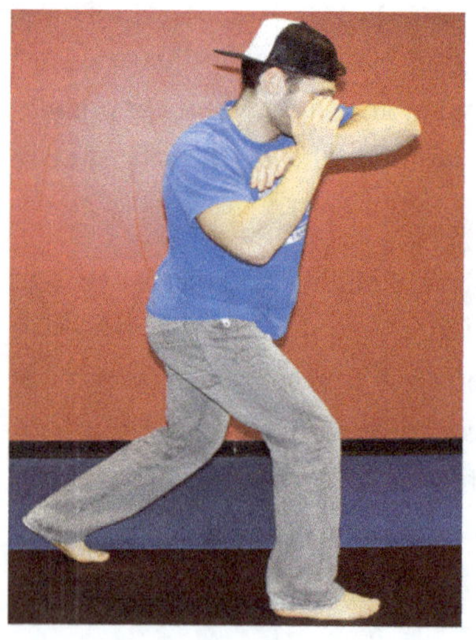
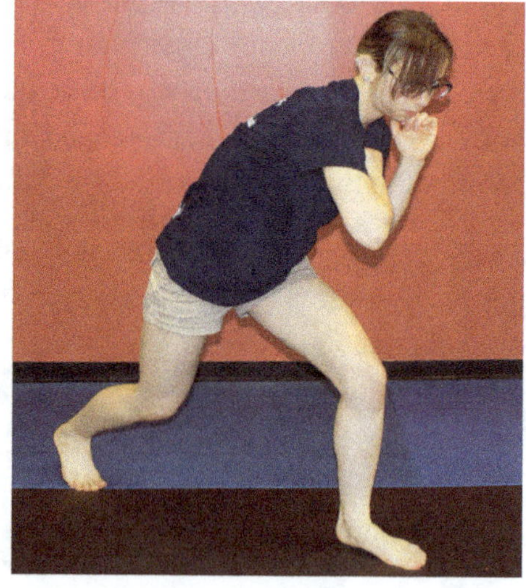

The elbow is an extremely devastating weapon. MMA legend Jon "Bones" Jones has mastered the art of the elbow in the sport of cage fighting. He has destroyed opponents with slashing downward elbows, upward elbows, elbows from the Ground and Pound, spinning elbows, etc. The elbow is very, very hard and is close to the power base of the body. Experiment on a heavy bag. Throw a punch at it, then hit the bag with an elbow, and see which strike yields the greater amount of power. You may never throw another punch again! Additionally, the thick elbow bone is much more durable than the multitude of bones (there are 27, to be precise) available to break in one's hand.

THE FOREARM

Ask any football player if they like using the forearm as a method to strike or block and how well it works. One of the core movements for an interior lineman is the Forearm Shiver. Step into your opponent with one hand open and the other fist clenched while you deliver a stiff forearm shot to the chest. The forearm and side of the wrist can be used to choke or levy pressure on an opponent. Blocking and deflecting blows, as well as striking the clavicle and neck of your adversary, is met with favorable results.

THE WRIST

As an implement of striking, the wrist is often overlooked. Proper execution of a Stick Punch yields one of the most powerful strikes that can be delivered by the upper body.

Back in the early 1990s, power meter striking pads were very popular. One year *Karate International Magazine* was hosting a very large karate tournament in the New York metro area (Hackensack, NJ), and I entered my student into the Impact-Pad Striking competition. He was a seventeen-year-old, new Black Belt who weighed approximately 175 pounds. There were over 30 adult Black Belts in the competition. Several were master-level instructors, many of them quite a bit larger than my young Black Belt student. They attempted Reverse Punches, Ridge hands, Boxer's Cross, etc. My seventeen-year-old, 175-pound student beat them all, by quite a margin, with the Stick Punch technique. The judges and other participants were in utter disbelief (and a few masters were a little irked) and made him perform his strikes a few more times. He still won with the Back-of-the-Wrist Stick Punch. Handily. In one sparring competition, I witnessed a fight where one combatant almost tore another one's jaw off with the Stick Punch. Roy "Big Country" Nelson knocked Cheick Kongo with a stick punch in their televised UFC bout.

The back of the wrist may be used at close quarters as well. We routinely break boards with the back of our wrists at very close distances of one to three inches. Not only can offensive strikes be delivered with the wrist, but it's great for blocking and deflecting blows as well.

THE FIST

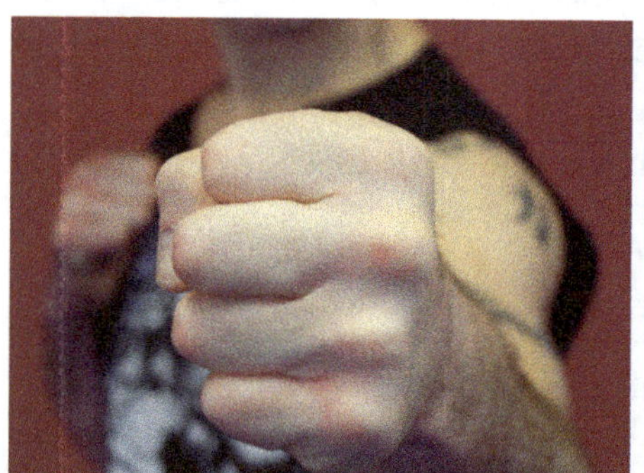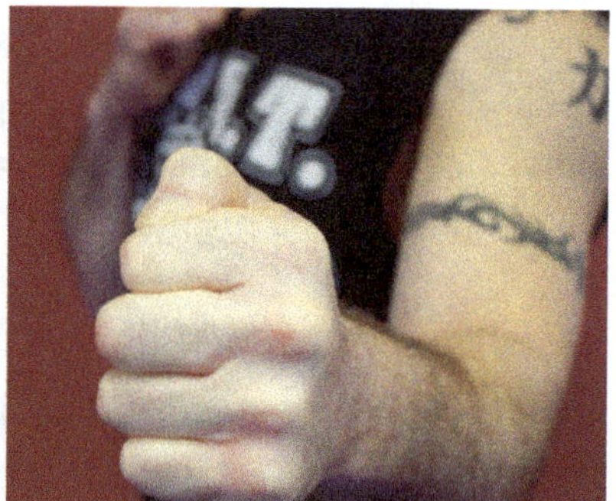

Standard configuration | Thumb stacked.

The Fist is the universal demonstration of power, might, defiance and defense. The clenched fist is almost an autonomic response when angered or threatened. One of the most powerful upper-body strikes is the straight cross. The whole martial art of boxing was developed with only the fists as weapons.

You may have noticed that I referred to boxing as a martial art. It is. A uniform and a ranking system are not necessary precursors for being considered a martial art. *Martial* is derived from warring; therefore, it applies to all combat sports and training.

THE HAND

The hand can assume a multitude of configurations for striking and defending. Open palms for both thrusting and slapping techniques work best for striking the "hard" targets, such as the head. Open hands are for parries and redirecting strikes coming at you while you are defending yourself.

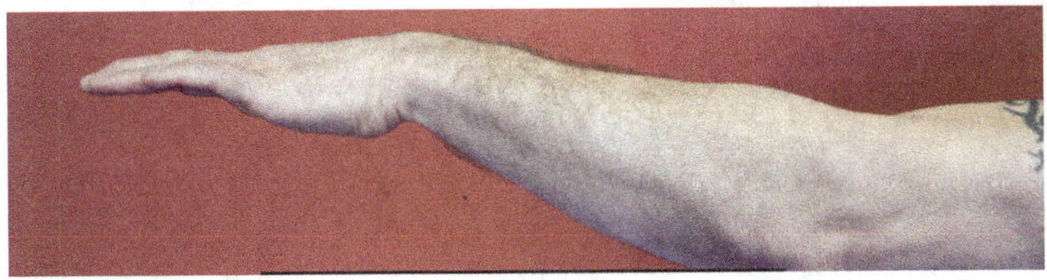

Knifehand strike.

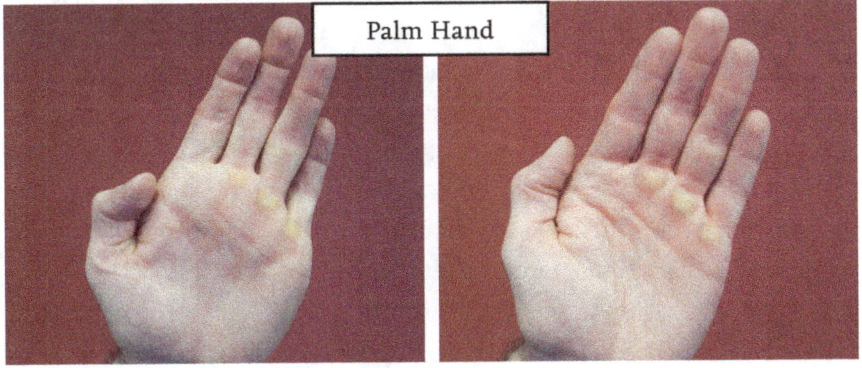

Correct | Incorrect.

THE FINGERS

Finger techniques may not "finish" your opponent, but they will certainly provide the opportunity for you to do so. Fish Hooks, Finger Jabs, Flicks and Eye Gouges applied to pressure points and nerve centers are on the list, and all can be devastatingly effective.

Attacking the eyes with your fingers yields the greatest results; permanently or temporarily blinding your assailant enables you to escape or provides a distraction to deliver a more lethal counterattack. Have you ever witnessed a fighter receive an eye-poke in the cage? They are incapacitated, temporarily anyway.

THE HEAD

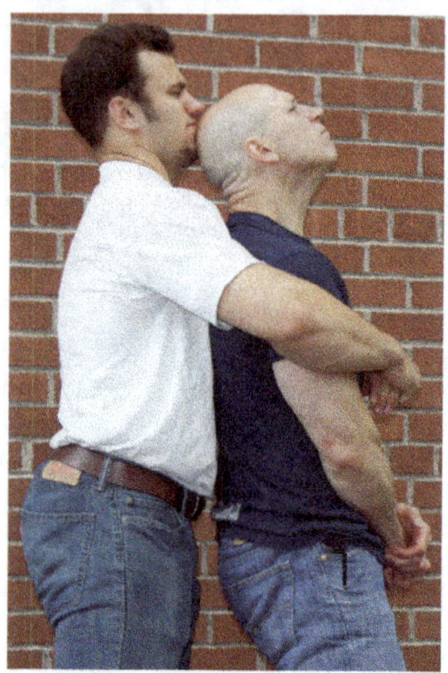

Headbutt.

Head Butts delivered by the front, side and top of the back of the head are both shocking and potentially devastating. So is dropping your head down to deflect a blow directed toward your face.

THE MOUTH

Mike Tyson does not have the corner on the use of bicuspids for fighting. If you choose to assume the role of Hannibal Lecter, there are many places to target. You may sink your teeth into one of several available, fleshy areas to inflict damage or to create a release from a grip or hold. The nose, ears, lips and neck offer up sensitive targets for levying a bite. The inside of the thigh, groin and fingers are also effective targets for the teeth.

Chapter 6
Targets of The Human Body

Unfortunately for us, we humans have a cornucopia of vital and semi-vital targets to attack. But fortunately, this goes both ways, meaning the body of someone attacking us has multiple areas to target as well. What is a curse is also a blessing, as our knowledge of these target areas enables us to both protect ourselves and exploit the weaknesses of our adversaries.

Most of our vital and semi-vital target areas are located along the center lines of the body. We need to both protect ours and attack the opponents at the same time, focusing primarily in this section.

Let's peruse the available areas to focus our attacks on. Starting at the top:

THE EYES

A poke, gouge, punch, scratch or strike will either permanently or temporarily incapacitate or blind your opponent. The toughest guy in the world has eyes that are no stronger than a baby's eyes. Animals instinctually squint during combat to help protect their eyes, knowing their vulnerability.

THE EARS

A cupping slap, especially a dual one, will disrupt the balance and cause a great deal of pain, potentially perforating the eardrum. The dual slap is also an excellent entry technique to gouging both eyes with your thumbs.

An authoritative single slap to the ear can knock out an assailant or render them incapacitated. In the worst case, delivering a slap to the ear is quite effective and will act as a significant disruption technique.

THE NOSE

This is one of my favorite spots to strike for several reasons. For one, it's located smack-dab in the middle of the face. Striking the nose hard can cause it to break and allow blood to flow, and smashing the nose will cause your opponent's eyes to water. The whole notion of "sending the nose back into the brain" is a lot of garbage. The nose will fracture and collapse and the cartilage will bend well before anything reaches the brain.

THE THROAT

Regardless of how big, strong or nasty they are, everyone has a throat. One cannot develop muscle to cover and protect the front of the wind-pipe. It's a great target.

The best techniques to use on the throat are the Scissor Punch, Axehands and Thumbs. If you strike the throat with a Scissor Punch, you can crush the windpipe and cause blood to fill that area, essentially causing the opponent to drown in their own blood. You are also set up to grab the windpipe and crush it. To properly grab the windpipe, use your index and middle fingers and your thumb. Try to make them meet each other behind the windpipe, squeeze, and pull.

There are also a variety of less-lethal attacks for this area. Jamming a thumb or index and middle finger into the Episternal notch will invoke the gag reflex and act as an effective technique of distraction.

THE NECK

Some people have necks the size of a Rottweiler's, so direct attacks to the thick areas of the neck will not work on everyone. However, the carotid arteries running up either side of the throat are a great target.

If someone were to grab you with a Front Bear-Hug (arms-free version), you could take your thumbs and drive them into the carotid arteries. This would send a nasty shock and cause their grip to release. I've also found that the more muscular someone is, the closer the nerves are to the skin's surface. This makes the application of this technique more effective.

There is an area of the neck where MMA (Mixed Martial Arts), karate and boxing all prohibit strikes. It's the spot directly below the skull where the spine and skull meet. An attack to the C1 vertebra can result in paralysis or death, which is why it isn't appropriate for sporting competitions. But for self-defense anything goes, and even if you do not kill your opponent with a blow there you could still knock them out or temporarily disable them.

THE TRAPEZIUS

If you ever watched the original Star Trek, you undoubtedly remember Mr. Spock pinching his adversary's trapezius between his thumb and forefinger, rendering them instantly unconscious. Unfortunately this is unlikely to work for you, as the best way to attack the traps is with a downward Hammerfist or Chop. Attacking from the rear works best, if you attack from the front the collar bone is more easily accessible.

THE STERNUM

The sternum is located in the center of the chest and often referred to as the breastbone. There are nerves very close to the surface of the skin here, and striking with a closed fist may result in cracking the sternum and potentially stopping the heart. An open palm strike is less lethal but will also stop an assailant in his tracks. Your striking technique must be strong and sound if you are to gain the desired result with either of these techniques.

THE ABDOMEN AND TRUNK

The solar plexus, liver, kidneys, floating ribs and bladder are the primary targets of the trunk. The solar plexus, or xiphoid process, is located directly below the sternum and is where the soft tissue begins on the abdomen. Striking this area with a closed fist will "take the wind" out of your opponent.

The liver is located on the front, lower-right side of the body. A well-placed shot will drop an opponent in their tracks. My favorite techniques to use in this area are Knee Drives and a short Vertical Punch or Uppercut.

The kidneys are located in the back on either side of the lumbar spine. Elbows, Knees and Vertical Punches are my techniques of choice when addressing these areas.

The floating ribs are the last ribs located on the bottom of the rib cage, easy to identify because only one side of the rib is attached to the rib cage. Vertical Strikes, Knee Drives and Side Bear-Hugs with the wrist cutting into the area are very effective attacks.

The bladder is generally a weak area for most people. The muscle wall is thinner than that of the "six-pack" abs, which are located directly above. The bladder is located two inches below the navel and above the groin. This is the area common to hernias. Any thrusting attacks with the knee or foot or an uppercut with a balled fist work well here. Your opponent may even wet themselves as they double over in pain after being on the receiving end of a well-placed powerful shot!

THE SPINE

The complete central nervous system (CNS) is encased in the vertebrae of your spine. Spinal cord injuries are debilitating and potentially lethal. The spine includes the area from the bottom of your skull to the end of your coccyx (tailbone). The most devastating areas to strike are the C1, as described before; the T1, where the thoracic and cervical sections meet; and the coccyx.

We have previously addressed the C1 and T1 regions, the latter being the area between the top of the shoulder blades. Downward Elbow Strikes work best here, and are sometimes called the "Death Elbow" when focused on this spot.

A Knee Drive from behind delivered to the coccyx is extremely effective. A kick to this area does not offer nearly as much impact as the knee offers.

THE GROIN

Everyone has groins, and they all hurt when struck. It is quite evident that a strike delivered to a male's groin is more devastating, but a well-placed kick, strike, or knee to a female's genital region can cause some significant pain and act as an effective distraction. Kicks, open-hand strikes, fist strikes, or a slap, grab and twist are all effective attacks directed at a man's groin.

THE THIGHS

There are many parts of the thigh to attack. The ones that provide the best results are the peroneal nerve and the femoral artery. A well-placed Shin-or Cut-Kick delivered to the outside of the leg at approximately mid-thigh will cause the leg to buckle or worse. The best spot to strike is the space between the quadriceps and hamstrings. There is not much muscle between the skin and the bone in this area. A strike there will pinch the nerve between your shin bone and the femur of your opponent, which crushes the peroneal nerve and is thus incredibly effective.

The femoral artery supplies oxygen-filled blood to the lower body. Kicks, strikes, slaps and horse bites (a slap followed by a grabbing and twisting of the flesh) are very effective when directed at this sensitive area. A Roundhouse Kick with the foot or instep is more effective than that of a shin blow when directed to the inside of the thigh. The snapping strike will cause more damage in this area than a "thudding" attack.

KNEES

To destroy a knee only requires a blow with 30 pounds of pressure directed against the joint. It takes less force to cause significant pain and temporary incapacitation. Front Kicks, Side Kicks, Cross Stomps and Oblique Kicks work best when attacking the knee. Roundhouse Kicks work well to the inside of the knee, but for destruction the thrusting kicks against the joint will yield the desired result most effectively.

Roundhouse Kicks or Cut Kicks delivered to the inside of the knee are very effective. Generally, the result is not as devastating as the attacks levied to the outside and front of the knee, but these strikes can cause some damage and disrupt or distract your adversary.

THE SHIN AND CALVES

A well-placed Ball-of-the-Foot Front Kick, when applied to either the shin or the calf, is a great distraction technique and may even temporarily disable your assailant.

Have you ever banged your shin into the coffee table in the middle of the night? Man, does that ever smart! Now imagine a well-placed kick with the tip of a boot or hard shoe. You can just imagine the effectiveness.

The spot to attack in the calf is located directly below the lower insertion point of the gastric (upper calf), where the sural nerve and the muscle meet. This is a great spot to attack someone from behind as you immediately grab your opponent by the trapezius and yank them to the ground.

THE ANKLES AND FEET

A well-placed strike to the talus or stomp to the foot and toes can provide temporary incapacitation or, at the very least, act as an effective disruption technique.

The talus is found where the instep of the foot and the ankle meet, the section of the foot where the crease forms when you bend your ankle. A Ball-of-the-Foot or a kick using the point of a boot or shoe tip to this area could dislocate the ankle. Whether that occurs or not, the strike is still very effective and difficult to defend against.

Foot and toe stomps are painful, effective and easy to apply. A case of "Turf Toe" can sideline a 245-pound NFL Running Back for several weeks, showing how vulnerable the toes are! You should dorsiflex your foot and drive the heel into the top of the target's instep or toes. These stomps will affect the nerves and potentially crush any number of the 26 bones in the human foot.

STANCES: HOW SHOULD ONE STAND?

STANCES

There are many different stances you can adopt when getting ready to attack or defend yourself. However, you should know that most of the stances used in most martial arts classes are useless for actual combat.

That *"Crouching Tiger, Hidden Dragon"* type of nonsense will get you killed in a real fight. Nevertheless, these stances are beneficial to strengthening your legs, developing balance and learning how to take root in the ground. Please bear in mind that these types of stances are simply transitory and should only be used as you move from position to position.

In actual combat you are better served to position yourself in a boxing or kickboxing stance. We refer to this as a "Walking Stance." To enter it, start with your feet together and simply walk. Stop at full stride, put your hands above your head and then drop your elbows down so that your fists are next to your jaw. Turn your body slightly sideways. Once you have become comfortable with this stance, you may vary it in accordance with the distance from your assailant and the aspects of the terrain.

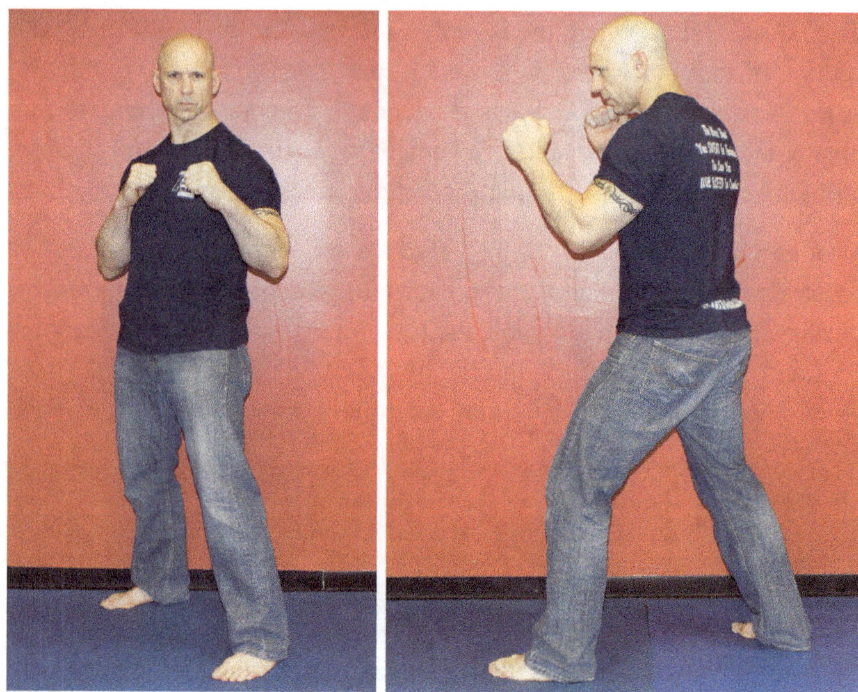

Orthodox stance.

The Targets of the Human Body

- Temple Eyes, Nose Mandibular
- Carotid
- Sternum
- Floating Ribs
- Solar Plexus Liver Bladder
- Groin
- Peroneal Nerve Knee Shin Ankle
- Foot/Toes Episternal Notch

- Occipital
- Ears
- Cervical Spine
- L1
- Trapezius
- Thoracic Spine
- Elbow
- Kidneys
- Radial Nerve
- Coccyx
- Hamstring
- Back of the Knee
- Gastroc Nerve
- Achilles

Once you are in your stance, you will either have your left or right foot forward. Bruce Lee espoused fighting with your dominant side forward, but maintaining the ability to switch is also vital. Traditional boxing proclaims that your power hand should be the rear hand. There are valid arguments for both.

Personally, my belief is that you should start with whatever side you feel more comfortable with and then work with the less dominant side. I like to start with my left side forward. I am left-eye dominant, and my left foot delivers better kicks than my right, yet my right-hand hits harder than my left. Since the first thing that meets my opponent will be my left foot, I prefer to have my left forward. However, when you throw a kick with your back leg and move forward, your stance will change. So, it would behoove you to be able to fight from either side.

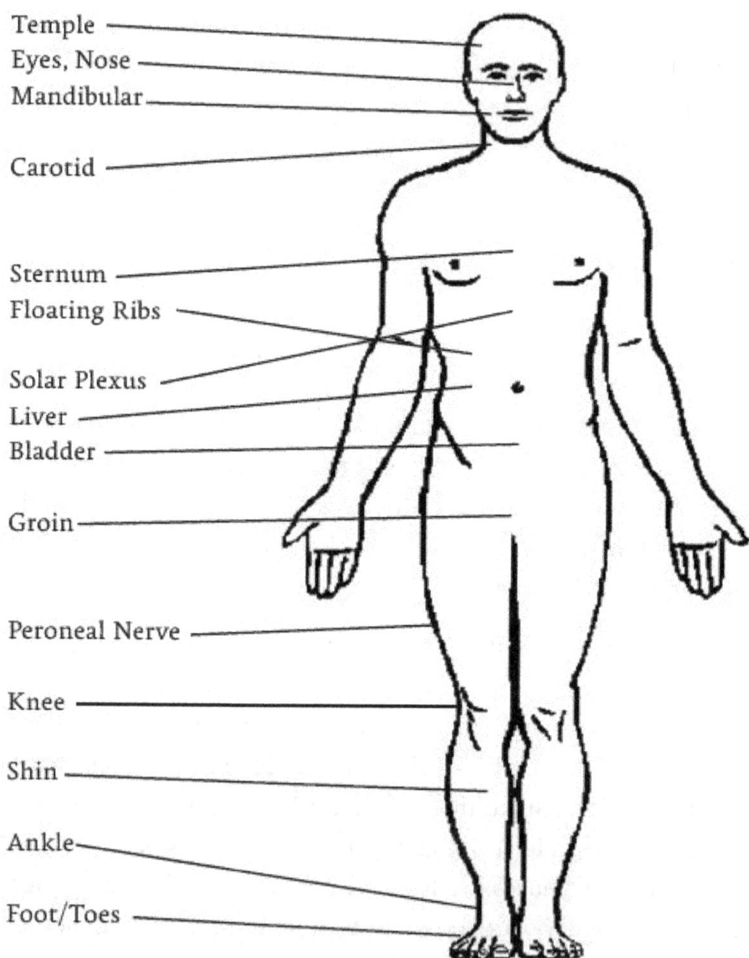

Temple
Eyes, Nose
Mandibular
Carotid
Sternum
Floating Ribs
Solar Plexus
Liver
Bladder
Groin
Peroneal Nerve
Knee
Shin
Ankle
Foot/Toes

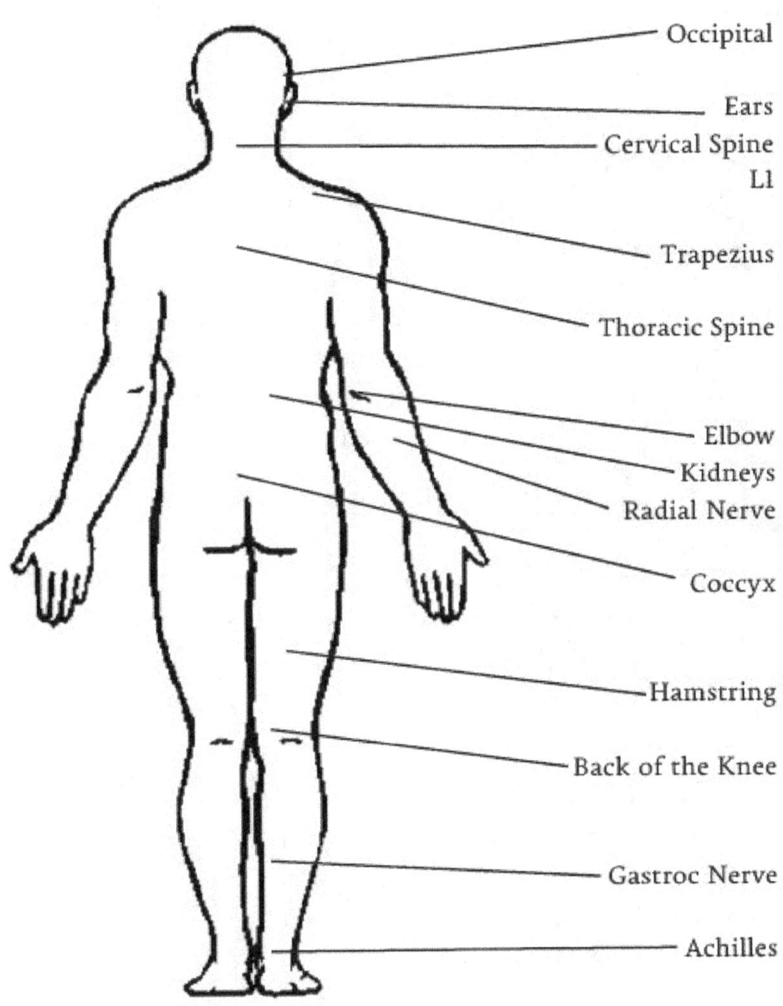

Occipital
Ears
Cervical Spine
L1
Trapezius
Thoracic Spine
Elbow
Kidneys
Radial Nerve
Coccyx
Hamstring
Back of the Knee
Gastroc Nerve
Achilles

STANCES AND FIGHTING POSITIONS EXPLAINED

ORTHODOX

Right hand and right foot are in the back while the left hand and foot are forward. People are predominantly right-handed, therefore this is the most popular stance.

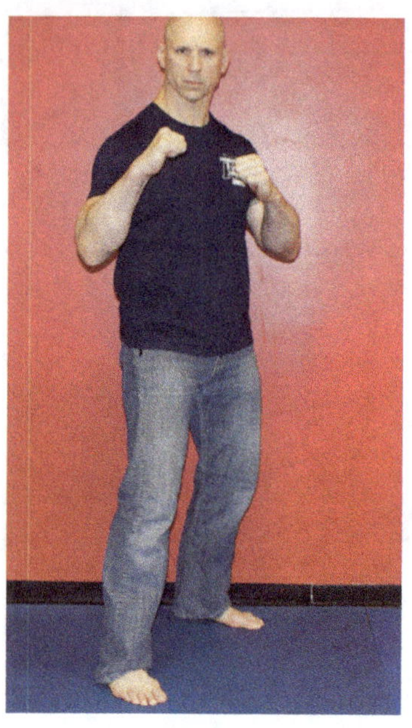

SOUTHPAW

Your left hand is in the back and your right hand and foot are forward. The term *southpaw* originally came from the game of baseball. Due to the alignment of baseball fields, a lefty's dominant hand faced the south side of the stadium.

If both fighters are in an orthodox stance, they will be *chest-to-chest*. If one of them is in an orthodox stance and the other is a southpaw, they will create a *mirror Image*. It is important to train with different stances and different looks.

When you are fighting someone with a different stance, it's important to "own the outside." What I mean by that is if you are an Orthodox fighter facing a Southpaw, your left foot needs to be on the outside of their right foot. This keeps you farther from their power hand and gives the advantage to your power side.

X-STANCE OR CROSS-STANCE

You start out like you would for your walking stance, and then you make it more compact. This is an unorthodox fighting stance and may throw your opponent off.

Round your shoulders, lower your head, and have your hands in an Axehand configuration and crossed in front of you. Turn your toes slightly inward and bring your knees closer together, drawing your genitals back so that they are provided some protection from an initial attack. This stance may be practiced from both the Orthodox and Southpaw postures.

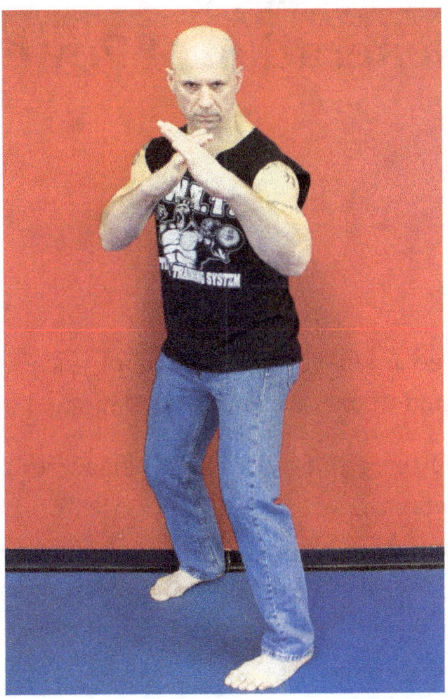

Cross stance.

Chapter 7
Generation of Power

These are the three main components of physical combat, and they must all be generated to maximize your striking and throwing power.

The mixture of the three must achieve a balance to ensure the highest level of implementation, with no exceptions. Too many practitioners try to apply too much power and too much speed to the techniques prior to learning how to perform the movements properly. They ultimately cheat themselves of power and speed, plus they leave themselves exposed to counterattacks.

You must always focus on proper technique execution. To achieve ultimate power and speed, you have to master the techniques. Work your movements slowly at first, paying particular attention to the position of your body during the execution of the movement. Employ the adage, *fast is slow and slow is fast.* Practice your movements slowly until they flow. This holds true for combinations as well.

Efficiency of movement and no wasted motion, that is the end point. Take your time and master the basics, you'll benefit tremendously from doing so later on.

TECHNIQUE, SPEED, AND POWER

If I sound redundant, it's on purpose. These tenets must be followed to the letter if you are to be successful. Fast is slow; slow is fast. Practice proper execution of your techniques and speed will come. Efficiency and fluidity of movement are crucial to the successful implementation of your techniques. Once you are able to perform your strike, block, movement, throw, submission or combination with technical fluidity, you will become faster and faster. Once speed has been added to technique, power naturally will come. Remember, *speed kills*. You will not have speed without technique. You will not have power without speed. All of these attributes of fighting technique must be added in order.

HIPS

All power is generated from the hips. Pick a sport, any sport (even golf, which is an activity, not a sport) where real movement is critical. Watch an NFL running back carry the football and elude defenders as he runs downfield, observe a professional baseball player drives a ball over the deep wall, or witness a knockout blow delivered by the middleweight champion. The limbs are mere delivery mechanisms for the power and movement generated by the hips. Torque, explosive power and incredible force are generated from our hips.

For eons, Asian cultures have revered the notion of "Ki" or "Chi" energy. (*Chi* is Chinese, and *Ki* is Japanese). Ki, in my opinion, is not some mythical notion, or at least it didn't start that way. The center of your body is where your "Ki" generates from. I do not subscribe to the mystical concept of "using someone's Ki against them" or having Ki wars (the thought makes me chuckle). I've seen far too many of these so-called "masters" debunked. However, the notion originated from somewhere and undoubtedly has some validity.

I will assert that the notion of Ki energy is a direct result of the application of hip power in movement. Using the hips adds incredible power to any movement, although your legs, glutes and back come into play here as well.

Try to throw someone twice your weight using your arms and shoulders, and you will not be successful and will most likely tear a shoulder muscle. However, incorporate the hips and you will be surprised and amazed with the results you achieve.

RELAXATION/TENSION

If your muscles are tensed up and tight, you cannot move. Try it; flex your arm then see how slowly it moves. If it's completely tight and rigid, it won't budge. This is why having incredible "weight-lifting" strength does not translate to being a good fighter. One has to relax the muscle to be able to move it. The tension and locking of the muscles occur at the moment of impact.

Practicing tension and relaxation are crucial to developing power. This is because your movements must be relaxed in order to be quick. As we have stated before, Speed leads to *POWER*. Power enables you to deliver meaningful blows that will incapacitate your opponent.

ROOTING IN THE GROUND

The most powerful force in your surroundings is the ground. There are times, especially when delivering hand strikes, when we will have our feet planted firmly at the exact point that our strike contacts the assailant. Using the force that you generate when driving from the floor or ground increases your power, stability and balance. Do not confuse this with immobility. This rooting is quick in coordination with the delivery of a strike. However, when training to develop this power, you will need to be stationary. Once you have developed this skill, incorporate movement.

FRICTION REDUCTION

Friction slows down your movement, period. You will notice this particularly when you kick. When executing your kicks, one needs to turn their foot on the floor. This will incorporate the power of your hip. To make this kick even more effective, add a slight jump so that your foot is off of the ground. Your kick will be faster and thus more powerful.

FORWARD MOVEMENT

Your forward motion will add power and speed to your technique. Straight lines and multiple motions close the gap quicker. As an example, if you throw a jab and do not step forward it will not be as powerful as one that includes the forward movement. Even if it's only a small step, there will be a significant addition of power. Additionally, if you don't have to step in to hit someone, you are so close that you should already be hitting them! If they're that close, they'll surely be hitting you.

ECONOMY OF MOTION

The shortest distance between two points is a straight line. You lose speed, power and accuracy when you "loop" punches. Even a Hook Punch or an Uppercut does not "loop." A punch follows this path: hip, shoulder, elbow and fist. This will keep your technique in line and maximize your alignment which will yield more power and speed.

The same is true for blocking. You should not overextend your blocks. The hands should be four to five inches wide, and you don't need to extend your blocks and parries much beyond your own body. Plus, when you reach too far out, it takes longer to get the limb back to the guarding position and leaves you exposed to another attack. In fact we have techniques designed to take advantage of blocks on which the defender overextends.

DELIVERY MECHANISMS

Reduced surface area provides more power per square inch. Therefore, striking with the knuckles or the edge of the hand will have a greater effect than an open-hand strike, given the same force applied to the blow. This is simple physics.

However, one must consider what target you are striking. Ponder the notion of yin and yang, the dualities of nature. Hard versus soft. Dark versus light. Good versus evil, etc. The defining line is not straight, but curved. There can be neither without the other, and everything includes some of both elements.

You may be asking yourself, what does this have to do with striking? Well, a great deal. Have you ever seen anyone with broken knuckles or wrists from punching another person in the head? That is because they used a hard implement to strike a hard surface. If you want to punch someone in the head with a closed fist and avoid injury, your hands need to be extremely well-conditioned. You are better off using a soft striking implement to strike a hard area and a hard implement to attack the soft portions of your assailant.

EXAMPLES

Use a clenched fist to deliver a blow to the stomach or kidneys. Use an open-hand strike to hit the head. Try this experiment if you dare. Walk up to a wall and slap it as hard as you can. Your hand will probably sting a bit. Now, address the same wall with a straight punch. What do you think will happen to your hand? If you do so (not recommended), you will most likely experience severe damage to your phalanges and metacarpals ... and it will hurt like hell.

Chapter 8
Grips and Locks

There are some basic locks, grips and holds that can be learned with relative ease. They are essential, because the biggest mistake that people make is practicing individual movements without rehearsing their entry to the submission or choke as well.

How do you get there? In Brazilian Jiu Jitsu or grappling training, there are many excellent flow drills that teach you how to position yourself properly and move from position to position as you attempt to secure a submission, all while avoiding your opponent's attempts to score a submission against you. This is an art unto itself and should be treated as such.

Here, we will be focusing primarily on the street application of Locks, Grips, and Chokes.

SMALL-JOINT MANIPULATION

Finger locks can be extremely effective and very painful. The fingers are filled with nerves and are sensitive. My favorite way to apply one when someone pokes me in the chest or puts a finger in my face is to place my thumb against their finger-tip as I grab the rest of their finger with my hand.

When grabbed, especially from behind, as would occur within a Full-Nelson attack, isolate two fingers and pull them back¬ward in a twisting motion. This method is best applied when your opponent attacks you from behind and you put your arm over theirs as you pull their fingers backward. Grab their fingers from the backside of their hand with the pinky side of your hand facing upward. It's best to grab two fingers; if you only grab one, it may snap. You want to maintain control through pain compliance.

WRIST LOCKS

There are many, many Wrist Locks that can be effective. We will focus on just a few techniques that work for most people in most situations. Please note that in order to "Earn the right to use jiu jitsu," meaning locks and holds, the opponent must be "dummied up" prior to their application. You must deliver powerful strikes prior to even attempting to apply a lock or hold. This is especially prevalent when performing Wrist Locks. We also must understand that the holds are placed on the hands, not the wrists. However, it is the wrist that experiences the pain.

It is particularly important to note that there needs to be three directions of pressure in all locks. Two directions do not supply enough power to cause pain compliance and balance disruption. Additionally, NEVER bend your back on any of these (as with most) techniques; bend from your knees, and maintain a neutral spine.

The terminology of the techniques varies among styles and instructors. Below are the names I was taught and how they are referred to while training

KOTEGAESHI (OR THE LOOKING GLASS)

In this position you gain control of the opponent's hand by twisting it so that their fingers are facing upward with your thumbs directly in the middle of the back of their hand. You will grab the inside of their palm with your thumb with one hand and pinky with the other. You apply pressure by pulling your fingers toward you, pushing your thumbs toward them as you step to the outside, rotating on a downward angle and towards their thumb.

Also, be sure to keep their hand on your chest. This will add pressure to the wrist of the assailant. If you are quite a bit smaller than your opponent or don't have a great deal of comfort with the technique, the application of chest pressure will be invaluable.

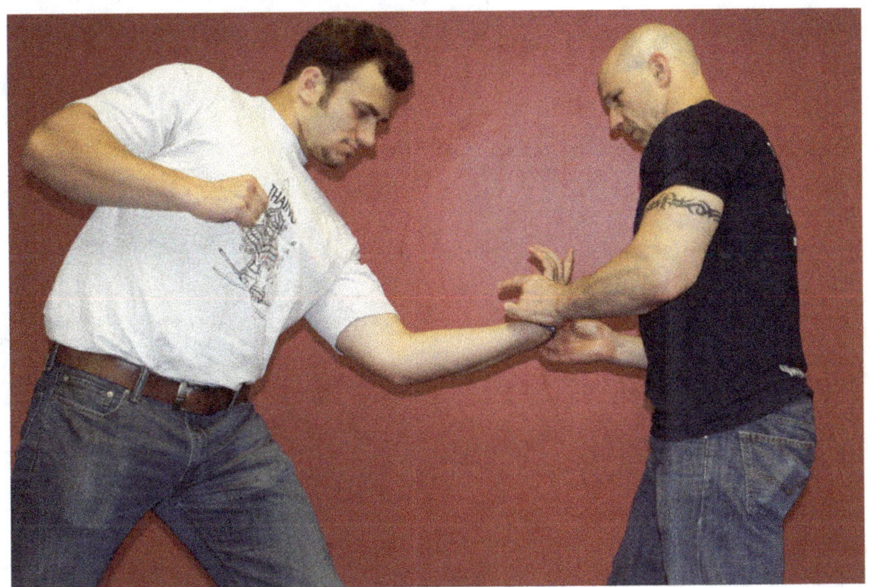

Kotegaeshi.

GAN KUN

One of the best ways to apply this move occurs when you get grabbed at the lapel. If someone grabs you with his right hand on your left lapel, reach across with your right hand while keeping your elbow high to protect your face from getting punched. Apply an overgrip so that your fingers grab the hand at the section below the pinky, then insert your thumb into the thenar muscle (the spot between the thumb and forefinger). Rotate your left shoulder inward as you shift back and raise your left arm high enough to clear the hand. You will rotate their hand so that their pinky is facing upward, then push upward with your right thumb and drive your left elbow downward into their forearm as you step and drag your foot backward. Be sure to keep your back straight and bend from the knees.

There are other versions of this move as well. All will be the same as in the above-described defense, except you will grab the assailant's arm with your left hand so that your fingers access the radial nerve. You will employ a "C" Grip on the arm, with your thumb under and fingers over, thus resembling a "C." Rotate their wrist to the right and their arm to the left as you push their wrist toward them on a downward angle. This is also referred to as the "Washrag" technique, due to the motion resembling the wringing out of a wet rag.

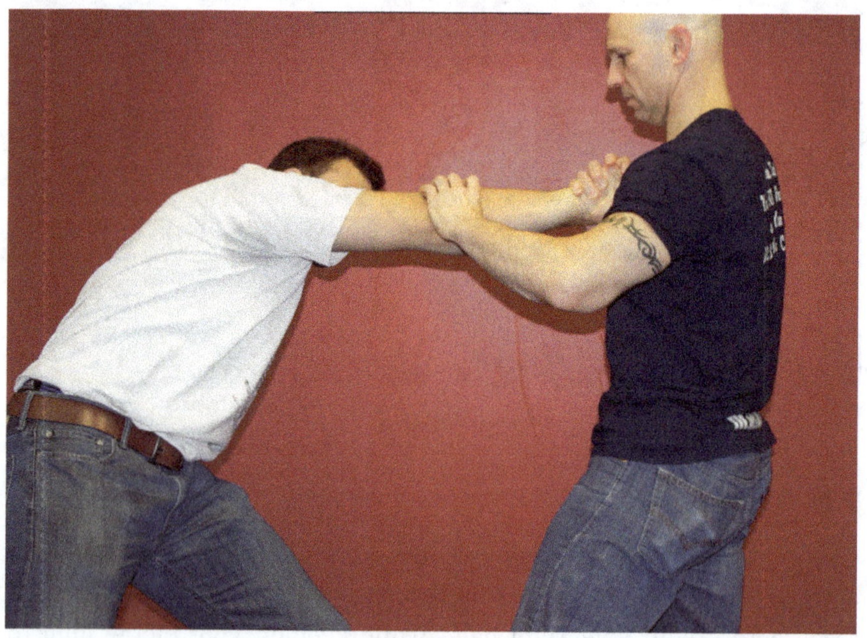

Gan Kun.

GOOSENECKS

These are very popular amongst law enforcement and security personnel. Often referred to as "Come-Alongs," the Gooseneck enables the person applying the technique to move or direct the other person from one place to another by using pain compliance. Hence the name "Come-Alongs."

There are several variations, but they all stem from the same base lock. To apply this you take your right hand and grab their right hand. This is generally done from a standing position but can be done from the ground as well. Thread your left arm under their right and apply a reverse chop to their bicep's insertion causing the elbow to bend. With your right hand, you should grip their thumb with your fingers. The thumb of your right hand should be aligned with their middle finger. Pull up on their thumb, put pressure down on the back of their hand with the palm of your thumb, and place your left hand on top of your right as you apply pressure.

You can also hinder their movement by stepping on their right foot with your left. By being on the side of the arm that you are controlling, you will have removed yourself from a potential strike from their left hand.

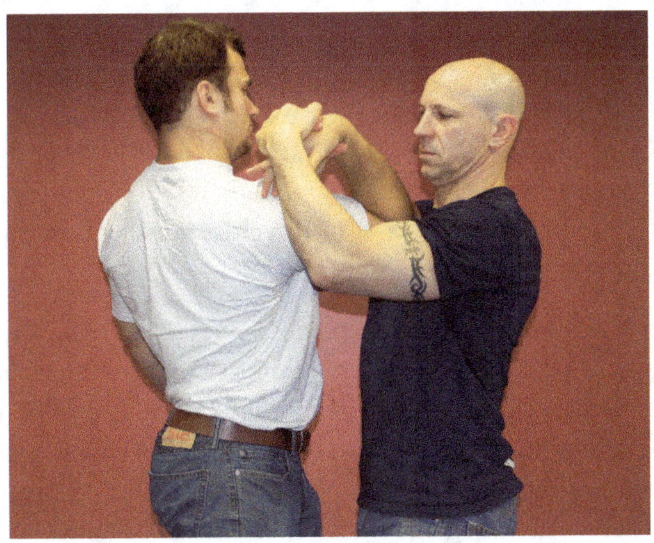

Gooseneck.

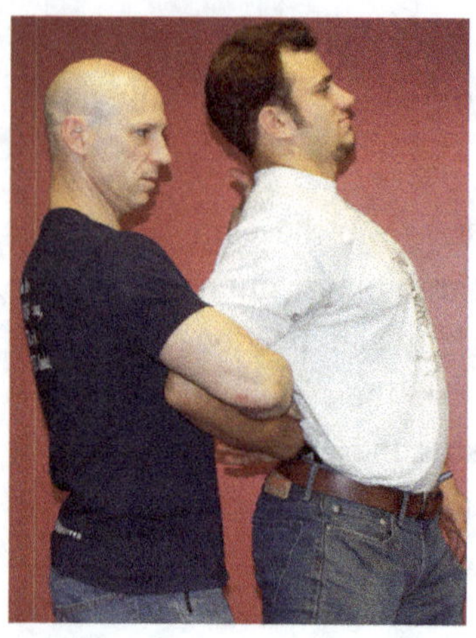
Walk the dog.

WALK THE DOG

This is another excellent "Come-Along" technique. I like this one best because you are behind the opponent. There are many ways to attain this position, but we'll focus on one method.

Reach for your opponent's right hand with yours. Step to their right side as you pull down on their wrist, and chop the inside of their right arm with your left hand so that their arm bends at a right angle. Slide your right hand over the back of their right hand so that you are able to bend their right wrist and their elbow is in the crook of your right arm (inside of the elbow). Take your left hand and grab their trapezius to prevent them from spinning to face you. Pull the fingers of your right hand toward you as if you were a baby waving "bye-bye." This will induce a great amount of pain in your subject.

ARM LOCKS

There are many variations of Armlocks, Armbars and other associated painful compliance and submission techniques that may be applied. The locks listed below are some of the most universal, meaning they can be utilized by the majority of people.

Please note that in a street confrontation, I never recommend that you go to the ground. Period. However, it must be understood that if the action lasts more than 10 seconds or so, the chances that the fight will end up on the ground are dramatically increased. As I have stated, I'd rather keep a street fight standing, but you'd better be prepared to unleash a hellish ground game if you fall or get taken down.

The application of the movements listed below are many. You will find the best methods of securing these positions through training with your partner. It's also good to practice transitioning from one position to another. Rarely will you ever simply end up in a lock; you will get it from an opportunity presenting itself during a scramble.

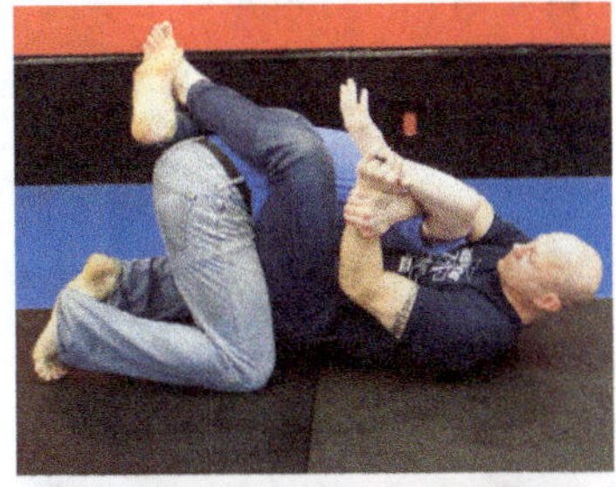

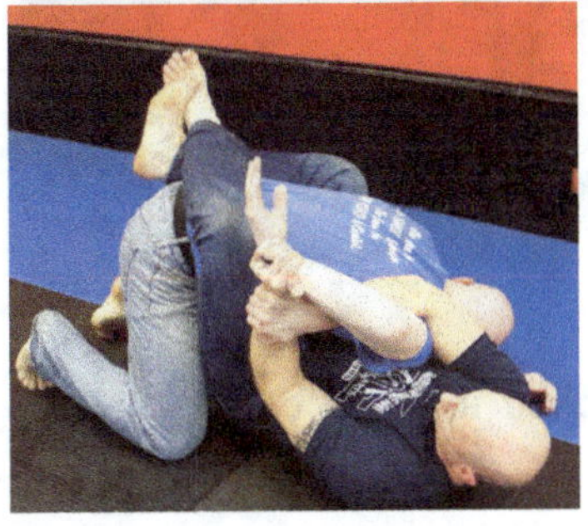

KIMURA (HAMMER LOCK)

One of the reasons I like the Kimura (aka the Hammer Lock) is that it can be applied from a variety of offensive and defensive positions. If someone is behind you and has their left arm around your waist, you can take your left arm and go over their arm. Then you take your right hand and grab their left wrist, then grab your right wrist with your left hand. Next you will pivot on your left foot and step around toward the side with your right foot. During the application of the Kimura, be sure to employ the thumb-less Gable Grip.

You may also apply the Kimura while on top or from the bottom while you are facing an opponent. If you are on the bottom and have your opponent in the Closed Guard (the Closed Guard occurs when you are on your back and have your legs wrapped around their waist with your feet locked at the ankles), as you sit up and unlock your legs position your left shoulder to theirs as you loop your left arm around their left arm. Grab their left wrist with your right hand. Thread your left arm through and grab your right wrist with your left hand. Relock your legs and scoot your hips to the right as you drive their left hand behind their back and toward their right shoulder.

When you find yourself in the top position, in either a full or side mount, grab your opponent's right wrist with your right hand, thread your left arm around their right arm above the elbow and then under the arm as you secure the lock by grabbing your right wrist with your left hand. If you are in a Side Mount, slide your right knee over their belly to assume the Full Mount. Once there, pivot on your right knee as you step your right foot toward their head while running their wrist toward their left shoulder and lifting their elbow to their head.

ARMBAR

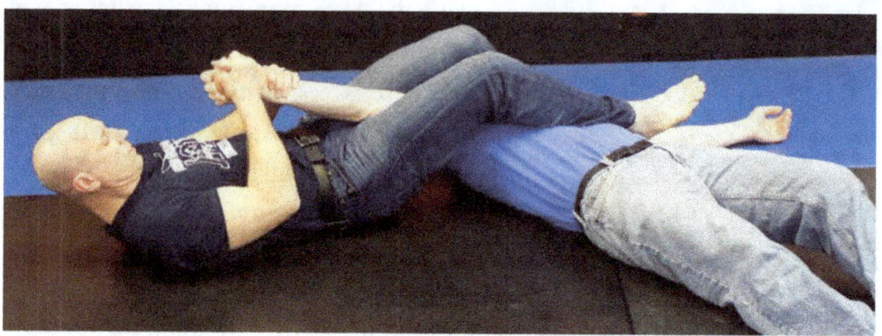

There are many Armbars that may be applied in street combat. Some are better suited for grappling competitions and not the best for the street. However, when you are on your back and faced with a last-resort situation, you have to do what you can.

When considering self-defense, the BJJ Guard (Closed Guard) is not a position that is recommended as a street combat position. Your groin, center line and face are exposed. Additionally, a strong opponent will be able to lift you up and smash you off the pavement. However, if you do get knocked to the ground and find yourself on your back with an enraged attacker on you, you had better have an answer.

Let's consider that you have been knocked to the ground, and your assailant is on top of you and is raining punches down on you. What are you to do? If you happen to be fortunate enough to wrap your legs around their waist and pull them into your guard, we will proceed as follows (if they have you in a Full Mount position, we will cover what you can do in Chapter 13).

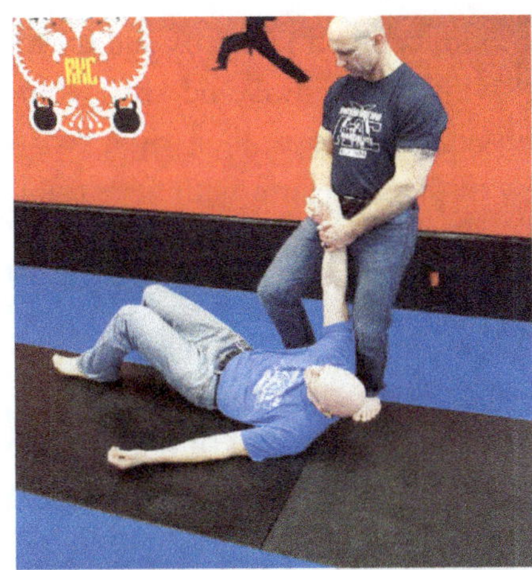 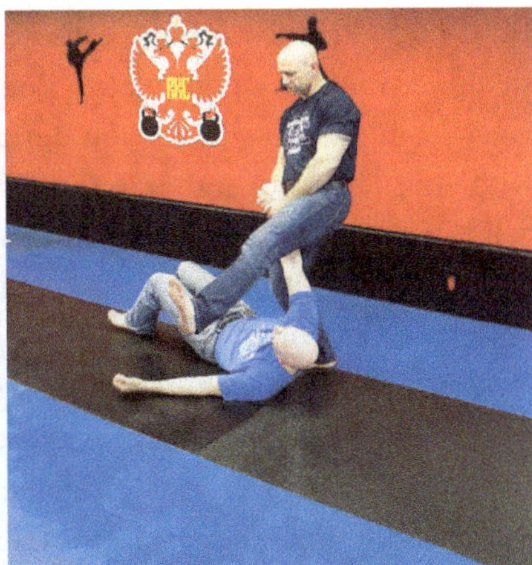

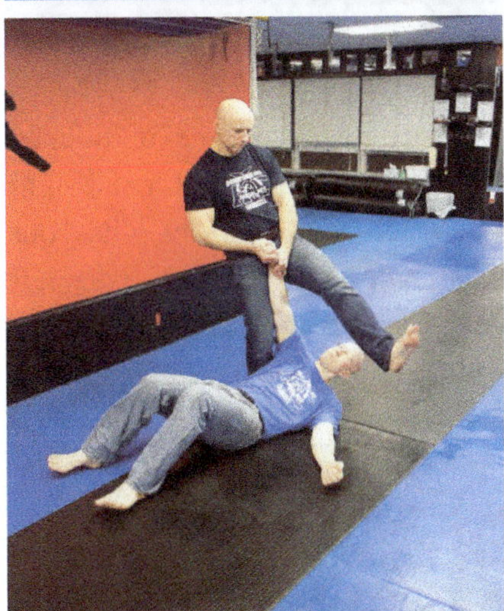 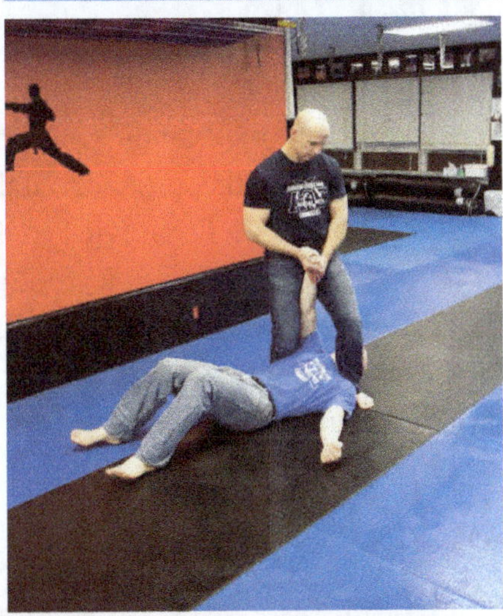

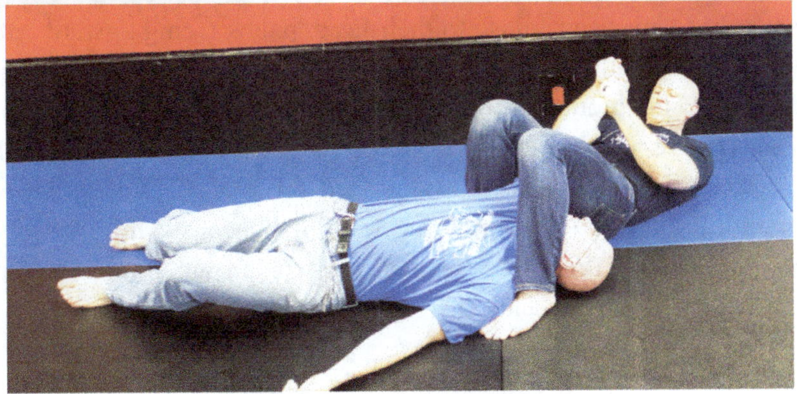

Now, on to the move. First, tuck your chin, contract your abs and try to sit up as much as possible as you "swim" your arms and shift your body from side to side as you deflect punches. Secure their right wrist with your left hand and grab the elbow of the same arm with your right hand in the thumb down (pointing toward you) position. Pivot on your back toward your right and assume a perpendicular position and place your right leg high on their back so that their arm is located on the inside of your leg. Hold on to their arm with your right hand, then shove their head to the side with your left hand as you bring your left leg over their head. Drive your heels to the ground as your arch the back driving your hips into the elbow joint while you are pulling on their wrist. And this is not a tournament, so don't stop until the arm snaps.

When we apply the Standing version, it means you will have knocked your assailant to the ground. Grab their right wrist with your right hand, then deliver a Front Kick to the downed attacker's ribs with your right foot, thus wedging your foot underneath their back. Lift your left foot up and over their head and bring your heel down to the left side of the head of the supine attacker. Sit your butt to your heel as you land on the ground with your head up and extending the opponent's arm. Again, apply quick, strong pressure until a snap results.

AMERICANA (KEY-LOCK)

Think of this as a "Reverse Kimura." When in the Side Mount, if the attacker has their hands close to their head, palms facing upward, grab their left wrist with your left hand and press down hard, thus pinning their hand to the ground. Slip your right hand underneath their arm and thread your wrist through and grab your own left wrist. Roll the knuckles of your left hand down toward the ground as if you were operating the throttle on a motorcycle. Simultaneously lift your right elbow up as you drag their pinned wrist in an arc downward and toward you. Do not stop until there is a snap heard.

PYTHON GRIP

This is my favorite move for the street. This technique may be utilized from either a standing position or with the aggressor on the ground. If the antagonist throws a right-handed punch, block their arm with your left hand, then chop and loop yours over theirs at the elbow and snake your arm through. At the same time, hit them in the throat with a right Scissors Punch and squeeze their throat as you place your left hand on your right elbow. Straighten your right and left in unison. From this position, slam the attacker into the wall or take them to the ground. Snap their arm and/or choke them out.

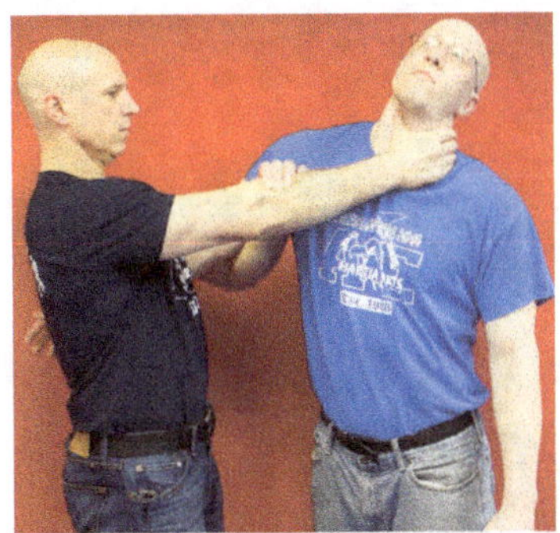

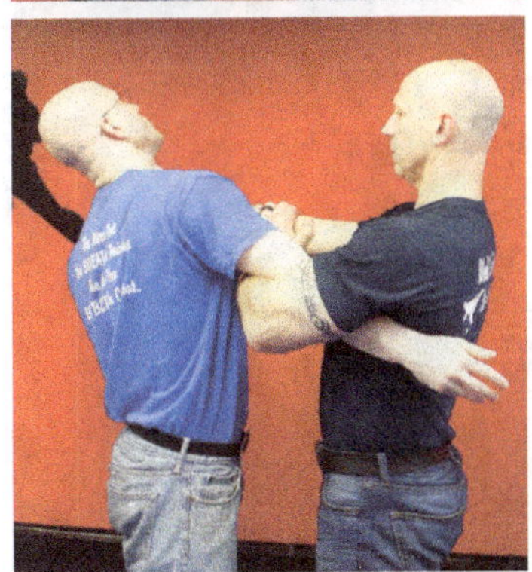

Python grip.

You can use the same move on a downed opponent, provided you are able to thread your arm around theirs as you take them down. This is not as difficult as you may think, provided you practice.

There are a few other standing locks that you may be able to apply from the standing position. I like these better for the street because you are not compromised by going to the ground.

STRAIGHT-ARM LOCK WITH WRIST

If you practice Brazilian Jiu-jitsu, think of it as a Kimura that you straighten out and apply a wrist lock to. This position is usually utilized when someone grabs you around the waist from behind. As with all self-defense movements, employ one of the loosening-up techniques: foot stomps, shin kicks, groin strikes, etc. If you are attacking the opponent's left arm, hook your left arm around their elbow and grab their left wrist with your right hand. Step 180 degrees toward the left with your right foot as you straighten their arm and pin it at the elbow against your chest with your left arm. Bend their right wrist downward. Apply knees to their head, if necessary.

STANDING WHIZZER

This position is a temporary one. You will need to begin striking or take the opponent to the ground once you've initially applied the hold. One of the best ways to get into the position is when the attacker grabs you by the shoulder. If your left shoulder is attacked, immediately place your left arm over their arm and scoop your elbow behind theirs as you point your elbow to the ceiling and put the back of your hand against their chest.

You will need to launch your counterattack now. Send a knee into their midsection and groin, then move into the Python Grip position or Chin Jab them in the face.

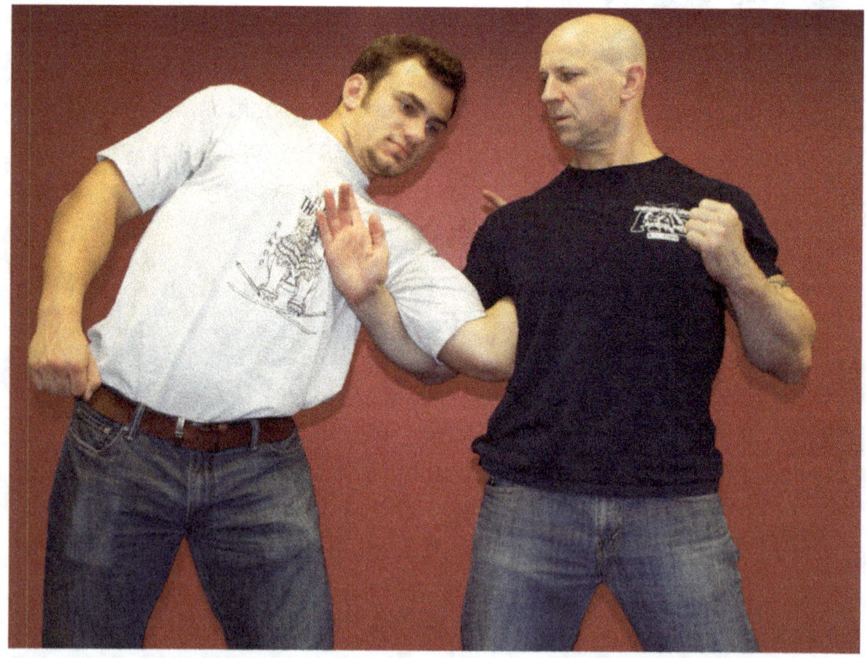

CHOKE HOLDS

No one loves MMA more than I do. It's the best sport on the planet, bar none and no-holds-barred (pun intended). But some of the chokes take too long to apply in a "street-level life or death" predicament.

You don't have five or even three seconds for a choke to take effect. A Street Choke needs to provide immediate results. Imagine if the guy has a knife in his pocket or boot and your choke takes three seconds to garner results? He could easily draw the knife and stab you several times in three seconds.

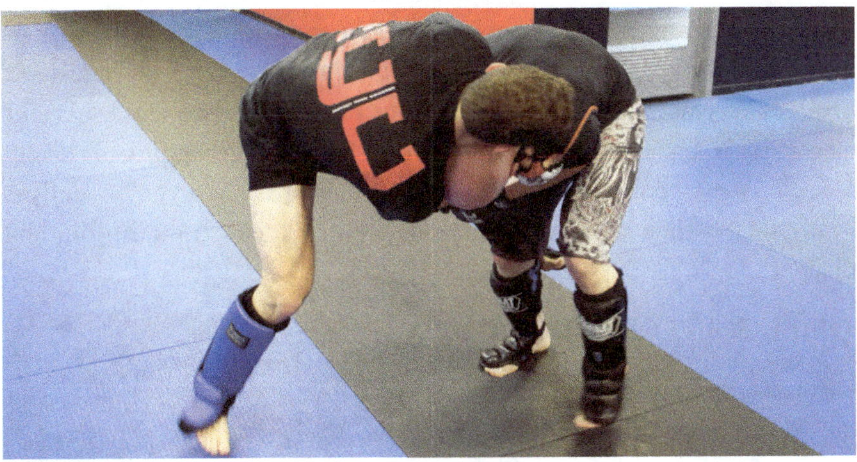

The notion of No Gaps is never more evident than when using Chokes. You do not want to leave any "wiggle room" available to someone you have in a choke. You will only rid yourself of these gaps when you practice, practice, practice these chokes over and over, getting feedback from your partner.

I have been practicing these chokes since the mid-1980s, so my terminology is based on what the chokes were referred to then:

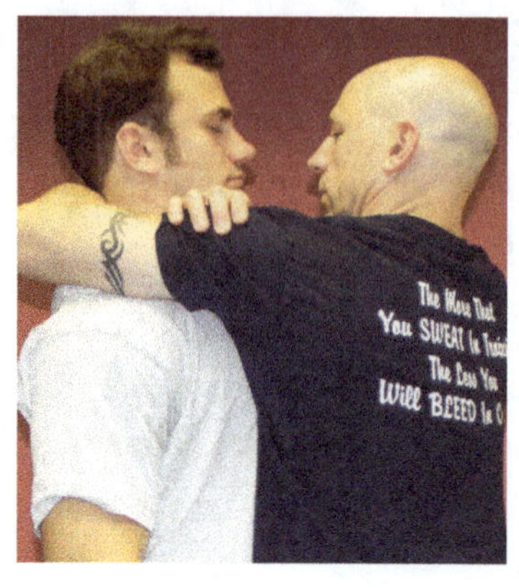

TWO-POINT CHOKE

This choke is very similar to the Ezekiel Choke. I will typically employ this choke when someone has me in an Arms-Free Bear-Hug from the front or as a strike defense.

Take your right arm and slide it on a 45-degree angle upward with your palm down. The hard edge of your wrist needs to be against their throat, with your fingers reaching back over their right trapezius. Shoot your left arm under your right hand and then quickly wrap it around their neck. Take your left hand and grip your fingers into the crook of your elbow. This choke may or may not result in your aggressor losing consciousness, but it's a great distraction and allows you to deliver head butts to their nose and mouth as well as knees to their groin and bladder.

THREE-POINT CHOKE

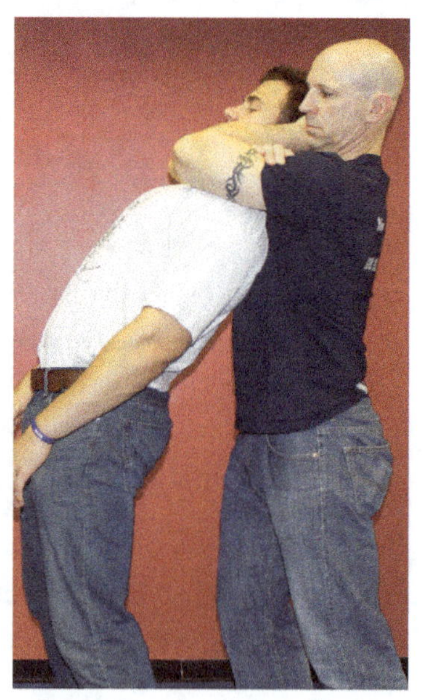

Our next choke is often referred to as the RNC, Rear Naked Choke, and is applied from behind. You will want to begin this move with a left Biceps Punch to the left side of their head as you wrap your left arm around their throat. Be sure to have your arm under their chin as you slide your arm back so that the back of your hand is against the right side of their face. This position is extremely important because with your hand in this position, it ensures that your wrist is planted firmly against the trachea. Next, slide your right arm over their right trapezius with your palm up.

You will secure the choke by grasping your right bicep with your left hand and then bending your elbow to allow placing your right hand on the top of the left side of their head.

There should be no gaps in the execution of these maneuvers whatsoever. To finish the assailant off, roll your left wrist into their throat and upward and drive your right elbow down into their chest as you push their head on a downward angle and to the right by curling your wrist. When done properly, the result will be an immediate loss of air and a crushing effect on the trachea.

FOUR-POINT CHOKE

This is the most devastating choke of them all. This is my preferred method to choke someone from behind.

The entry is shorter and quicker than on the Three-Point Choke. Take your right hand, with your thumb facing up, and ride downward along their right clavicle and then snake your hand onto the left side of their face and position the back of your hand against the left side of their face. Your right hand will be palm down and set to meet the left.

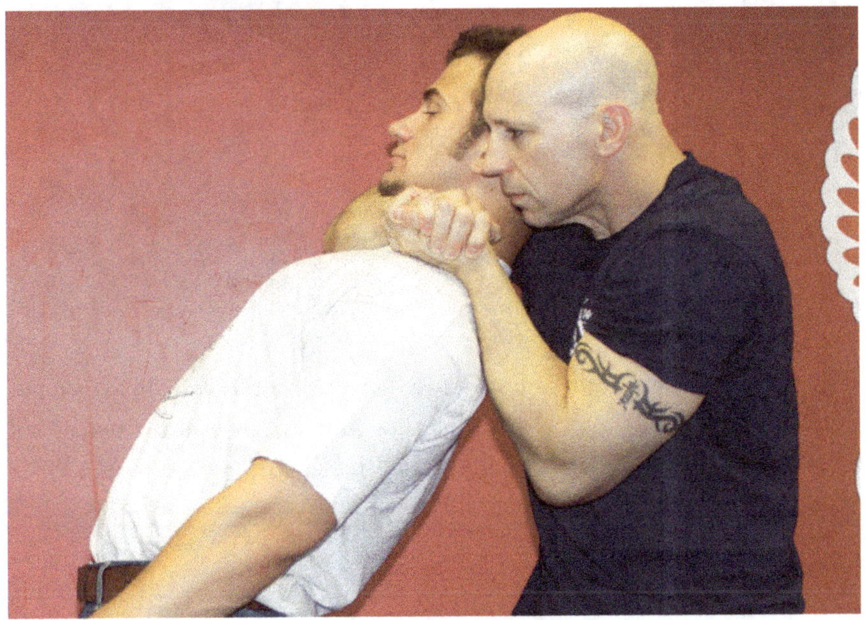

Now take your left hand in a palm-up position and secure a Gable Grip as you place the top-right portion of your head to the back of the left side of their head. Situate your left elbow in their back as you pull your right elbow back behind their shoulder and roll your right wrist upward and inward into their throat. This will provide you with four points of pressure. If applied correctly, the choke will yield the desired result in less than one second. Yes, I did say one second or less. This choke is the quickest, nastiest and most devastating method of applying a choke from the rear position.

FRONT CHOKE, STANDING

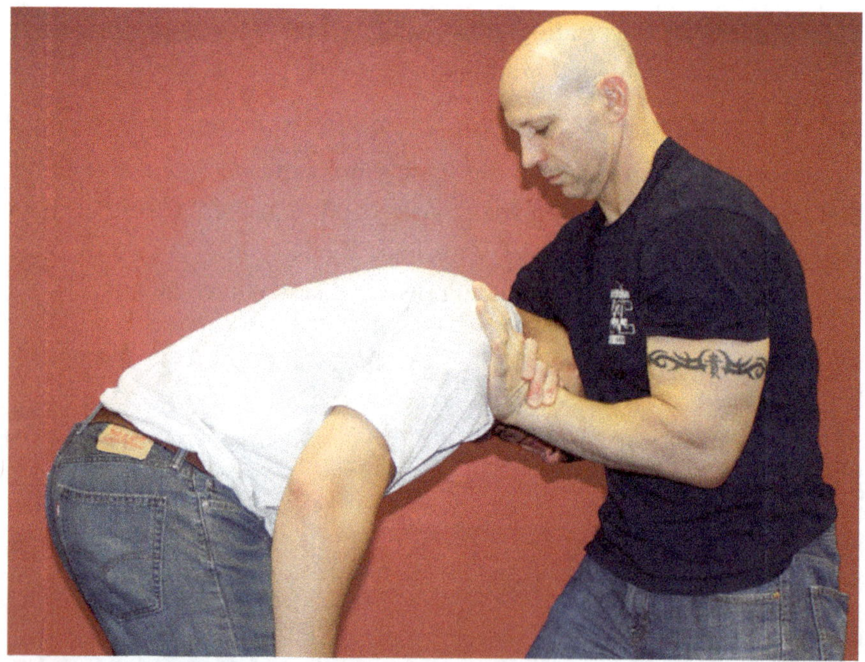

If you have struck your opponent in the groin or given them a head snap and brought them down so that they are bent over at the waist, it's a good time to apply this extremely effective choke.

Loop your right arm over their neck so that the bicep is against their face and the back of your wrist is against their throat. Your hand should be dorsiflexed, thus bringing the back of your hand against the side of their face. Smash into their shoulder with your left hand and then grab your left wrist with your right hand. Apply pressure by dropping your right elbow and shoulder downward, pushing into their shoulder with your left hand and driving your hips toward them in an upward and inward motion. Be cautious if practicing this with your training partner, as this movement places a great deal of stress on the neck.

LEG LOCKS

Leg locks are a great deal of fun and very devastating, but extremely difficult to apply in a street situation. For starters, you have to be on the ground to administer it. As discussed before, going to the ground in the street is not recommended. This limits the number of choices that we are able to utilize because we must remain on our feet for most moves. Additionally, certain footwear makes it difficult to apply a pressure lock; only the twisting locks will be effective.

ACHILLES LOCK

There are several methods to get to the position where we can implement the Achilles Lock. One is for a downed opponent that tries to kick up at you. Another is when you apply a single-leg takedown. Yet another will result from an opponent throwing a kick at you.

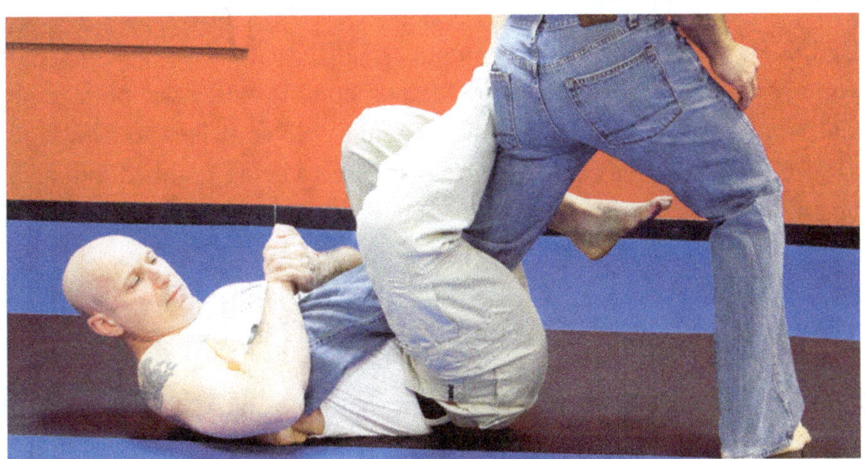

With any of these, secure his right leg by wrapping your left arm around it so that his foot is in your armpit and the back of your arm is against his Achilles. Thread your right arm under your left hand and then place it on top of his leg at the shin. Roll your shoulder back and down, then roll your wrists into the technique as you extend your arms. This is referred to as the Python Grip.

Next, kick him in the groin with your right foot as you arch upward. Sweep the remaining leg and step on it when it's on the ground. To finish him, hold this grip and execute a forward roll directly on top of the downed attacker. This will wreak havoc on his hip, knee and ankle.

HEEL HOOK

Let us assume that you begin from the basic position of the Achilles Lock with the assailant on the ground and you in control of their right foot. With them in the supine position with their toes pointing upward, slide your left arm in so that you can place the crook of your elbow firmly on their heel. Bring your left hand over the top of their foot with your palm down while you firmly grasp with your right hand employing the Gable Grip. Pivot on your right foot and step in a semi-circle toward the downed opponent with your left foot while you twist their ankle. The knee will receive the brunt of the damage.

BREAKING GRIPS AND LOCKS

Evil doers may grab you in a number of different ways. Especially if you are a smaller individual, larger perpetrators will attempt to grab and control you. Instinctively, you should deliver strikes to vital and semi-vital target areas as your first response to being grabbed, but also be prepared to pursue other methods of escape or self-defense.

SMALL CIRCLE (JIU JIT SU):

This was developed by Professor Wally Jay and focuses on small joint manipulation and the application of small circular movements to gain an advantage in leverage. This is based on the principle of using much of your body to control a small portion of theirs. By bringing a limb, joint or hand close to your body and away from theirs, you have created a power and balance advantage for yourself. Here is an example: If someone grabs your left wrist, they are most likely going to pull you toward them. Let them and then strike them in the face with a Palm Heel strike. Keeping your elbows tucked into your body, rotate your left hand in a small circle and slip your right hand underneath, grabbing their right hand. Place the Axehand edge of your left hand in the palm of their right hand and pressure down. Next, step off on an angle to their right side with your left foot and then your right. All the while, you are using your wrist.

It is important to note that the hip drives your power a hundred percent. This should be an effortless motion, no matter what the size differential.

GRAB, RE-GRAB

One of the most effective methods of practicing your grips, locks and escapes is with the Grab, Re-Grab drill. This is a flow drill.

Start off slowly and then add speed and power to your practice. Start in the standing position. One partner grabs the other by the wrist, hand or collar. Apply one of the Wrist Lock techniques, Gan Kun, Kotegaeshi, or one of the variations. Your partner will "go with flow" and move in the direction that you are taking them. They will counter with a Wrist Lock of their own. Now you are to move with this pressure and perform a counter-lock. This lock-counter-and-lock continues until the drill is over. We usually do it for time, two to three minutes at a clip. This will exhaust your grip, so be pre¬pared to work. When you have two people who are very experienced at this drill, it's amazing to watch them roll, counter, and apply one lock after another with speed and fluidity.

LEG-LOCK DEFENSE

I love the fact that MMA has become mainstream. It's a dream come true for me. Back in the early 80s, we yearned for a venue such as the

UFC to compete in. You younger guys (and gals) have no idea of how lucky you are!

As with all great things, there are some drawbacks. Untrained knuckle-heads see this stuff on TV and in their video games and try to emulate it. There is one positive aspect in our favor that can counter this, and that's that it's reasonably difficult to successfully apply a potent Leg Lock.

Again, we will focus on the principals. You need to step into the defensive technique by bending your leg, dorsiflexing your toes and moving toward the assailant. If you attempt to pull away, you will only succeed in making the lock tighter. Once you have accomplished this, secure a top position and rain down strikes on your opponent.

Chapter 9
Entry and Single Techniques

Entry Techniques: As conveyed to me by one of the American pioneers of jiu jitsu, Dr. Tony Palminteri, "You have to earn the right to use jiu jitsu."

What does that mean? In a nutshell, there is no way you are simply going to walk up to someone and apply a Wrist Lock on them. It just won't work. They will strike you and resist. The idea is to accomplish your goal while sustaining a minimal amount of damage to yourself. A well-placed strike (either by you OR your adversary) can render one helpless. This works both for and against you. A powerful punch in the nose can turn a BJJ Black Belt into a White Belt. Whereas a well-placed loosening-up technique will dramatically increase your chances of successfully applying a choke or lock. You won't be able to properly administer your techniques until you "dummy the opponent up."

So, we need to consider our entry or loosening up techniques. The below-listed moves, along with other single strikes and techniques, are extremely effective.

ENTRY TECHNIQUES

These techniques must be applied very quickly and with purpose. There can be no hesitation or holding back whatsoever.

You may also implement them in multiples. There is no rule that states these techniques are only designed to be entry strikes. In actuality, their application demonstrates quite the contrary. Many of these tactics may be used to temporarily or permanently disable an attacker. Your proximity to the assailant will determine what techniques are available to you.

FINGER-JAB TO EYES

The Three Stooges were a great comedy trio, but the manner in which they delivered eye pokes wasn't the best for street combat.

When done right, this maneuver is extremely quick and effective. Take all four fingers and aim for the bridge of the nose with the full intention of striking the eyes. Flick the fingers out quickly while they are slightly bent. It does not matter how big, tough, or strong your opponent is; everyone has eyes, and they all feel the same amount of pain. If they are wearing glasses, rake the glasses down and simultaneously strike.

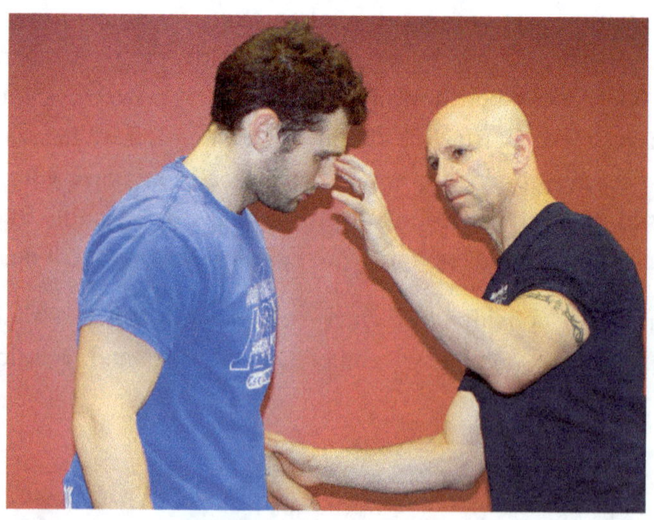

SHORT AXEHAND

This technique protects your head and face and serves as a powerful, unorthodox strike. This technique may be delivered via a variety of methods.

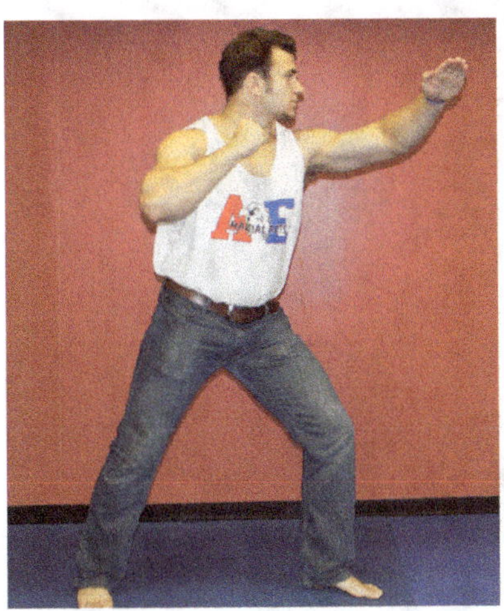 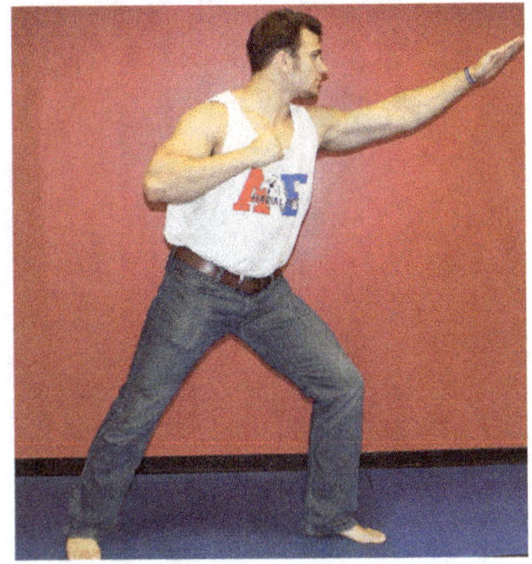

For instance, you may launch your attack from a Cross Stance (Chapter 6), Interview Stance or from a Fig-Leaf Stance with your hands folded one over the other in front of your groin. From the Fig-Leaf Stance, have your right hand over your left. Apply pressure and tension to both hands with your right hand pulling back on your left and your left providing counter-pressure. You are creating a "spring effect" very similar to a Jack-in-the-box. When you are ready, release your left hand and launch forward with your left foot, stomping hard on the ground as your Axehand hits any of the targets (eyes, nose, throat, ear, mouth, carotid artery, or neck) from the neck to the ear. Your striking implement will be the fleshy part of your hand located directly below your pinky. Your hand must be flexed and with tension. Practice "making your hand big" by forcing your metacarpophalangeal joints (knuckles) outward while pulling your fingers back.

Practice this movement, it will add strength and flexibility to your hands. In fact it is one of the easiest and most effective methods for developing the intrinsic muscles of your hand. Axehands are the only hand techniques where the hip moves in the same direction as the strike. All other hand techniques require the rotation of the hip inward of the striking limb.

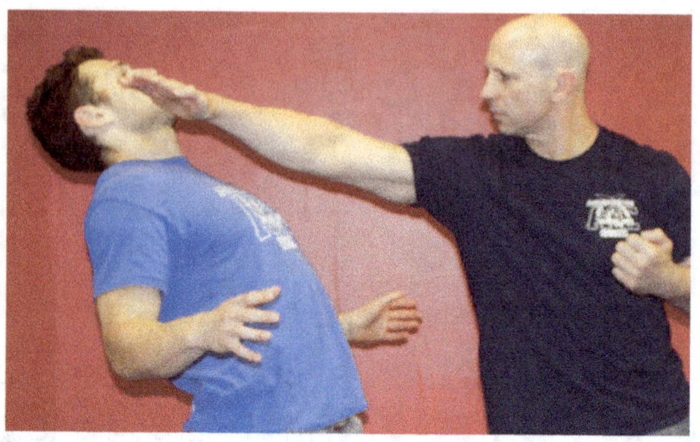

PALM-HEEL STRIKE

This technique is excellent when delivering strikes to the face, mouth and especially the nose. The motion is very similar to a straight punch, except that your hand is open. You pull your fingers back, and your contact point is the heel (lower section) of your palm. Since this is considered a "soft" striking area, it is perfect for striking the harder sections of the body. However, this technique is very successful when applied to the sternum, which can be fleshy on larger individuals.

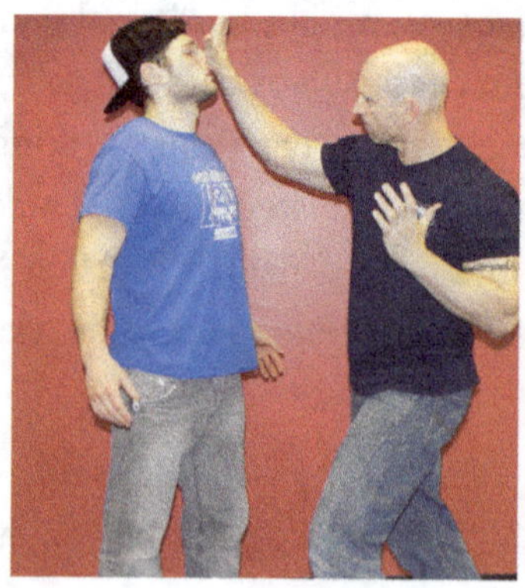
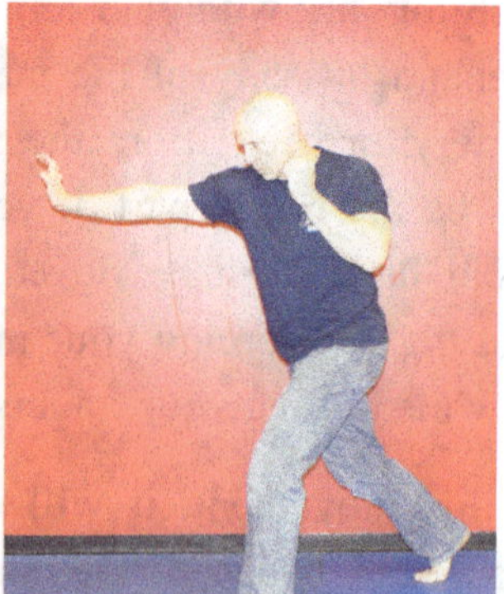

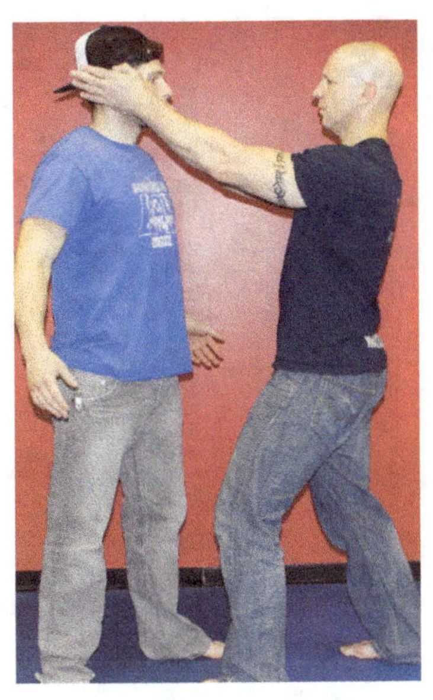

SLAPS

Your slap should be brought up from the hip out of the opponent's line of sight, then quickly and powerfully placed on the ear of the target. The strike is delivered with an upside-down "L" pattern, straight up and then straight across as you rotate your hip into the strike. To increase the effectiveness of the strike, slightly cup your hand thus forcing air into the eardrum of the attacker.

Slaps are a great means employed to loosen up or distract, enabling you to deliver a more potent knock-out or disabling technique. Slaps, as well as other open-hand strikes, are the best methods to deliver head blows in street defense.

HEAD-BUTTS

There are four basic Head-Butts to use to defend yourself. All are extremely effective and carry relatively low risk of injury to you.

FOREWORD

When face to face and at very close range, you attack your opponent's nose or mouth with your forehead. Drive your head forward and down toward the target while contracting your abs and moving your whole upper body forward.

Many people are under the false belief that the power of the technique comes solely from the neck. As described, the whole upper body is involved in the power generation, and the forehead is simply the delivery mechanism.

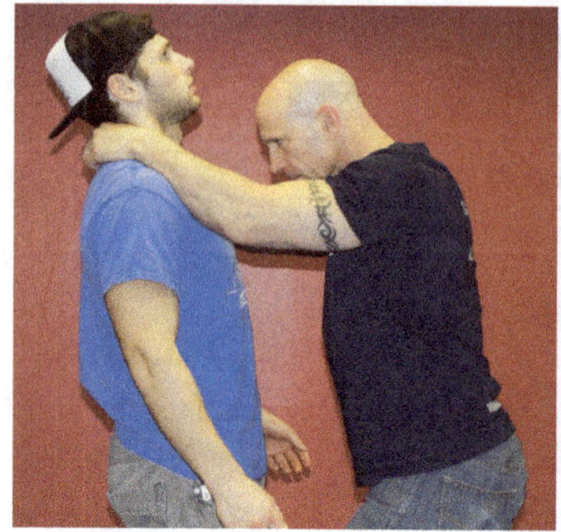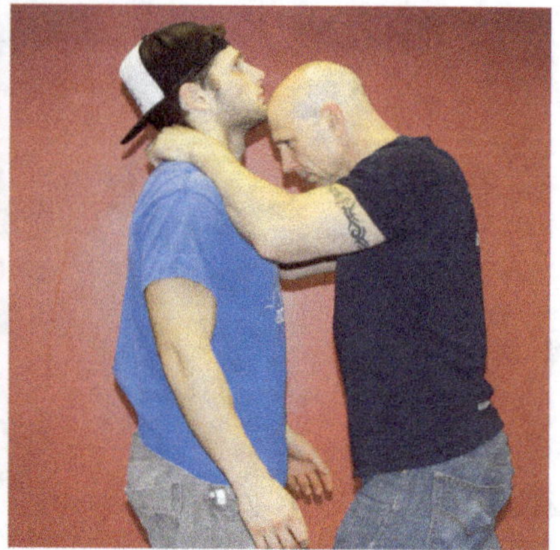

Foreward head-butt.

BACKWARD

When you are attacked from behind, bring your head forward and then back - *hard*. It's tough to see where their nose is from this position, so it's recommended that you incorporate a butt smash into them coupled with foot stomps.

UPWARD

You may be facing each other, but with your head lower than theirs. If this is the case, bring your head upward into their chin. If they are positioned properly, you can apply a Forward Head-Butt when their head comes back down. Generally, it's best to strike an open target or knock them to the ground.

SIDEWAYS

If you are Bear Hugged from the side, immediately bring your head sideways, banging the upper back corner of your head into their face. The targets of the nose and mouth should be utilized again.

This movement, as with most Head-Butts, will not result in a knockout. You'll want to immediately Hammerfist- Smash them in the groin and stomp their foot. In most instances, this will be enough for you to get them to loosen their grip so you may escape.

ADDITIONAL SINGLE TECHNIQUES

These will be your core striking techniques. You should practice these movements with regularity, focus and intensity. Muscle memory and neural patterning will only be developed through this type of practice. Knowing how to do something and being able to execute under pressure are two completely different animals.

Consider an MMA fighter. They practice a plethora of strikes and kicks, submissions, takedowns and combinations for hours on end. Striking pads, drilling and sparring with partners, and working on sequencing and transitions.

But what percentage of the moves practiced do they pull off in a combat situation? As a general rule, somewhere between 10 and 15 percent of the trained movements. That seems amazingly small, but when you consider the time that you have to react and respond to a specific situation, there are only so many techniques that you will be able to execute. Bear this fact in mind when training. As we have pointed out beforehand, the magic number is seven, plus or minus two.

LONG AXEHAND

Form your hand as you would for a Short Axehand. Next, draw your right hand back past your ear with your elbow in front of your face. Step toward your target with your right foot, landing with a stomp as you deliver the Axehand to the side of your opponent's neck or head. You should make a full motion through to the end.

While practicing in the air or on a pad, bring your right hand back far enough to pass your right shoulder. As with all strikes, the incorporation of your hips and engagement of your complete body in the movement is essential for maximal results. As with the Short Axehand, Long Axehands require the hip to move in the same direction as the strike.

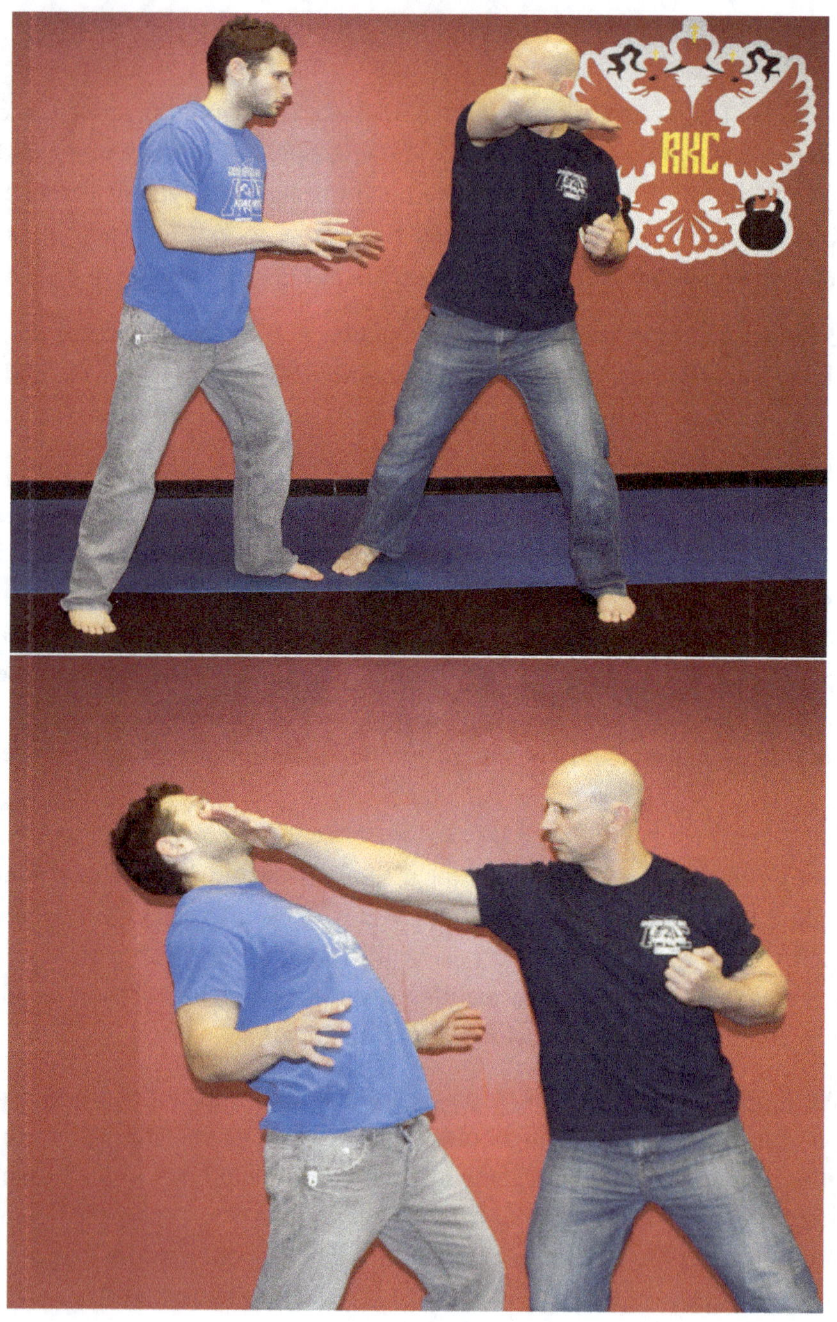

Long axehead.

CHIN JAB

This is an incredibly powerful strike, generally resulting in a knockout. Your hand is positioned like it would be for a Palm-Heel Strike, with your fingers pulled back and your hand flexed so that the heel of your palm will land first on the designated target. Your forearm slides up their chest at an angle as the radial and ulna bones drive into the chin of the assailant. Follow through with the upward-angled motion snapping their head backward.

This motion will induce "Referral Shock." This quick shot will cause the brain to move in its fluid cushion and crash into the surrounding skull.

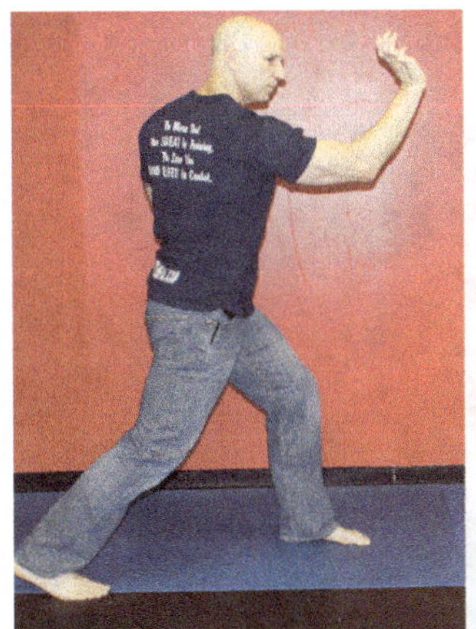
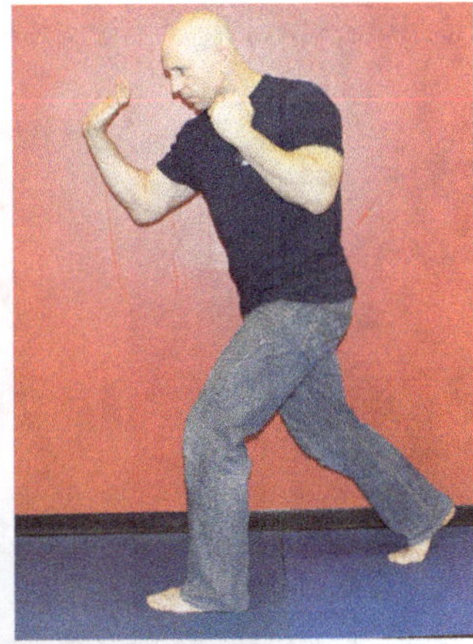
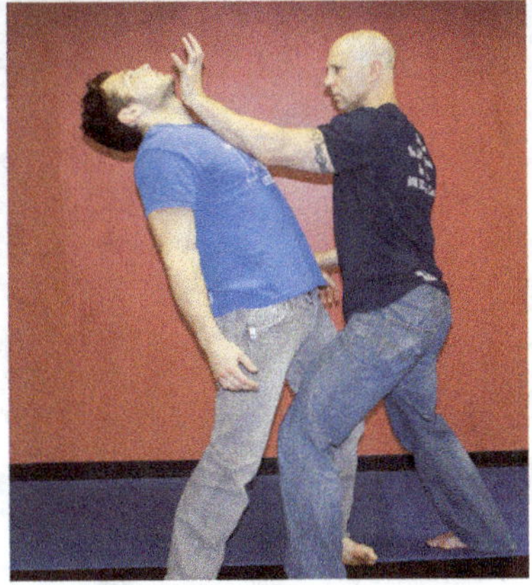

VERTICAL FIST

This technique is best suited for Bare Knuckle applications or while wearing MMA gloves. Due to the size and configuration of boxing gloves, the strike is not as effective with large 10-16-ounce gloves on. The fist is clenched with the thumb at the top and pinky facing the ground. Generally, this punch is

delivered at close range and the arm is not fully extended, meaning that the elbow is not locked out. This blow is delivered to the targets of the center line: bladder, solar plexus, sternum, chin or nose. The arm is slightly bent, the lats are locked, and the body tightens completely upon contact. Prior to that, as with virtually all strikes, the body is loose. This strike is based on Bruce's Lee one- and three-inch punches, which he delivered with unprecedented verve.

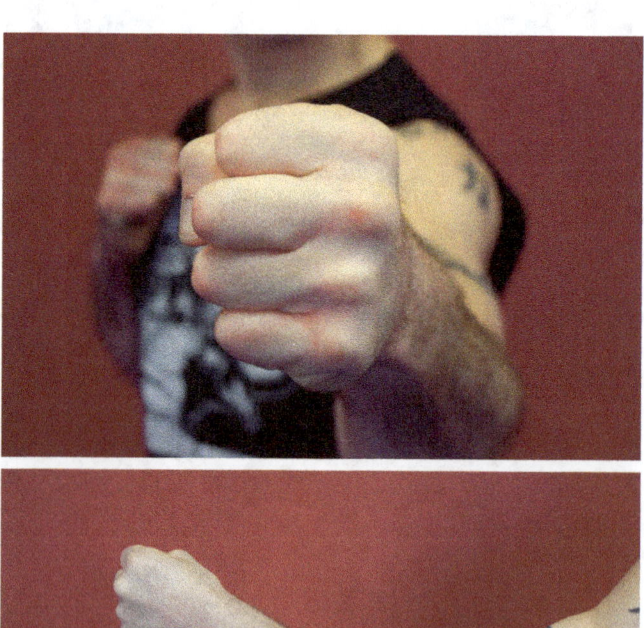

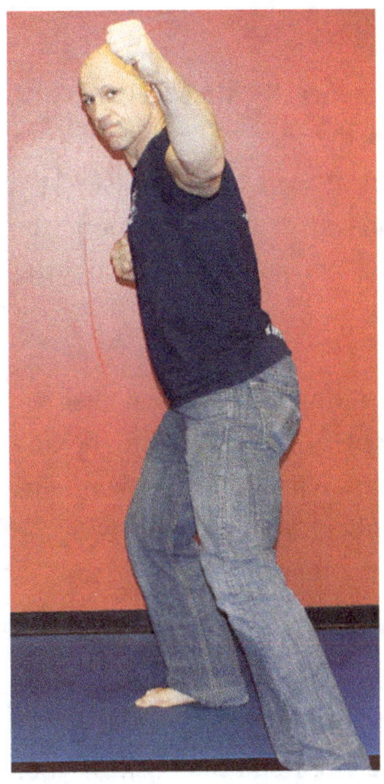

Backfist.

BACKFIST

This strike was made popular in the 70s by the most innovative martial artist of all time, once again the indomitable Bruce Lee. This lead-hand technique is efficient and very quick. The angle that the technique presents varies from the standard straight lead-hand techniques. Keep your hand high, step in with your lead leg, and rotate your lead hip inward as your fist is directed in the opposite motion and toward the target. Keep your other hand high next to your head. Even though the technique is effective, it is not generally considered a knockout blow, but more of a set-up strike.

SCISSOR PUNCH

Slightly curve and press your fingers together and separate your thumb from your forefinger as far as possible, so that the webbing between your thumb and forefinger is taut. Deliver a straight shot to the throat, striking with the crotch of your thumb and forefinger. Immediately grab the windpipe of the perpetrator and wrap your thumb and fingers tightly around it attempting to crush it in your hand.

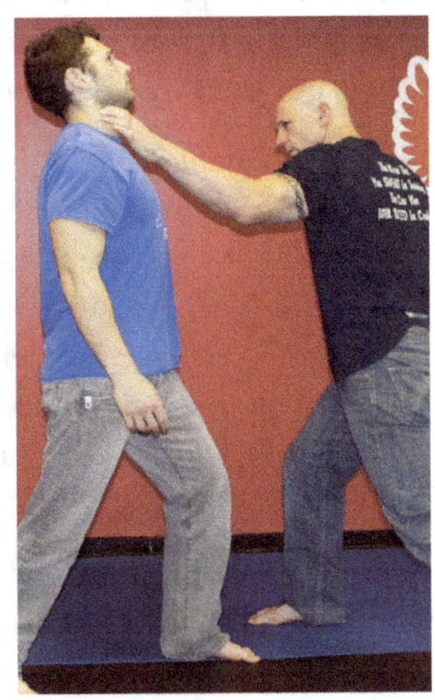

EYE GOUGE

The best method to apply an Eye Gouge is generally after a Head Butt, Groin Strike or a Double Ear Slap. Grasp the sides of the attacker's head and stick your thumbs into the section of their eyes closest to the bridge of their nose. Then dig your thumbs in deep and "scoop" the eyeballs out toward their ears as you grip the sides of their head tightly.

PUNCHES

There are six Basic Punches. This is the numbering system that we employ in our kickboxing training. There are some Western boxing systems that use the same numbers; others vary slightly from this particular numbering system. The odd numbers are delivered with the lead hand, and the even numbers represent the rear-hand techniques.

The path that all punches follow is hip, shoulder, elbow and fist. The hip generates the punch and then it goes to the shoulder. Shoot the elbow straight-forward, keeping it in line with your hip as you rotate your fist, positioning your thumb facing the floor and the back of your hand at the ceiling. Your arm is loose and quick as you step forward into the technique, only momentarily tensing upon impact. Retract the hand quickly to diminish "dead time." The dead time is the period of time that it takes for your hand to get back to your head.

We want to employ one of two tactics when considering the retraction of punches. You will either bring your hand to your head or your head to your hand. If you are using angle steps forward, bring your head to your hand. If you're more or less stationary, bring your hand back to your head. When using either method, imagine a rubber band attached between your fist and shoulder. Once you throw the punch, snap it back to its original position. You should remember to always use head movement, as moving targets are more difficult to hit.

Whenever you throw a punch with a lead hand technique, the lead hip rotates inward. When throwing a punch with the rear hand, the rear hip moves inward. This axiom holds true for all for all Punches, Jabs, Crosses, Hooks, Uppercuts, Backfists, etc...

With no further ado, here are the six types of basic punches:

1. **Jab:** This straight punch is thrown off of the lead hand. Step in slightly and time the landing of your step with the fist's contact with the desired target. Not only is this strike a great set-up tool for your other techniques, but you can knock someone out with a good stiff jab, especially if they are moving into you. Muhammad Ali was famous for his jab, and George Foreman's first title was won almost exclusively with it.

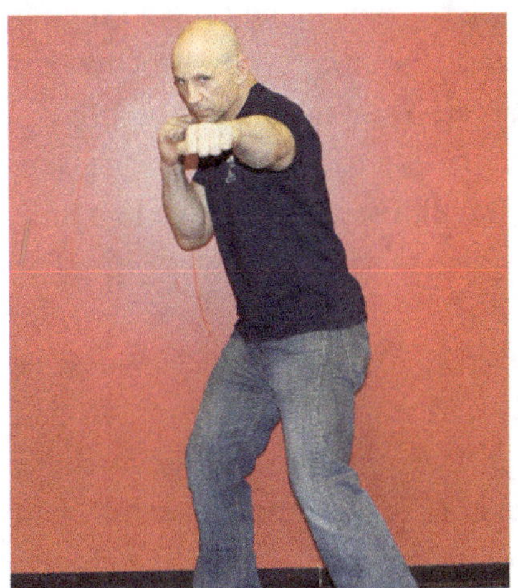 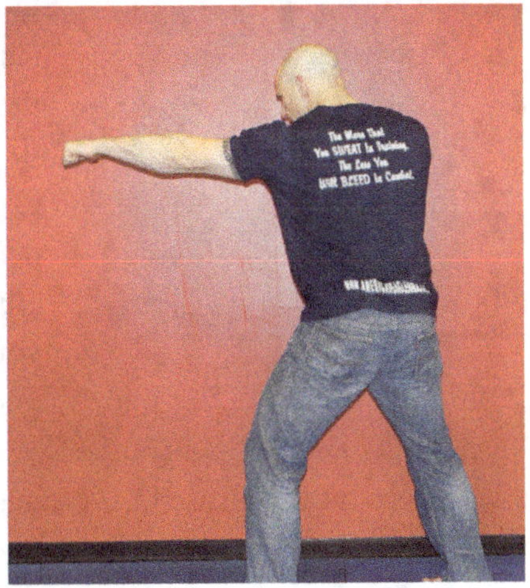

2. **Cross:** Or "Big Bertha," as we often refer to it. "The Knockout Punch" is also a straight punch but thrown from the rear side of the body. In karate, it's referred to as a "Reverse Punch" for this reason. In boxing the term "Cross" is applied because it crosses your body. This enables you to generate more power from the increased rotation of your hips. Slide the foot of the punching hand forward and slightly to the side as you deliver the strike. The rear foot moves up to keep your feet equidistant. Be sure NOT to rise up onto your toes, but to keep the balls of your feet on the ground, pivoting them as the punch is thrown. Your hand assumes the same position as with the jab, and the retraction strategy is also consistent.

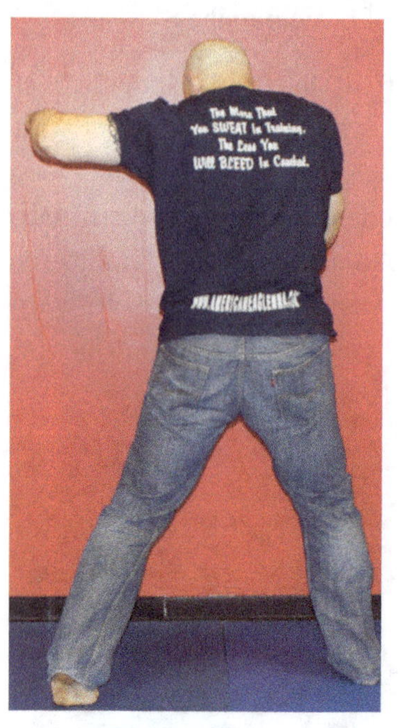

3. **Lead Hook:** This technique requires more athleticism to throw than any other punch. When done well it carries tremendous knockout power, and in fact the legendary Joe Frazier won a world title with it! The lead hook is a great counter-punching weapon. To execute this punch, start out as if you were throwing a jab and then rotate your hip and pivot on your lead foot, pointing your heel toward the target. Your fist should be in relatively the same position as the jab, except with the thumb rotated slightly down and the pinky slightly up. The elbow is bent at a 90-degree angle, your lat is locked in place and your shoulder is packed. The punch is delivered across (into the target) and on a slight angle downward. The foot work employed is generally a slight step to the outside to avoid a straight punch. A hook that lands on the side of the jaw can easily drop an opponent. By hitting the chin at this angle, more than 50 percent of your target's neck muscles will be unavailable to stabilize the head.

4. **Rear Hook:** This athletic maneuver is an exceptionally effective means to attack the body. I like to use this to attack the floating ribs, solar plexus and liver. You want to take advantage of your leg power when delivering this blow. Be certain to bend your knees and synchronize landing your shot as you come up. Your fist is almost vertical when it lands, the thumb is at approximately 80 degrees, and the pinky is facing the ground.

5. **Lead Uppercut:** This punch is generally used to strike either under the chin or at the solar plexus. As with the Hook, you want to have your arm bent at a 90-degree angle, your shoulder packed, and your lat locked. Use your legs and hips while you drive the strike upward and

inward into the target. The fist is positioned with the palm facing you as you twist your hand with a quarter turn en route to impact. The Uppercut also works well if someone is diving for your legs and trying to take you down.

6. **Rear Uppercut:** This strike is used primarily as a body shot. You throw it as you would the Lead Uppercut, except with more potential power because it's off of your rear hand and enlists more leg and hip power. The targets for the Rear Uppercut are the floating ribs, bladder, solar plexus and groin.

OVERHAND RIGHT

This is a derivation of the Cross. I also refer to it as the "Bar-room Punch." Think of combining a Hook and a Cross together. This punch is best delivered after either a Jab or a Fake

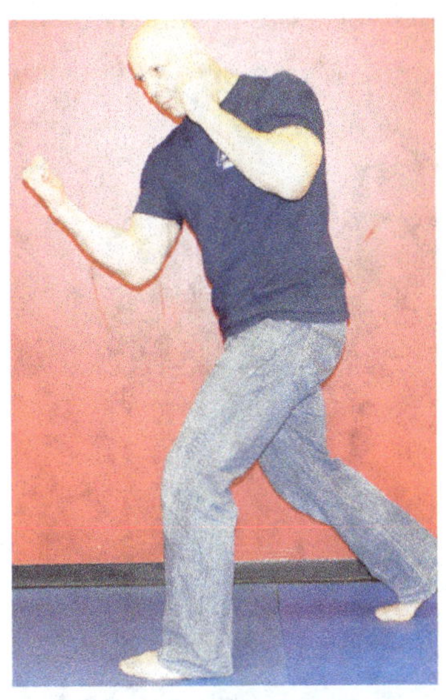

Rear uppercut.

Jab, and you'll release it by sliding your lead leg inward and on a 45-degree angle to the outside as you bring your rear foot in. The fist will travel in a slight arch, going upward and then downward. At the point of impact, your elbow will be slightly higher than your fist.

ELBOW VARIATIONS

Throwing an elbow is an extremely effective striking technique. I like to use the elbow, if possible.

Why? For starters, the elbow is closer to your power base, so you are able to deliver more power than with a conventional punch. Second, the chance of injuring your elbow is very slim when compared to what can happen to your hand when striking. Most Elbow Strikes thrown to the face and head are of a slashing nature, so you will want to keep your hand open. This will aid the slashing movement and maximize the damage when ripping the skin of the enemy's face or head. When you are attacking the body, you want to employ a closed fist. This will deliver more power to the intended target. The clenched fist will deliver more power when thrusting or smashing with the elbow.

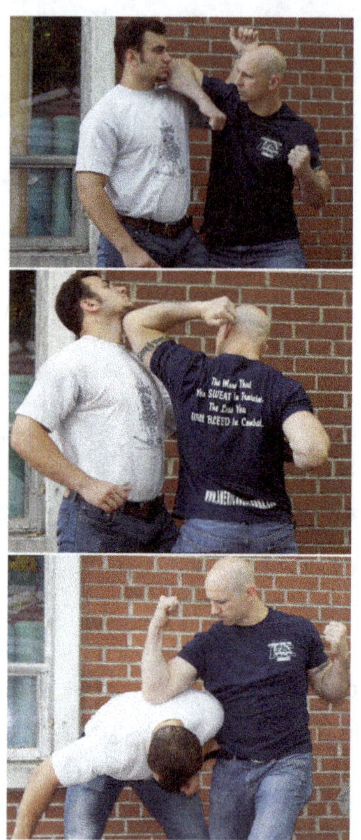

Elbow hook across | Elbow upward | Elbow downward.

ACROSS

If you are throwing a right elbow, step into the target with the right foot. Your forearm will be parallel to the floor with your palm facing down, your hand loose as you bring your elbow across the face of the assailant. Aim for the side of the head at the temple and go all the way across the head.

UPWARD

The Upward Elbow Strike is another strike that we perform with a loose, open hand. This blow is directed straight upward into the chin of the attacker. This is the main target area of this technique. It's not very effective with any other targets.

DOWNWARD

This strike begins with an open hand and then ends with a closed fist upon impact. Often referred to as "The Death Elbow," this technique is delivered to the cervical or thoracic spine. The Downward Elbow was deemed so damaging that the UFC banned fighters from using it in the top position. Once you have doubled your opponent over with a strike to the bladder or groin, rise up on the balls of your feet, twist your hips to the right, and then drop the right elbow downward, smashing it into the attacker's spine with full force. Deliver this downward blow with speed and power as you drop your weight into it.

SIDE AND BACK

Elbow Strikes directed to the side and the back are thrown the same way. Make a fist with the hand of the striking elbow, and place the open palm of your opposite hand on the knuckles of the closed fist. Step into the technique, bend your knees, and twist your hips into the strike while pushing on the clenched fist with the open hand. These elbow strikes should be delivered specifically to the ribs, stomach or bladder.

ANGULAR

Elbows thrown on an angle, either upward or downward, are delivered

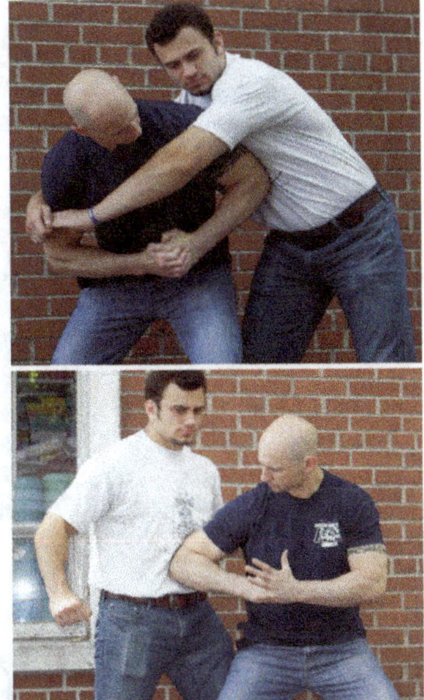

Side and back.

with an open, loose hand. The open hand accentuates the ripping of the skin and maximizes the trauma. Loop the elbow upward then down-ward and across the target, generally the head or face. As the strike comes downward, drop your weight by bending your knees and turning your hip into the technique.

Upward Elbows require you to bend your knees and then partially straighten them, as the elbow is thrown on an angle upward into the chin or side of the head, if the head is turned.

FOREARM SHIVER

Step into your opponent with one hand open and the other fist clenched while you deliver a stiff forearm shot to the chest. The forearm and side of the wrist can be used to choke or levy pressure on an opponent.

Blocking and deflecting blows as well as striking the clavicle and neck of your adversary will lead to favorable results.

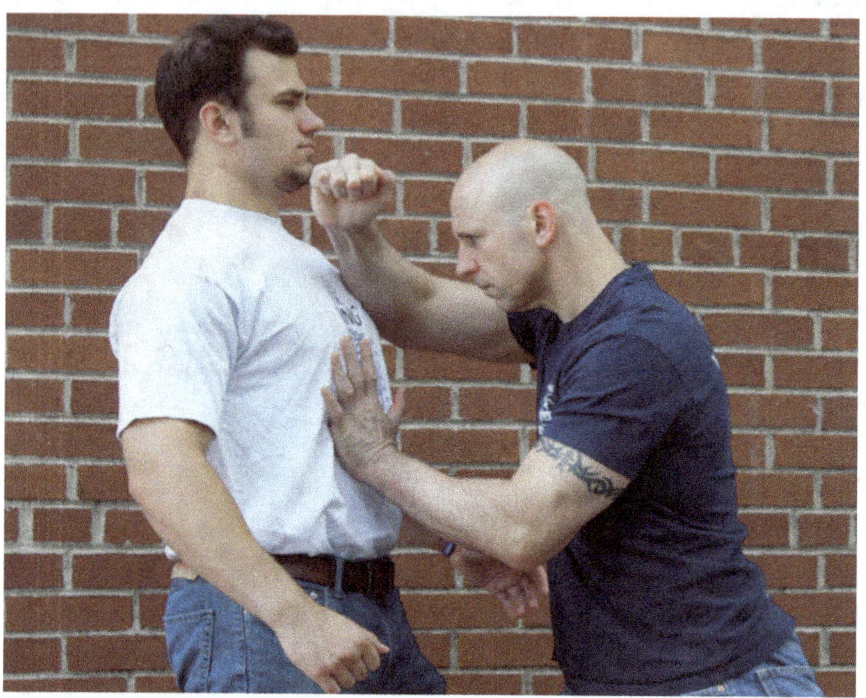

FOREARM SMASH DOWNWARD

Once your opponent is bent over, rise up on the balls of your feet, rotate your hip first upward and then downward as you smash your forearm down upon their back, neck or head. When delivering the blow, position your forearm parallel to the ground.

Most blocks double as strikes and may be used as a push or shove. The blocks that we list are both defensive and offensive weapons.

1. **High Block:** Synonymous with most basic karate standards. This image is of a karateka in a Horse Stance with one hand over their head in a High Block and the other in a fist in chamber at the hip. To practice this movement, take your left fist and place it in your right armpit as you twist your left hip to the right. Then rotate your hip back in the

other direction as your arm is positioned above your head. Your arm should be on a 45-degree angle, with your palm slightly rotated toward the ceiling. This is the typical block. You need to bear in mind that if you attempt to stand in front of someone and execute this block, you will be hit. You need to step back to allow for the time necessary to execute the block successfully. In Bando, we use this block more as a means to shove the opponent back. You assume the same basic position and then lower your level and use a front stance with the foot of the blocking hand forward as you launch the forearm into the assailant.

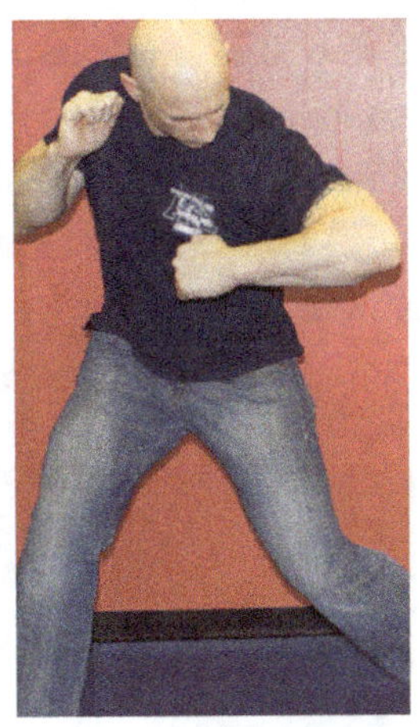

Forearm smash downward.

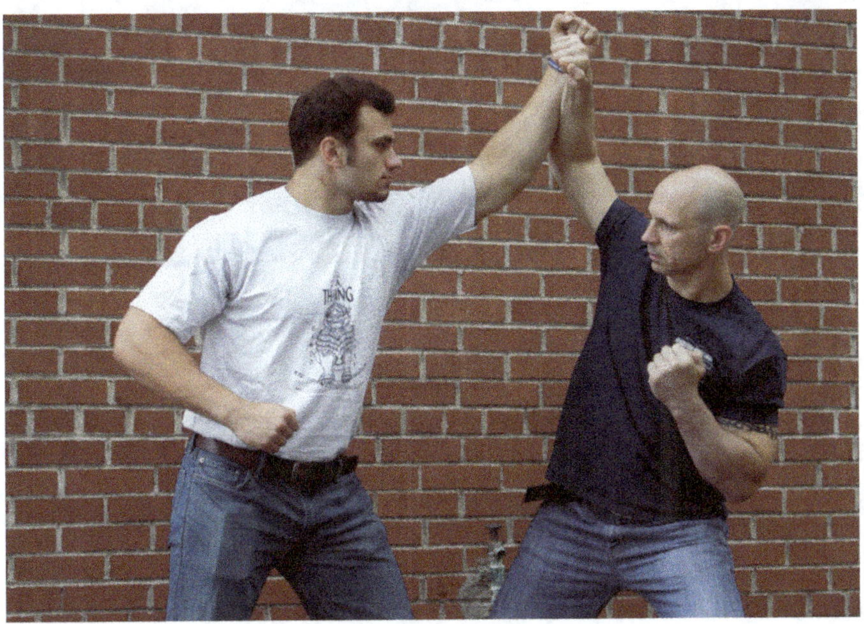

2. **Hammerfist Block:** That this movement can be used as both a block and a strike is very evident. When performing the blocking application, you'll need to move backward. Step in and attack with the technique

when you are on the offensive. Place your clenched fist up to your ear, with your pinky facing the ceiling and your thumb facing the floor. Bring the hand across your face as you rotate the fist so that your knuckles are facing the ceiling and the palm side of your hand is facing you. Make certain that your fist travels all the way across your head with both the block and the strike. The Hammerfist is used against a straight punch directed toward your face, and it's used to attack the side of the head or neck of the assailant.

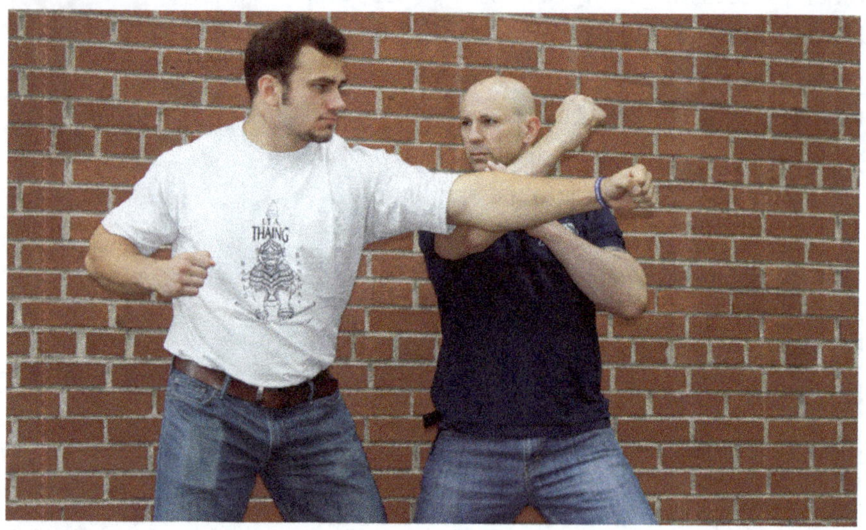

3. **Outside Middle Block:** This movement is primarily a block, but a grab may be employed as well. Do you remember the old "wax on, wax off" from the Karate Kid? Well, it's that block, more or less. Take your right hand and reach under your left arm touching the back of your right hand against your left triceps. Twisting your hips to the right, bend your elbow at a 45-degree angle as your open hand is brought across your body. Your fingertips should be at approximately eye level. Use this technique to block a straight attack to your midsection.

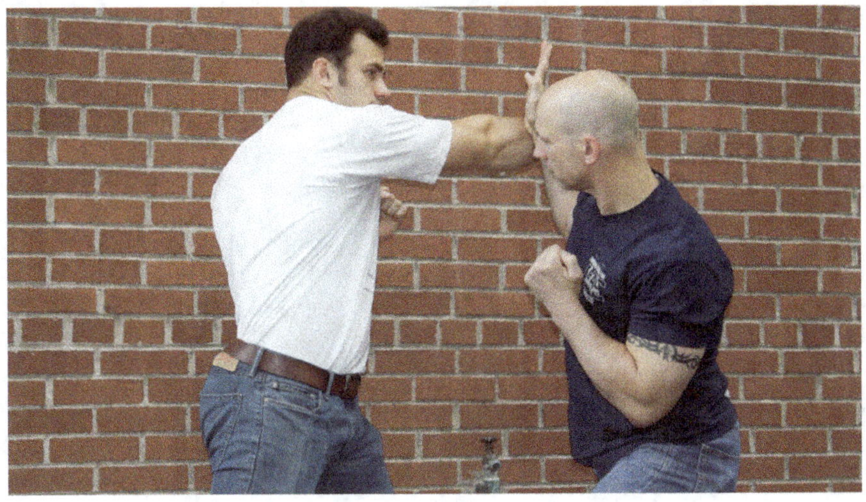

Outside middle block.

KNEE DRIVES

How many techniques elicit a better result than a well-placed knee strike to the groin or a lunging knee to someone's head? On the straight knees that are driven upward, the Straight and Springboard Knees, dorsiflex your foot. This engages the hip flexors to a greater degree and enables you to lift your knee higher and faster. When performing the Roundhouse Knee, it's preferable to point the toe in the event that your opponent moves back, so you may easily turn the Knee into a Roundhouse Kick.

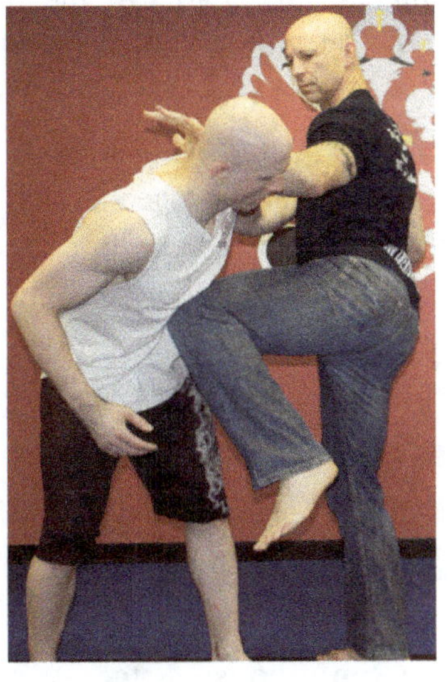

1. **Straight Knee:** Deliver a quick strike upward to the opponent's groin, quadriceps, peroneal nerve, solar plexus or bladder. You may also throw this to the face of a doubled-over opponent, usually after a knee to the groin or bladder.

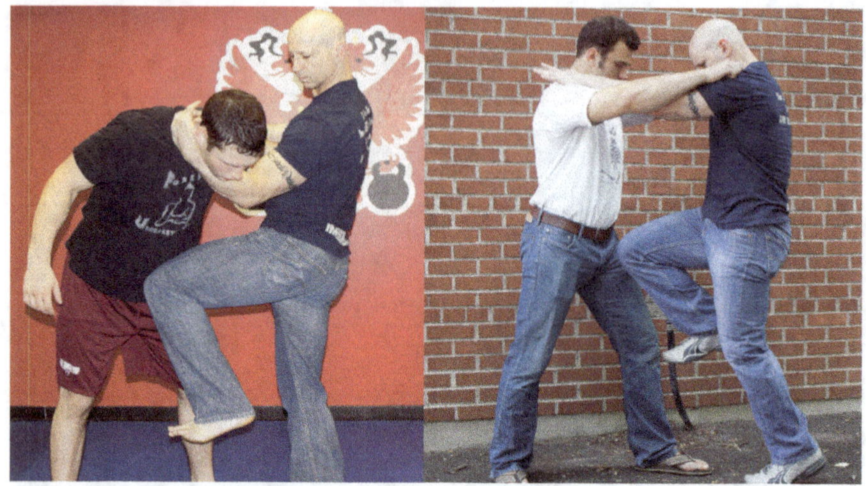

2. **Springboard Knee:** This is an extremely powerful blow delivered to almost any part of the body, but primarily directed to the same leg regions of the aforementioned Knee Strike: groin, solar plexus, sternum, ribcage, face or head. This strike is done after the initial loosening-up techniques and is used as a finisher. If you deliver the Knee Strike with your left knee, stomp your right foot on the ground and simultaneously bring your knee upward into the intended target. Repeat this strike as many times as possible until your assailant falls.

3. **Roundhouse Knee:** We generally direct this technique to the peroneal nerve, IT (Iliotibial) Band, floating

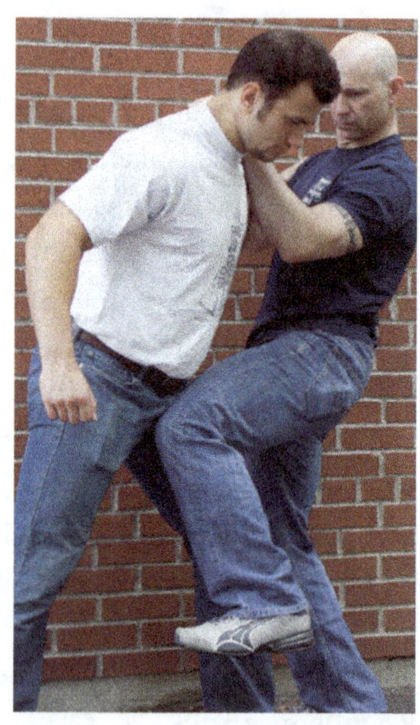

Straight knee.

ribs or the side of the head to a doubled-over opponent. If you are throwing a left knee, step toward your opponent on a 45-degree angle with your right foot. As you step, pivot your foot on the floor and bring your left knee into one of the aforementioned targets.

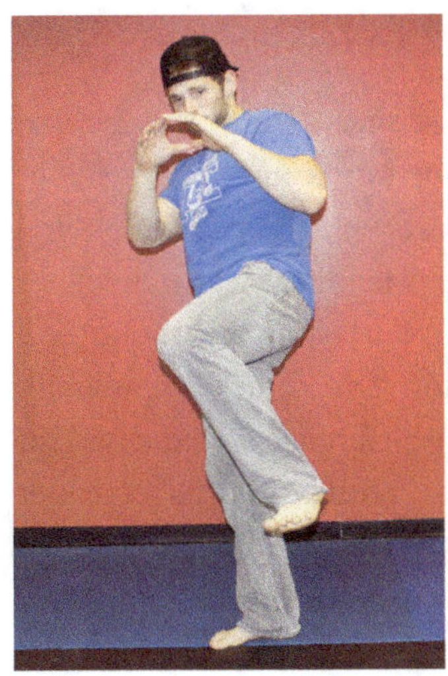 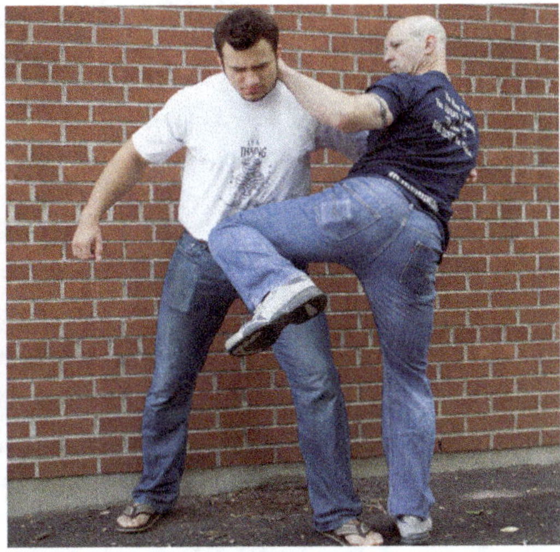

FOOT STOMPS

This counterattack maneuver can be applied in several combat situations. If you are grabbed from behind, are face-to-face, or grabbed from the side, draw your knee up as high as possible and dorsiflex your foot. Drive your heel down into their foot with as much force as possible. Repeat this movement as many times as is required.

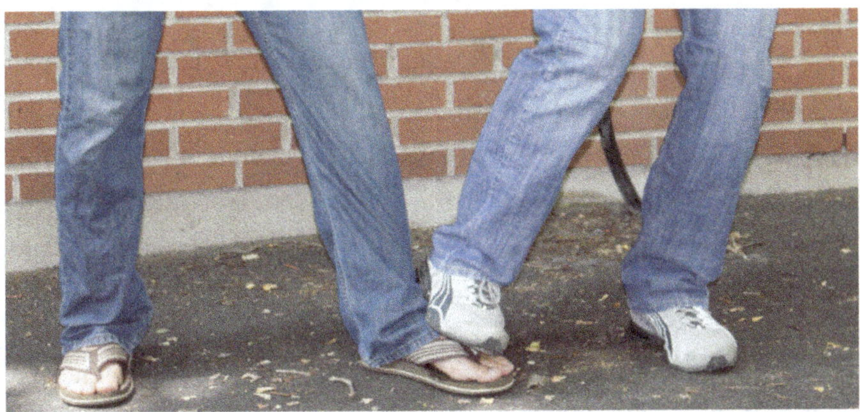

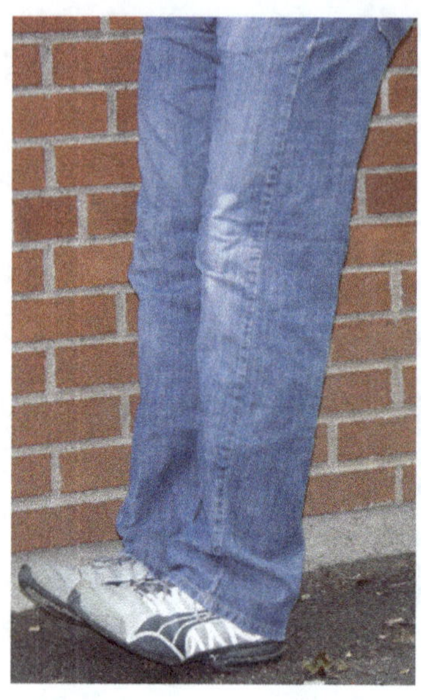

PARACHUTE STOMP

The name comes from the act of bending your knees and driving your legs very hard into the ground as you would when landing while using a parachute. We use this technique as a finishing blow to a downed opponent. It makes no difference if the assailant is supine or prone. Let us consider that our opponent is in the supine position. Place your feet together and jump into the air while bringing your knees up to your chest and dorsiflexing your feet as you drive your heels into the downed assailant's groin, abdomen, chest or head. This should put an immediate end to the situation.

This next group of Kicks is performed from the Fighting Stance or at least while you have some distance from your opponent.

ROUNDHOUSE KICK

This has to be my all-time favorite kick. When I look back at all of my fights, I don't think that I had one ring fight (that included kicking) when I didn't throw a Roundhouse Kick. It's quick, versatile and can be used to attack many areas. There are also many variations of this kick, all quite potent.

For now we will focus on the Lead-Leg Roundhouse Kick. There are four parts to this kick: the up, out, back and down. You bring the knee up into the chamber, kick the foot out, bring the foot back and then place it back on the floor. This is a chambered kick. When you first learn to do this kick, you step up with the rear foot and then lift the lead foot as you step into the kick. As you become adept at throwing this kick, you will replace the lead foot with the rear and almost "hop" into the kick.

Doing this will produce more speed and power due to the forward movement, the slight hop that reduces friction, and the power that you will get from having your foot land on the floor as your striking foot lands on the target. You will need to plantar-flex your foot by pointing your toes. The striking area of your foot will be the instep to the talus. You may direct this kick to many spots on the human body, including the shin, knee, femoral artery, quadriceps, groin, bladder, ribs, neck, and head, to name a few.

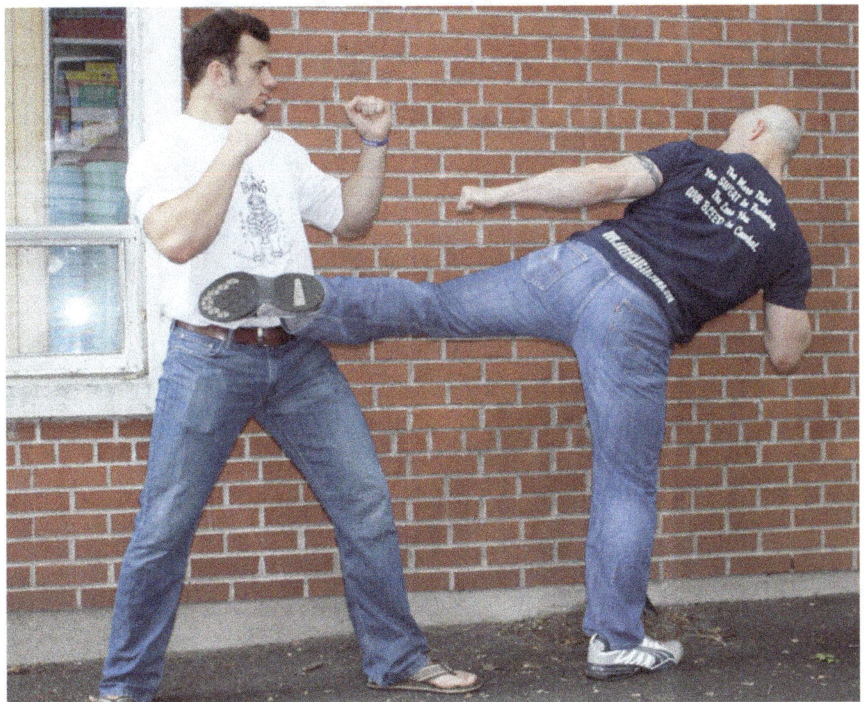

CUT KICK

This is a standard as far as kicks are concerned in Bando and Muay Thai. You will use the shin as the attacking implement. If you kick with your right leg, step at a 45-degree angle with your left foot into the opponent. You'll be throwing the kick from the hip, not a chambered kick but rather a kick delivered with the knee locked and only slightly bent. The primary targets are low: the shin, gastroc, peroneal nerve and hip joint.

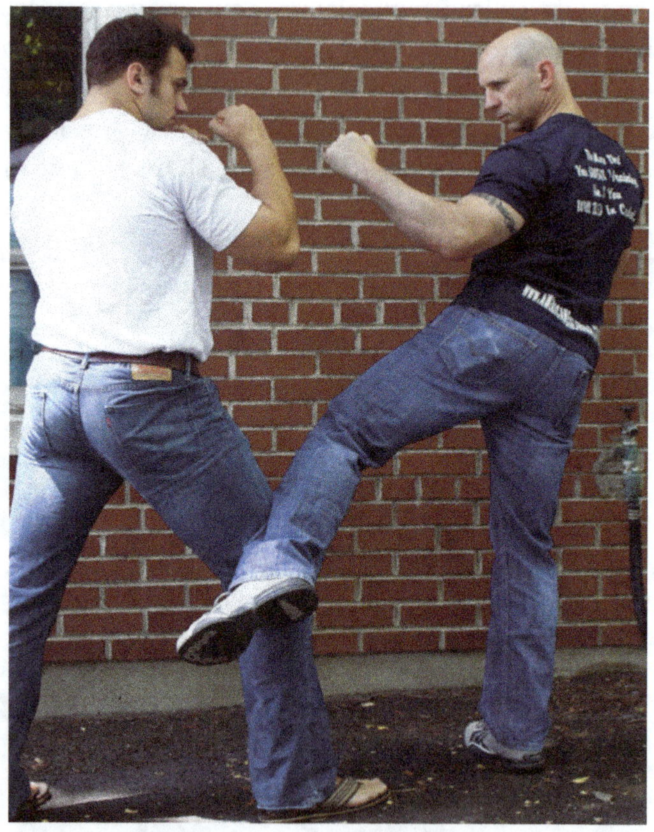

Cut kick.

Be cautious with the shin-to-shin kick. If your shins are not conditioned sufficiently, you may incur just as much trauma as your assailant! When you become more accomplished at this move, you can direct shots to the ribcage and even the head. However, for most street applications, you have no reason to kick someone higher than their abdominal region.

SHIN KICK

This close-quarter kick is an excellent, hard-hitting kick that can be thrown while you are in the Boxing Range. Bring your knee up high, dorsiflex your foot, and throw a sharp short hybrid Roundhouse Kick with your shin to their thigh or ribs. This kick may be extended into a Ball-of-the-Foot Roundhouse Kick if the opponent backs up out of Boxing Range and steps into Kicking Range. As with most of these kicks, turn your foot on the floor, rotating your hip over.

FRONT KICK

There are a great many varieties of this kick you can throw: Lead Leg, Lunging, Ball-of-the-Foot, Flat-of-the-Foot, Straight-Up with the shin and so on.

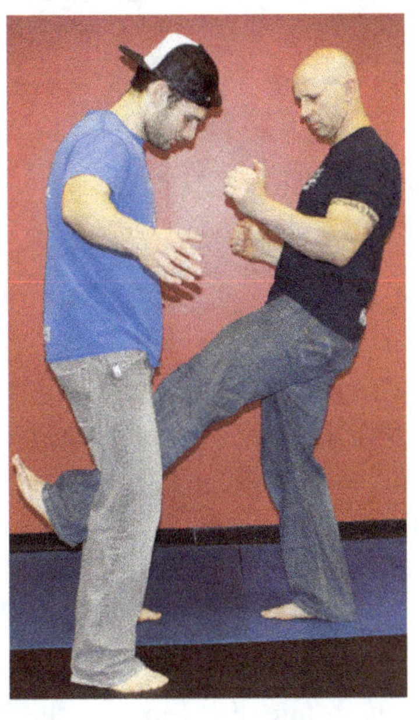

The Full (Rear-Leg) Ball-of-the-Foot version is applicable in most situations. This is a chambered, four-position kick. Bring the leg up, kick out, then bring it back and down to the floor. In a real situation, you will most likely be moving forward. Practice it both while stationary to aid with developing your balance and while moving forward, as you would do when driving your opponent backward. This is a straight kick; keep your hip, knee and foot on the kicking leg in one straight line. There is a slight rotation of the foot on the floor, but not nearly as dramatic as with the Roundhouse or Side Kicks. I like the Ball-of-the-Foot Kick best, there is a greater pound per square inch of force yielded with the reduced striking area. You also get extra distance in your kick with the extension of the foot, and this kick may be directed to virtually any part of the body.

SIDE KICK

This is a great striking technique that is underutilized in MMA competitions, but it remains a mainstay in taekwondo, karate, kung fu and many other striking based arts. I will attribute its lack of use in Mixed Martial Arts competitions to the overwhelming presence of Muay Thai as the preferred striking art. However, there are an increasing number of MMA Fighters who have added the Side Kick to their arsenal.

There are several methods for delivering a powerful Side Kick: Stepping, Skipping, Potochagi, Jumping and many more. Here we will focus on the Stepping Side Kick.

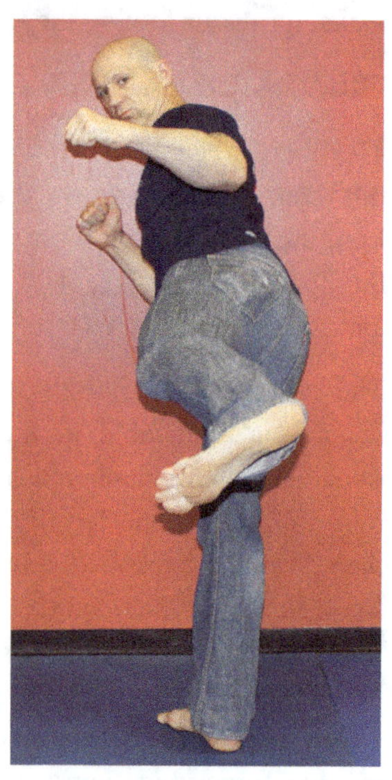

If you are in the Orthodox position in a Side Stance, your feet will be lined up evenly with your left side forward and at a right angle to your target. Attack with the lead foot by stepping up with the rear foot and replacing the lead foot as you pick up the lead foot to kick. This is another chambered kick that has the up, out, back,and down movements. As the kick comes out, rotate the foot on the floor and turn the toes of the kicking foot downward by rotating the hip.

Be certain not to over-rotate your upper body. You can ensure this by counter-rotating your left arm and shoulder. Your heel, knee, hip, and left shoulder should all be collinear and help you direct your energy through the target, not simply to the surface. Your foot will be dorsiflexed, and the area of the foot you hit with will be your heel. This kick may be delivered to the ankle, knee, quadriceps, hip, ribs, stomach, chest, throat or head. Unless you are particularly skilled at high kicks, however, do not try to kick your attacker above the waist.

MULE KICK

The delivery of this kick is how it attained its name. Imagine a mule throwing a kick with its hindquarters and there you have your kick. Pick your knee up high and toward your chest, bend your upper body forward at the hip, thrust your kick straight back with your foot dorsiflexed and strike with your heel. This kick is delivered to targets behind you.

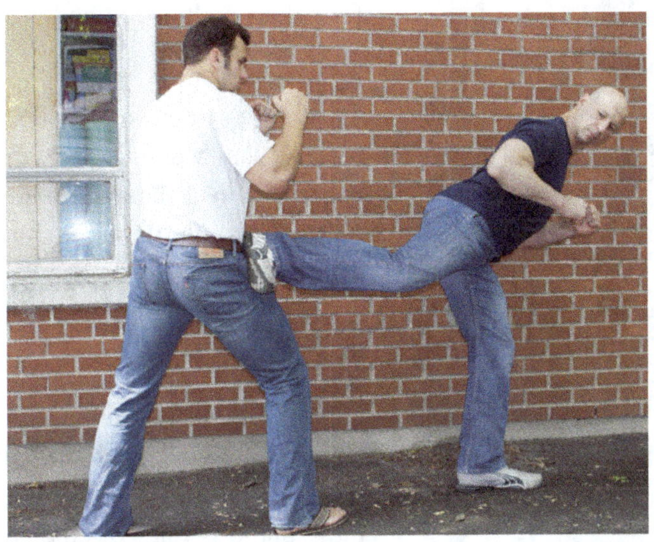

If your opponent is in front of you, make a quarter turn to your back so that your back is facing momentarily toward your target and then execute the kick. This move is often referred to as the Back Kick when thrown in this manner. There are many targets to hit with this kick, but it's a perfect counteroffensive technique when directed to the knees, groin or midsection of an assailant attacking you from behind.

Okay, so we have this great list of techniques. When and how do we use them to our advantage? This will depend upon the circumstances that you are facing. There are crucial elements that need to be considered. The most important of these are your proximity to the opponent, the number of assailants, who you are with, if there are weapons involved, the escape routes and the environmental conditions and constraints.

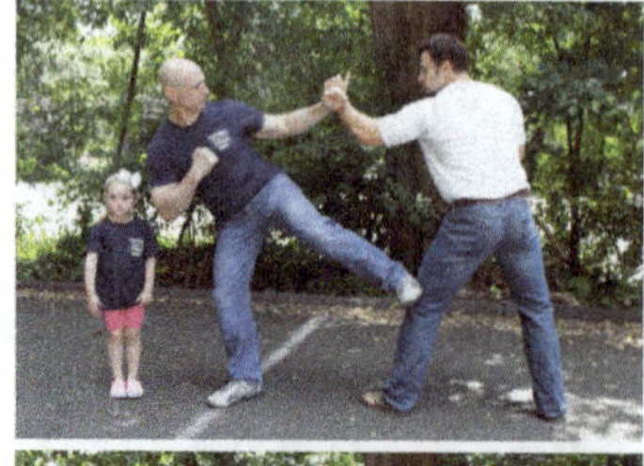

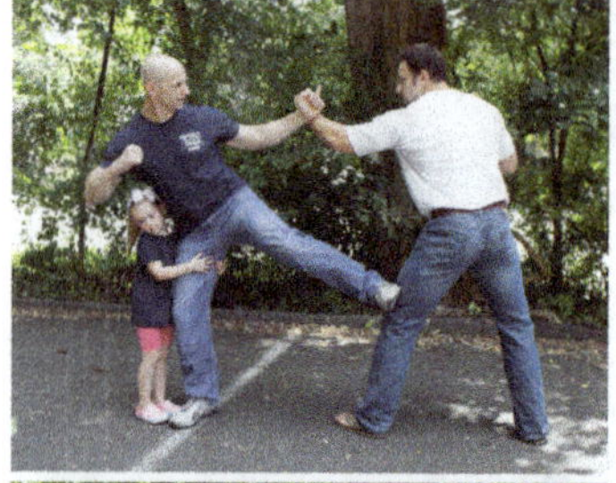

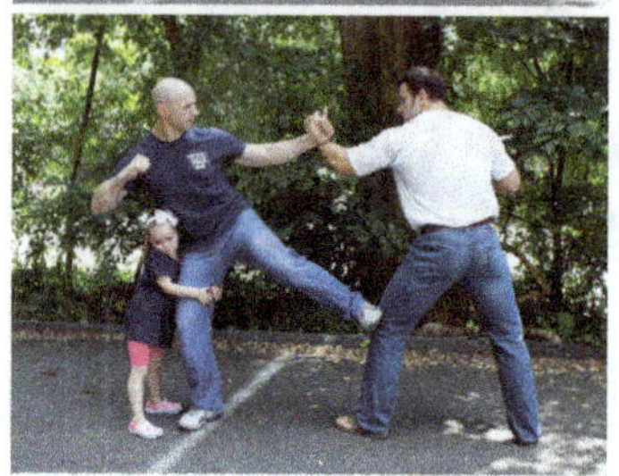

EXAMPLES

If there is ice and snow on the ground, it may not behoove you to relinquish 50 percent of your balance by delivering a kick. You could easily slip and fall, thus making defending yourself more difficult.

What if you have a child in your arms? What would you do first? You need to protect the child and yourself, plus deal with the imminent threat. You may have to put the child down on the floor behind you before you take any action.

What if there is a gang of assailants surrounding you? How do you choose the first one to hit? The biggest one, the smallest one or the perceived "ringleader"?

We must first acknowledge that action is faster than reaction. This means that if someone attacks you, there will be a delay before you respond. The movement must be recognized visually, and then it must register in your brain and then tell your body to move in the proper manner. That's a lot for you to accomplish in the time (between 200 and 400 milliseconds) that it takes when someone initiates an attack until the time you have been grabbed or struck. Therefore, it's best to strike first.

Despite what you may see in the movies, most street fights are won by the guy who lands the first blow. If you want to increase your odds of success in the street, strike first and do so with conviction. The bad karate Instructor from *The Karate Kid,* John Kreese, did have a valid mantra: "Strike first, and strike hard, no mercy SIR!" These are good words to live by if you want to survive a street encounter.

Now some of you may think that I am telling you to "run around punching people in the head." Not quite. I am, however, letting you know that unless you get the first shot in during a serious, real-world physical encounter, you will be at a distinct disadvantage. To have a better chance you have to rely on positioning and anticipation, which can put you in the driver's seat and put your villainous opponent on the defensive.

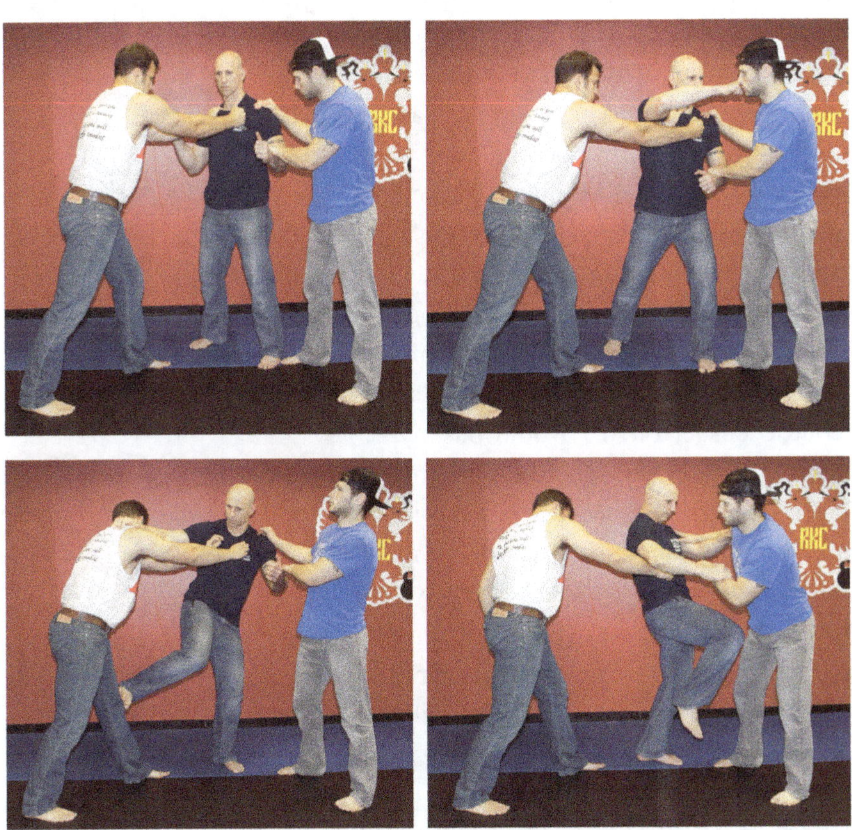

Most people who have been in a confrontation were aware that it was going to happen before the attack occurred. We will not address those who have been "set-up" by another person. If you did something bad in your past to the wrong person, you're probably going to have to spend a great deal of your time looking over your shoulder. In that case, you best handle your situation and bring it to a resolution. But that's enough said about that, so let's get back to situations that may actually happen to people simply minding their own business and/or those whose vocations may require them to resolve conflicts from time to time.

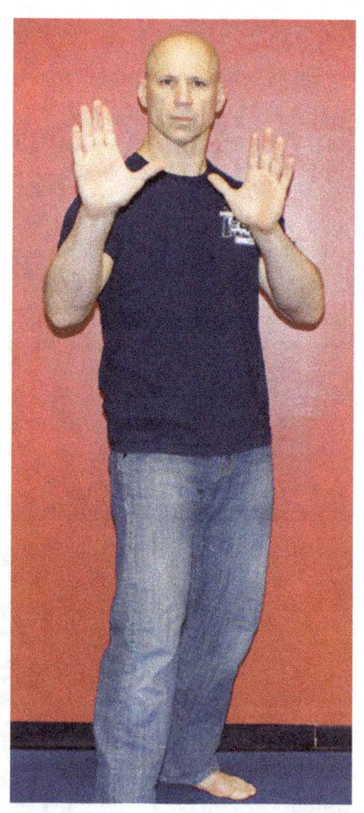

Interview stance.

Your chances of success in a situation can greatly be increased by the Stance that you adopt when the verbal portion of the confrontation occurs. When I was a young bouncer, we had quite a few confrontations on a nightly basis. The club that I worked at had previously been a biker club, and we were converting it into a dance club for the college crowd. The owner and my coworkers could tell simply by my stance that a confrontation was about to ensue. First, I would put my hands up in front of my face with my hands open (it's quite easy for me to talk with my hands due in part to my Italian-American heritage). I'd have one foot slightly back so that I was essentially in a "hidden" fighting stance. In this position, I could readily defend myself if an attack was launched. My hands were up to deflect an attack and deliver blows. My feet were positioned in a fighting stance, allowing me to move to avoid contact and then launch a counterattack.

Practice this position (the Interview Stance) and become comfortable with it. The life you save by doing so may be your own.

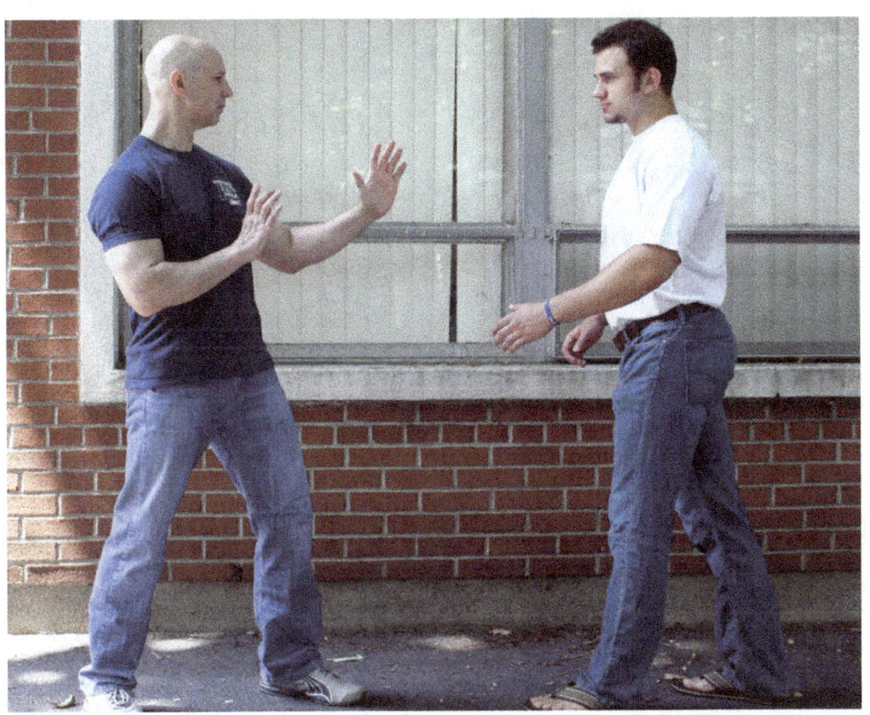

Chapter 10
Movement and Zones

Your knowledge of the various zones, your position relative to your assailant, the accessibility of your repertoire and your exposure to your opponent are essential, yet among unskilled fighters they are the most ignored components. Understanding movement, position and ranges will tilt the odds dramatically in your favor, which is why you should practice these skills during every training session.

Please bear in mind that if the assailant moves from the Green Zone to a Yellow Zone in an aggressive manner, it means they have initiated an attack. If you believe that you or someone you are with is in imminent danger, you may defend yourself. If you believe that your life or the life of a loved one is in peril, you have the right to protect yourself by whatever means necessary.

Green

This is your "safe" zone. The opponent can't reach you, but neither can you reach them without some type of overt movement.

Yellow

This is the "caution" distance. The opponent has entered your personal space. You are at the distance to strike, but also can be hit.

Red

This is the danger zone. You are in a hot spot, meaning your proximity to your assailant will give you no time to react if they lash out first. You must be fully engaged in combat at this distance, striking, moving and looking to finish.

MOVEMENT AND POSITIONING

Movement is key. You can't hurt what you can't hit, and you can't hit what you can't touch. It's best to MOVE and move with purpose. You will want to avoid the attack and position yourself to launch your counterattack. Practice economy of motion buoyed by fluid and purposeful movement. Practice your footwork religiously and keep your hands up!

PIE-STEPPING

Think of a large pizza, with eight slices. Other than jumping up and down, these are the only directions that you can move in. Any other direction is simply a variation of these eight.

When practicing Pie-Stepping, always step back to the center. Imagine the little "mouse table" on your pizza, which will represent the center of the pie. (The "mouse table" keeps the cheese from sticking to the top of the box.) During practice, your changes of direction will occur at this point. When repeating movements, the foot you use to step will remain the same throughout a sequence (right foot direction 1, right foot direction 7, and so on). Of course you should alternate so you're completing sequences with each foot.

Here's a starting sequence to practice:

1. Front

2. Back
3. Straight to the Right
4. .Straight to the Left
5. Up on a 45-degree angle to the Right
6. Up on a 45-degree angle to the Left
7. Back on a 45-degree angle to the Right
8. Back on a 45-degree angle to the Left

Keep your hands up the whole time, always keeping your lead hand forward which will require you to switch your hands according to which foot is forward. Move from one position to the next with a shuffle step. Place the majority of your weight on the stepping foot so that you would be able to throw a kick with the inside foot.

One (1) Step: moving forward and jamming the advance of the opponent. You will back them up by placing them on their heels.

Two (2) Step: move backward shifting your weight toward the back foot. This will draw the opponent toward you.

Three (3) Step: move straight to the right side and face the center.

Four (4) Step: repeat to the left.

Five (5) Step: on a 45-degree angle up and to the right. Parry with your left hand as you position yourself to the side of the opponent.

Six (6) Step: return to the center and do the same up and to the left side.

Seven (7) Step: fade back and to the right, avoiding the attack on an angle.

Eight (8) Step: do the same to the other side. While practicing, this foot will be the same one that you perform the One Step with.

JAMMING

Think of this as an extension of the One Step. Move into your assailant with your hands up and with your forearms at a 65-degree angle as you shove them backward. This puts them on their heels and makes it difficult for them to defend themselves.

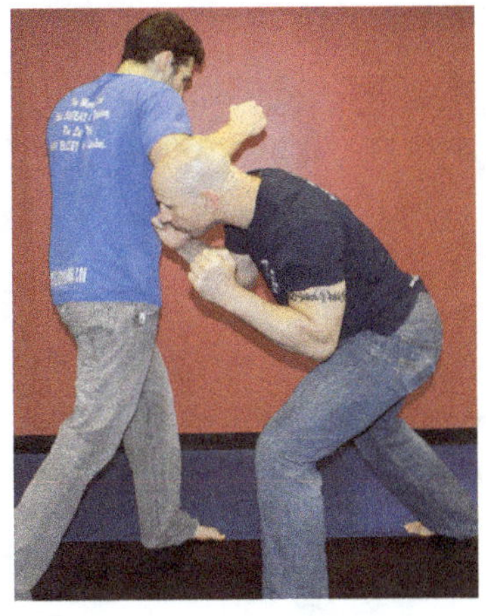

DUCKS (BOBS)

Imagine that you have a pencil in the middle of your forehead and that you are drawing a "U" with it. If someone throws a right punch at you, bend your knees and move your head from left to right in a "U" fashion, placing your head on the outside right of the opponent. You are now positioned to counterattack, usually with a right body shot and/or a left hook to the chin.

ANGLE FADE (DRAWS)

There are times that you will need to fade back to draw your opponent out so that they commit to a movement. Stay slightly out of range and follow up by applying a counterstrike.

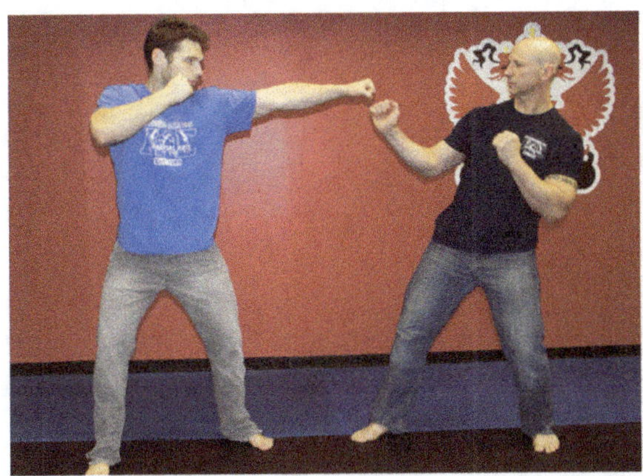

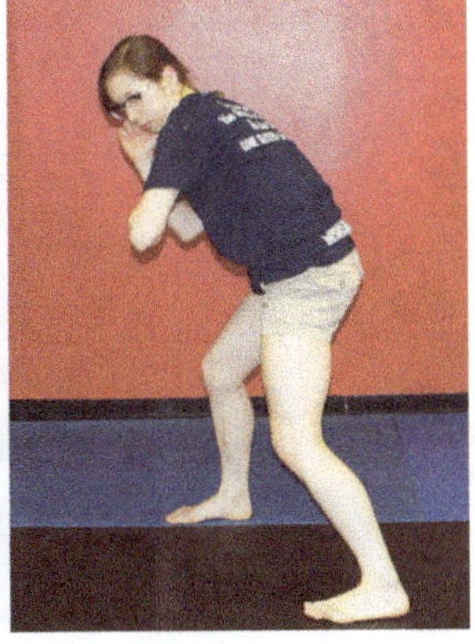

PARRIES

Using an open hand, slap a punch away as it comes at you. If a left strike is being thrown, parry with your right hand as you move to the right, avoiding the strike and positioning yourself to launch your counteroffensive.

Generally, there are two taps of your hand with the parry: the initial and the redirect. The motions used should only be large enough to redirect the strike. If you push it too far, you may compromise your ability to defend and counterattack.

BOX-STEPPING

This stepping method is very well suited for side stepping and maintaining a good stance. Pretend that there is a box on the floor and that you are in a fighting stance. It does not matter if you are in the Orthodox or Southpaw Stance. If you are in the Orthodox Stance, move to the left step with your left foot first and then your right. Lead foot then rear foot. When moving to the right, the right foot comes first, then the left. Rear foot and then lead.

Whatever stance you are in will make no difference. You will step with the foot that's closest to the direction that you need to move. This will now put you in an advantageous position to strike.

Chapter 11
Basic Grappling

I have made it quite clear that it is far better to stay on your feet during a confrontation. But you still need to know how to grapple, for several reasons.

To effectively combat an attack, you need to know how it works. If you are trying to defend against a take down or submission, you need to have a basic knowledge of how they are applied. As we have discussed in other sections of this book, if a fight lasts more than 10 seconds or so, the chances of it ending up on the ground increase dramatically. So you had better know what to do once you are on the ground, that's simple logic.

Proficiency in grappling must be gained through working with a partner, so secure a good one. The closer you are to each other in weight and size the better off you'll be, especially if you are a beginner.

The grappling arts are the most difficult to master. But by learning the basics, you'll increase your chances of success in a street fight dramatically.

Let's now delve into some basic grappling techniques:

BALANCE DISRUPTION

You can break the balance of an opponent by pushing, pulling and foot sweeps. You should try to gain the inside position by placing your hands on the insides of the attacker's arms at the biceps, since pushing and pulling are best applied from this position.

FOOT SWEEP

From the inside tie-position described above, push with your right hand and pull with your left. This will cause your opponent to pick up their right foot and step forward. Knowing this, as you perform the pushing/pulling action lift your left foot up and sweep their right foot as it moves forward to regain their balance. Continue the push-pull until they fall. If they regain their balance, immediately perform this movement to the other side. This will generally cause them to fall.

Another simple sweep you should practice starts by grabbing the opponent's wrist and pulling them toward you and across their body. Use the same side's foot to hook behind their heel and kick their foot in the direction that their toes are facing. This may or may not knock them down, but you will have succeeded in disrupting their balance and opening them up for follow-up attacks.

BASIC HIP TOSS

This is the mother of all throws. If done correctly, you will be able to effectively throw an adversary twice your weight, meeting no real resistance in the process. Throws are dynamic, so there must be movement involved to execute one. It is also easier to relinquish your space than it is to throw someone to another spot.

Foot placement, movement and hip pop are crucial to performing a successful throw. Thread your left arm under their right arm and have your head on the same side as your arm. This is called an Underhook. Slide your left hand across their back to their opposite trapezius. With your right hand, grab their left arm at the triceps. Next, step across with your right foot, and then your left will follow as you bring your hip in and your butt across.

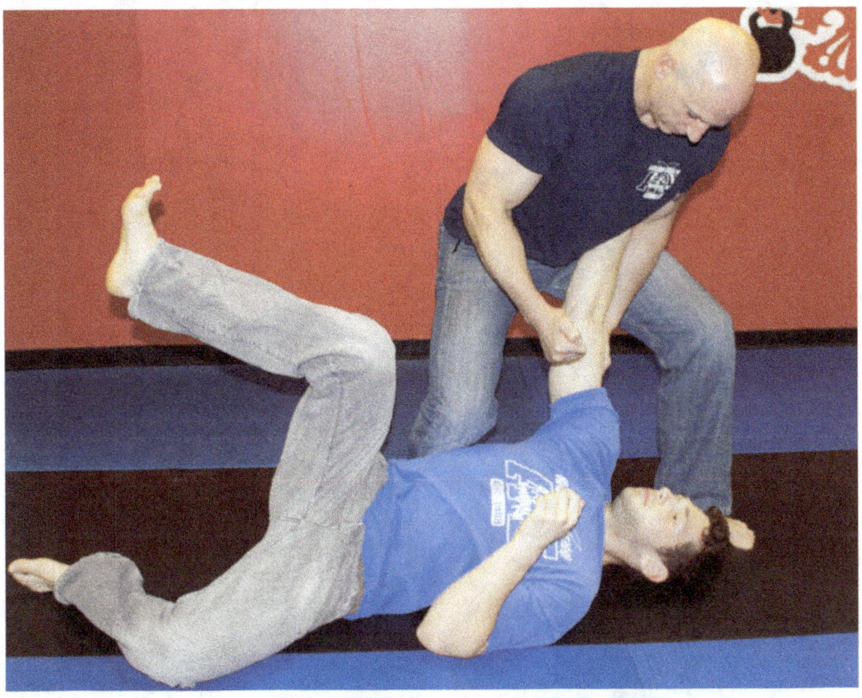

Make certain that your feet are close together; having them too far apart is the practitioner's biggest mistake. Flex your knees, pull on their left arm with your right, "punch" with your left as you pivot your feet and finish the throw. In combat situations, attempt to have your adversary land directly on the top of their head. This will immediately end most confrontations. If not, maintain control of their right arm when they hit the ground and apply a choke or pull up on their arm as you stomp their head with your right foot.

You'll need to repeat this move a thousand times to be able to execute it properly and it requires ten thousand repetitions to master it. Believe me, it's well worth the effort!

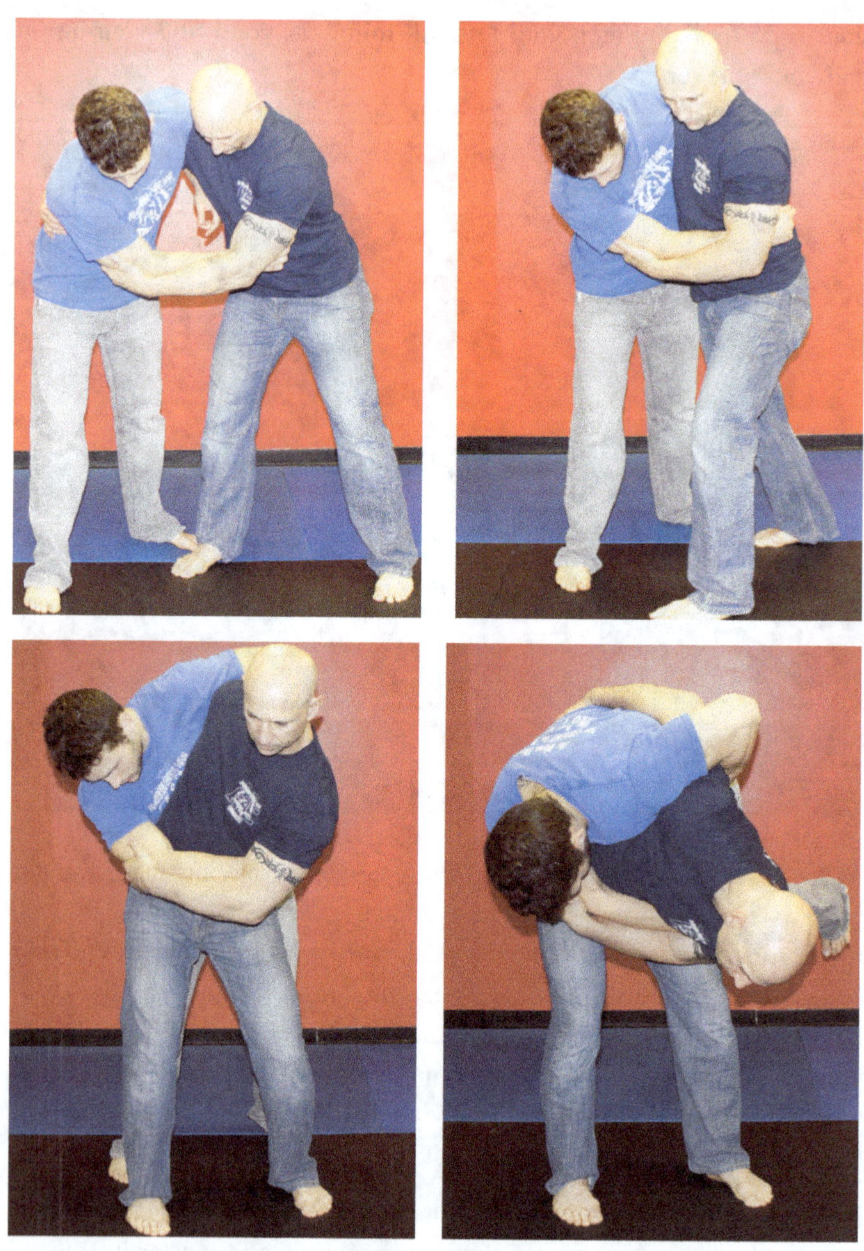

Basic hip toss.

SPRAWL

This one defensive maneuver is the single most important move to keep you on your feet when your legs get attacked by someone determined to score a takedown.

When you are attacked with a Double- or Single- Leg Takedown, do not give your adversary both of your hips. Drop your weight into your left hip as you drive your hip downward and throw your legs back. Take your left arm and loop it around their right arm as you are performing the sprawl. With your free hand, smash your arm across their face and turn their head away. Once you have secured this position and they can no longer take you down, strike the adversary in the head with your free hand. You may also force them to the ground and spin behind them and take their back. Deliver your Ground and Pound from here or apply a choke.

SPEAR DOUBLE-LEG TAKEDOWN

There are several immensely effective Double-Leg Takedowns. I chose this one because you don't have to go to the ground to perform it and your head remains in the middle, making it more difficult for your opponent to apply a choke to you.

You need to be close enough to touch your opponent to be able to take them down. In the street or in an MMA cage, delivering a solid strike to the face prior to the shot is a very effective means to gain entry. As you prepare to execute the takedown, lower your level by bending your knees as you shoot for a take-down. "Bull" your neck and aim your head at his solar plexus as you grab behind both of their knees. Thrust your head into them, pull with your arms and drive with your legs until they have hit the ground.

It's very important to make certain that you don't reach with your arms or put your head down when you shoot. You must get your body onto theirs. Be cautious following them onto the ground. You may get rolled or injure yourself on the pavement. It's better to knock them down and administer kicks to them.

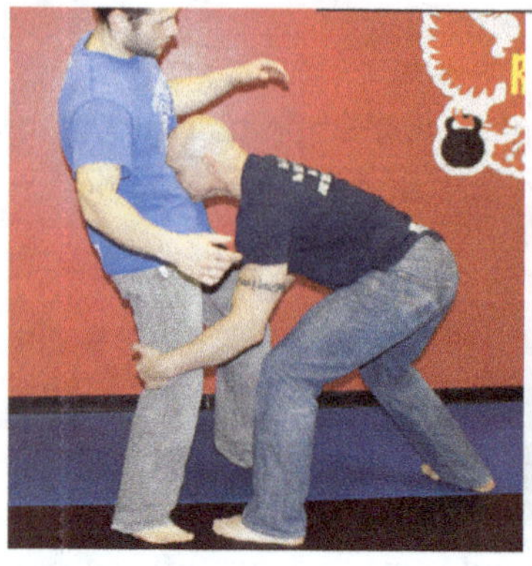 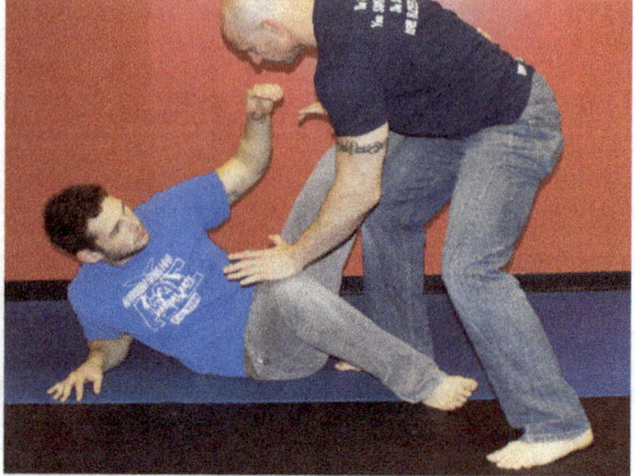

There are several extremely effective grappling systems. But wrestling (Folkstyle, Freestyle, Greco-Roman, Submission & Catch), Brazilian Jiu Jitsu, Judo, and Sambo are the most effective for combat training. They are some of the most effective forms of unarmed combat available, but also the most difficult to master. Seeking professional instruction in one of these arts will teach you a great deal about your body and how to move.

Chapter 12
Combinations and Series

The saying, "One strike, one kill" is actually a misinterpretation of the Japanese saying regarding strikes.

When karate started to become popular, people feared Black Belts. They knew the "Death Touch" and that they were trained to "kill you with one blow." This notion is nonsense and has since been debunked. The true saying was "To strike with killing intent."

Is it possible to kill someone with one shot? Yes, but death usually occurs when someone gets knocked out on their feet and hits their head on the ground as they fall. Nevertheless, our hands can be used as lethal weapons, if we have great techniques, which is what I'm introducing you to here.

How do we use our strikes? Mainly by using combinations. If you consider the punch statistics of a professional boxer, most fall far short of landing 50% of their strikes. These professionals throw thousands of punches a day and most of them only land a little over 1/3rd of them. This is one of the most important reasons for throwing multiple blows. In addition, multiple strikes are generally required to neutralize an assailant. So when you start punching it is best to stay busy.

Listed below are some very effective combinations you can practice. These should be performed in front of a mirror, on a heavy bag and with a partner. Use the mirror to check your technique, the heavy bag to develop power and your partner to work on distancing and timing.

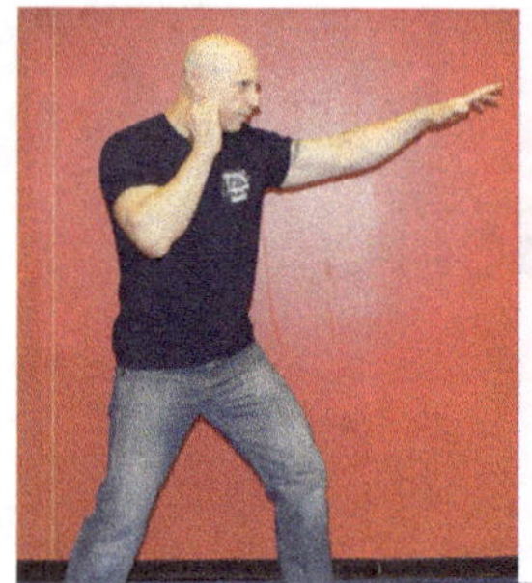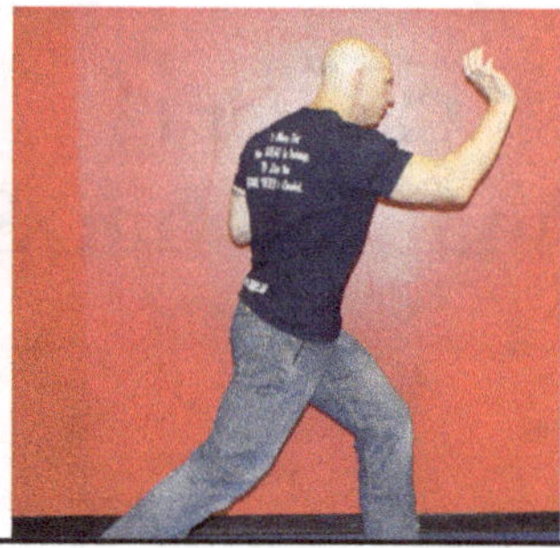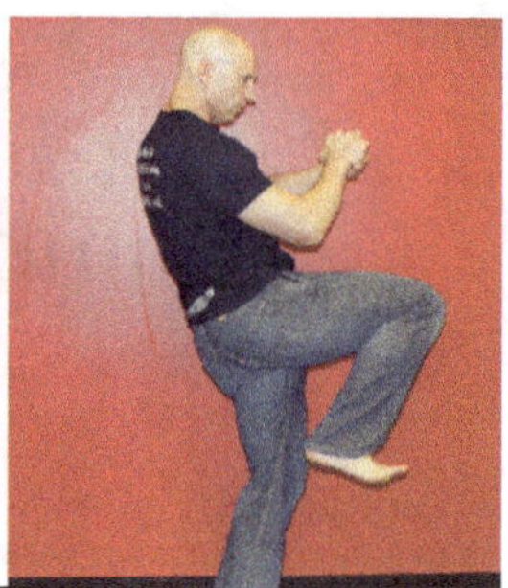

Axe-hand | Chin jab | Knee

HAND AND FOOT COMBINATIONS

1. 1, 2, Cut Kick
2. Short & Long Axe-hand, Chin Jab & Knee
3. Elbow Across, Elbow Upward, Straight Knee and Round Knee
4. Two Straight Knees, Downward Elbows
5. Sidekick, Backfist, Hammerfist Smash
6. Palm-heel, Elbow Downward, Knee Drives
7. Lead-leg Roundhouse Kick, Backfist, Elbow Smash
8. Elbow Across, Angle Down, Angle Up, Straight Knee
9. Strike and Subdue Drills
10. Finger-jab, Chin-jab, Knee Strike
11. Back-hand Slap, Low Side-kick, Elbow Smash
12. Duck, Side-step, Body-shot, Knee, Hook, Elbow
13. Lunge Front Kick (Big Boot), Knees, Redirect and/ or Smashes
14. (Rear Attack) Foot-stomp, Backward Head-butt, Back Elbow
15. Dual Ear Slap, Eye-Gouge, Springboard Knee to Groin

1. Parry, V-step, and Clothesline
2. Head-butt, Tracheal Choke, Knee Drives
3. Piet a te, Back-slap, Knife-hand Chop to neck
4. Skipping Side-kick, Knee Drive, Sweep
5. Sliding Lead-leg Front Kick, Shin Kicks & Foot Stomps

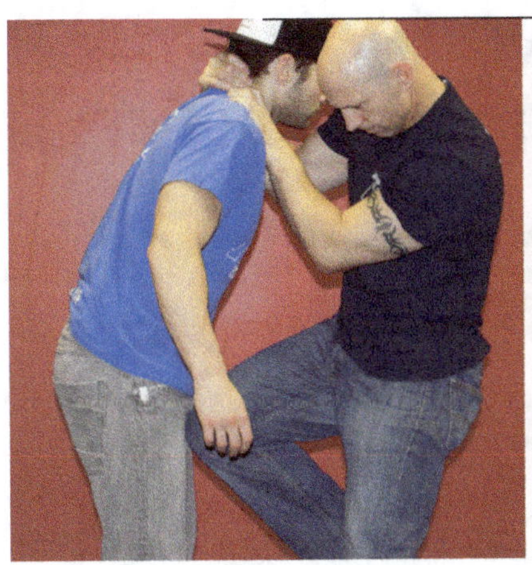 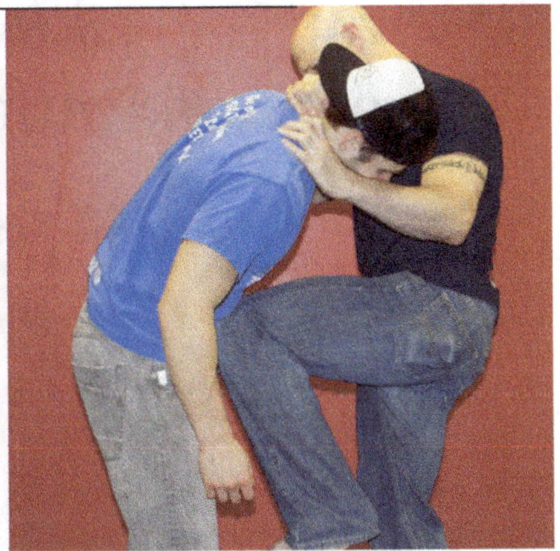

Episternal notch | Knee drive.

BLOCK AND ROCK

The complete Block-and-Rock Series is counteroffensive. Step back and shift your weight onto your back foot. Once you have engaged and deflected the attack, immediately fire back with a Straight Cross to your opponent's face.

Here is the series:

HIGH BLOCK AND STRIKE

1. Hammerfist Block and Strike
2. Outside Middle Block and Strike
3. Knifehand Front and Side
4. Hammerfist Front and Side
5. Episternal Notch, Knee Drive

Chapter 13
Street Applications and Tactics

Most of the incidents recounted in this book have men depicted in various situations. In fact there are quite a few women I have trained who defended themselves successfully in the street, and one event in particular stands out for its dramatic nature

I was sitting at the desk of my martial arts studio back in December of 1995, and in walked the mother of one of my students that was away at college. She began to kiss and hug me, not that I minded it, but I asked her why. She told me that I had saved her daughter's life.

"How?" I queried, and what her mom told me blew me away.

Elizabeth had trained with me from eighth grade through high school. She was 110 pounds, 5'4" and stunning, and she had just finished her first semester as a college freshman. Fortunately, she had trained hard and was very serious about self-defense.

She was attending American University in DC and left a party early to go home and study. She did break one of my rules, as she was traveling alone at night, but she was wearing the proper attire. While walking across the campus, she was accosted by a large knife-wielding assailant. Her reactions, choice of kicks and strikes, and knowledge of distancing, zones, and movement all came into play. This was the first time she had ever been in a street situation. Prior to this incident her only fighting experience had come in class and in a few tournaments.

Not hesitating, Elizabeth launched an attack. She Front Kicked him in the groin, applied a Side Kick to his knee, and then a Roundhouse Kick to his face when he hit the ground. She then booted the knife out of his hand and took off. All of the kicks and movements she applied were part of our daily basic training.

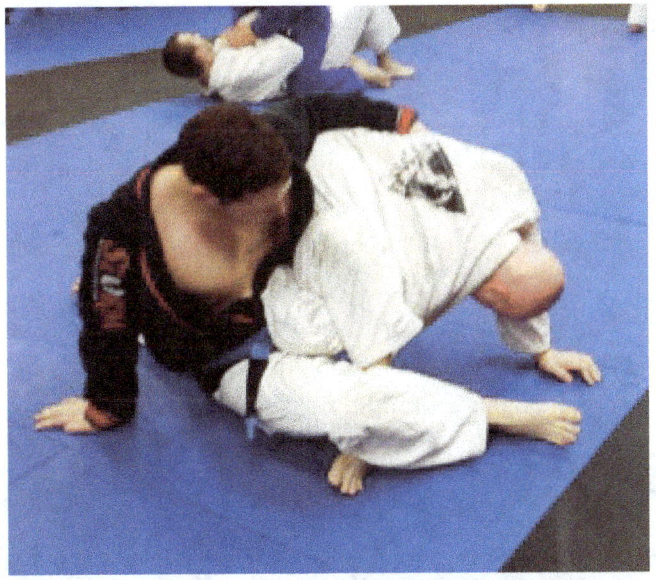

Brazilian Jiu Jitsu.

The result? He was arrested and hospitalized with ruptured testicles, a dislocated knee and a broken nose. When the DNA was taken, it matched the DNA present collected in connection with four sexual assaults that had occurred on campus. Elizabeth's training saved her from becoming number five.

There have always been debates about what "system" or "style" of fighting is best suited for the street. Martial arts can be broken down into three categories: Self-Perfection, Sport-Combat and Self-Preservation. Which works best for our purposes?

Self-Perfection arts include Aikido, Tai Chi, many Kung Fu Styles and any of the kata or forms-based karate styles. They are completely useless for street application. If people want to argue, fine. I'm judging this based on what I've seen work in the street and on sound training principles. The aforementioned arts are fantastic for peace of mind, learning stances, developing discipline and providing fitness as well as mobility. But knowing 57 different katas will not help you win a street fight. Consequently there is no need to discuss these arts any further in this book.

Sport Combat was created for practitioners to train against other humans. This art develops the reflexes and body awareness applicable to actual combat. There is nothing like drilling and training with a live person to help you develop your skills and a more functional type of strength for combat. From a street-fighting perspective the only drawback would be the rules applied to Sport Combat. The rules are implemented for the safety of the participants. Certain movements and target areas are disallowed. This, along with equipment, is geared to the safety of the participants and rightly so.

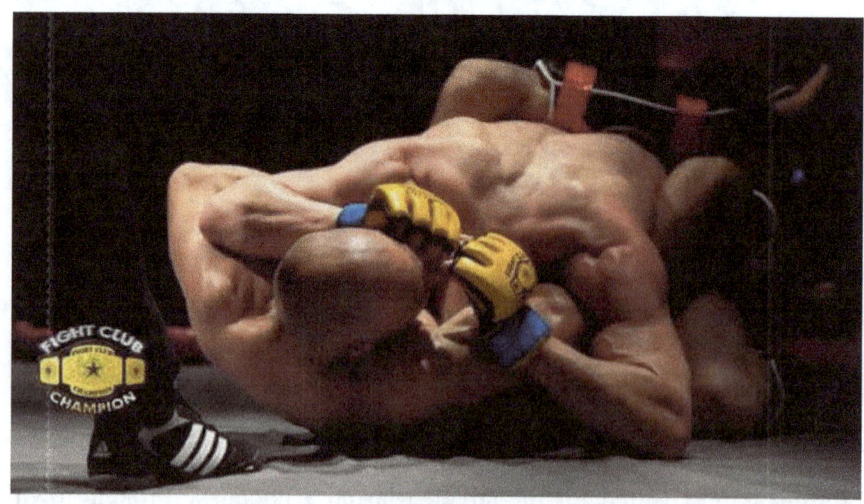

MMA fighters.

A number of years ago, I was training with the World Kickboxing Champion, Carl Moffett. He was watching my guys and me using virtually no equipment and beating the crap out of each other. He thought that we were nuts (maybe he was right) for "conditioning" our bodies for combat in that manner. He advised us to decrease our injury rate by padding up and to condition our bodies with methods other than full-contact, no-equipment sparring. As it turned out this was great advice. Combat is unpredictable, so you should take precautions while you are training.

Each of the sport combat arts has its drawbacks and limitations. At the onset, you may think that a Mixed Martial Artist has the immediate advantage. Maybe, maybe not. Most street fights last only 10 seconds or less. Most fights start standing up and all are without a referee. Usually, the guy who lands the first shot wins, regardless of what style they prefer. So in general, a boxer or accomplished striker would have an advantage over a grappler.

If the fight does not end in the first few blows, it will ultimately go to the ground. Under this scenario, you would think that an MMA Fighter or Brazilian Jiu Jitsu Black Belt would have the advantage. But this is not necessarily the case. In the street, generally, it's the guy who has the most friends who wins the ground fight. While you're attempting to apply an Armbar, his buddies will be kicking you in the head, which goes to show that in street battles fighting fair is a quaint notion.

Even if you are in a one-on-one street fight, submissions may not be the best option. If someone tries to apply a Triangle Choke in the street and the other guy picks him up and slams his head onto the concrete sidewalk, how practical were his ground-fighting techniques, really? You would be better off being a wrestler with a good Ground and Pound game. You could take him down with a solid Double-Leg Take-down and "Oil Rig" his face with a barrage of punches, open-hand strikes and elbows (oil rigging means holding down an opponent with one hand and punching them, usually in the head, repeatedly with the other fist).

A fighter with expertise in kicking-based arts such as Taekwondo, Muay Thai, Savate and various karate systems have their set of disadvantages as well. First of all, anytime you pick your foot up off of the ground, you sacrifice 50 percent of your balance. This makes you easier to take down. And what if the surface is slippery or unstable with gravel or loose footing? What if there is an obstacle, such as a pole or chair? You would not be able to apply your kicking techniques. What if you are seated in a chair?

Did you hear about what happened when Jean Claude van Damme fought Chuck Zito? As the legend goes, they got into a confrontation at a Gentlemen's Club in NYC and Chuck knocked Van Damme out cold with one punch. They were in punching range. So much for JCVD's kicks.

So does that mean boxing is the best? Maybe, maybe not. Most boxers train with gloves and wraps. The use of gloves was implemented for the protection of the boxer's hands, not to lessen the severity of a blow to the heads of the combatants. This method of fighting actually prolongs the combatants' exposure to mind-jarring blows. That being said, a boxer's hands are very quick and their movements are good, but most of the time their hands are not conditioned for street combat. A closed fist must be conditioned properly for Bare-Knuckle Fighting, and if you punch someone in the head and don't hit them perfectly your hand will break.

What if the boxer gets kneed in the groin? Or taken down to the ground or faced with a weapon? How about a kick to the knee? Most Boxers are not trained to deal with such attacks. Even if they bob and weave out of the way of a strike, they may get cracked in the head with a knee as they did down instinctively to avoid a blow.

Wow! You're probably asking yourself, "How the heck am I going to be able to defend myself when trouble comes? Boxing, wrestling, BJJ, Taekwondo?

They all have such apparent weaknesses. So what the heck do I do? How can I train to defend myself? Is this hopeless?

Have patience. The answers to your doubts will be coming. I'm just not ready to give them to you yet, so please keep reading …

Self-Preservation or pure Self-Defense systems: This eclectic category includes pressure point training, Krav Maga, Russian Systema, the various tactics practiced by Our Special Forces, etc. Some of these systems are excellent for fighting and some leave a lot to be desired.

I cannot speak for all systems, nor can I earnestly speak for all instructors. But for a Self-Preservation or Self-Defense system to have validity, they must involve some type of actual Sport Combat training against another human. If an instructor states, "We don't spar because we only practice "death techniques" and cannot spar for fear of the safety of our students and others that may come in" … you can dismiss this individual and his methodology immediately. Many of these guys have never been hit in the face or kicked in the groin and would wet themselves if they ever got cracked. They hide behind their "death techniques" because they are poor fighters and are, rightfully, so insecure about their ability to perform that they hide behind unsubstantiated nonsense. They lull their students into a false sense of security while setting them up for failure, lining their pockets with the hard-earned money of their pigeons in the process.

There is actually one type of Self-Defense fear-predator that I despise even more. They are the Internet Video Huckster, and that one misleads the unwary on a grand scale. These guys purport to have knowledge of "secret techniques" that are "banned by the government." They flood the Internet with false advertising and promises of street invincibility with their secret arsenal. They claim that their programs are so complete, so devastating, that simply by purchasing their DVDs and practicing the moves in your basement you will be able to defeat an MMA fighter in mere seconds! That's like saying to someone, "Watch this video on swimming, and you'll be able to beat Michael Phelps without ever getting into a pool!"

That's enough time spent exposing these phonies. I just wanted to give you a heads-up on what to watch out for. If it sounds too good to be true, you can assume that it is and quickly move on. Now let's get back to some useful material.

WHICH METHOD IS BEST?

"Now, some SF (Special Forces) guys have become expert martial artists. And most of them will tell you that your particular style or discipline is as good as any other, and that the thing that matters is the effort and heart you put into it. And they put as much time and effort as any other Black Belt in anything does, and they'll tell you they did it on their own time."

*— From the Weapons Man Blog, written by a former
Special Forces member*

There is no ideal choice. What you need to do is train in our system or a system akin to it while getting in the best of shape and making your body strong as possible. It is imperative to engage in some sort of real Sport Combat practice, to ensure you know what it feels like to be under the gun when the fists and feet are flying. This would include training in all or a combination of boxing, kickboxing, Brazilian Jiu Jitsu, Mixed Martial Arts, wrestling, Sambo, Judo or other Combat Sports where there is contact between you and your practice partner.

You must practice your Defensive Tactics with fluidity, purpose and control. For the safety of your partner and yourself, one cannot practice these techniques with full force.

WHAT TYPE OF TRAINING SHOULD I START WITH AND WHAT DO I NEED?

I am a hundred percent honest with my students and I have been a hundred percent honest in this book. So, I will not stop now. To be able to handle yourself in the street, you need to train in certain base arts.

This is because they are the most practical and translatable to real combat.

The best arts to learn first are boxing and wrestling. Here's why. Most fights occur within the punching range, so learning how to box is very important. Wrestling is important because you *don't* want to get taken down in the street. Wrestlers are trained to resist being taken down and develop great balance. Both boxing and wrestling are tough methods of combat and require getting hit, slammed and roughed up. The weight shifting, body conditioning, development of reflexes and footwork (movement) required in both of these Combat Sports will prepare you for fighting, unlike any other activities.

If you so choose, you may then add an art loaded with practical kicking moves and another with submissions and locks. I'm not trained in Sambo specifically, but I worked with a bunch of Sambo practitioners and that's another solid base art. There are others, but make sure that your choices include authentic combat components.

Next, you should learn how to use weapons. The more you know about a weapon, the better you are able to defend against it. It is important to know your own body and how to make it move *prior* to learning weapons training. Don't rush into using a weapon. If you're not good at it, you'll likely lose your weapon to your assailant, who will then use it against you! So be cautious (we will discuss the use of practical weapons in Chapter 16).

I come from a wrestling and boxing background. Most of my street fights started with me throwing punches and then landing a takedown. When I learned karate, I would kick, punch and then land a takedown.

As far as submissions, I would primarily use wrist locks and choke holds when I needed to subdue someone on the job.

A REAL-LIFE EXAMPLE

In the 1980s, I worked as a bouncer in several establishments. It was 1983 and there were three of us working as security at a bar called Quincy's in Greenbelt, MD. The bar was formerly a "biker bar" called Jimmy Comer's, and we were part of the crew that converted it from a biker bar to a dance/sports bar and restaurant. The three bouncers on duty that night were Kirk, Percy (who wrote a passage for this book) and me. It was "Beat the Clock" night, so patrons were encouraged to drink early and a lot.

Most bar fights start for very stupid reasons, and this incident was no exception. Kirk was about 6'4" but thin and wiry. He wound up getting into an argument with a patron about the video game *Ms Pacman*. Yes, that's right, *Ms Pacman*; not even the Original *Pacman*, but *Ms Pacman*! On the other side of the dispute there were three of them, and they were enormous. One was about 6'5", 270 pounds. The others were 6'2 and 6'3" and approximately 30 to 40 pounds lighter. Noticing the argument intensifying, Percy and I trotted over to see if we could help. Now Percy is only about 5'11", but he was tipping the scales at 250 pounds and his barrel chest arrived five minutes before he did. At the time, I was 5'10" and around 195.

As we stood there, Kirk and the big guy decided to step outside so they would not mess up the bar. We tried to keep the fights outside, to mini-mize damage to the bar and not incite more patrons.

Right at the beginning, Kirk made a crucial mistake – he turned his back on the foe to walk outside. Seizing the opportunity, the guy stepped up behind him and belted him in the jaw. Kirk did not fall to the ground, but his body bent at the waist, and he fell backward. By the time he regained his balance, I had the guy who hit him on the ground, and Percy had dropped one of the other guys by slamming him into the brick wall. The third guy put his hands up, stating "that he was cool and wasn't going to make trouble."

So how did this transpire? After the big guy hit Kirk, I ducked under his punch and hit him with a Right Hook (body shot) and then I got behind him, reached between his legs, and flipped him backward with a wrestling move known as a Suplay. This is a wrestling move used most often in Freestyle and Greco-Roman Wrestling. Once you are behind your adversary, you lock your arms around their waist, pop your hips in and lift them as you bridge backward. If you keep the bridge, they will land on their head or the back of their neck. If you turn at the last moment, you will land on top of them and they'll be prone.

Once I had him on the ground, I quickly scrambled to the top position and applied the Python Lock, securing one of his arms with my other hand wrapped around his windpipe. (I saw Percy's feet on either side of his head. His legs were shaking due to the adrenaline dump.) I then told the big guy I had on the ground to relax or I was going to bite his nose off. He relaxed fairly quickly and then I informed him I was going to let him up. I also advised him to not look back, say a word or do anything but walk out. He complied.

What's the importance of this story? One, I used boxing and wrestling to take out a much larger adversary. I was only able to use the Submission Hold after striking him hard and putting him in a disadvantageous situation.

WHAT ARE THE MOST IMPORTANT STRIKES AND KICKS TO LEARN?

"I fear not the man who has practiced ten thousand kicks once, but I fear the man who has practiced one kick ten thousand times."

— Bruce Lee proverb

There are dozens and dozens of striking techniques. How do we choose which ones to use? What are the most effective?

You can refer to the list of single techniques in Chapter 9 for a complete menu of recommended Kicks and Strikes in our system.

In Chapter 1, we spoke about the "The Magic Number Seven, plus or minus Two." In a stressful situation, the brain is able to respond to the immediate external stimulus with anywhere from five to nine movements. Given this fact, you may now be asking yourself, why learn all of these movements? I can only use nine moves at the most. Isn't training with those other movements a waste of time?

No, it's not. Here's why.

First of all, you have a different set of responses to different stimuli. A set for Grabs, Strikes, different weapons, etc. You must develop all of these sets of movements. You wouldn't perform a Double-Leg Takedown on someone with a gun to the head, but you'd shoot a Double if you just slipped a punch.

Second, how do you know which movements work best for you without having tried them? This is very akin to the little kid that only wants to eat macaroni and cheese and chicken nuggets. If you don't try the other foods, how are you going to know what suits you best? Unless you try a variety of movements, you'll never know which ones work best for you and your students.

Another point is that the better that you know a technique, the better able you are to defend against it. If you want to effectively defend a punch, you had better know the mechanics involved in throwing one. This holds true for kicks, grappling and especially for weapons. It's beneficial to become well-versed in various movements and strategies. Know thy enemy.

As stated before, the basic movements work best. You will use your basics 90 percent of the time. Once you have identified a basic set of movements that works for you, the other 10 percent of the movements will be those that work especially well for you (you feel most comfortable with them, in other words).

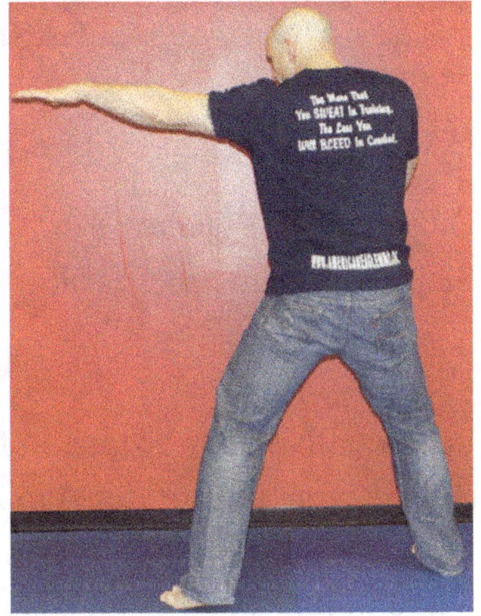

Spearhand.

Here's a sample case that makes the point. Let us suppose you have a fighter who uses a number of basic techniques quite effectively, like Front, Round, and Side Kicks, and the Jab, Cross and Hook. But he also has a great Jump Back-Kick, which he can use to devastating effect from time to time.

And now let's consider a grappler. Most of his Submissions may come from the Rear Naked Choke or the Armbar, but he also happens to have a nasty Peruvian Necktie in his tool chest, which he has used on occasion when an element of creativity or surprise was needed.

In these instances, these fighters had their basics, and used them often. But they rounded out their repertoire with techniques that were ideal for them as individuals.

One final word on this: even though I never recommend throwing a Jump Spinning-Kick in the street, it's beneficial for coordination, balance, and the development of stabilizers and intrinsic muscles and will have a positive impact on the performance of your technique set. You will most likely never use a Spear-Hand technique, either, but the practice of it increases the range of motion and strength of your hands.

BASIC TECHNIQUES

HANDS

Closed Fist, Punches 1-6. Open-hand strikes such as the Axehands, Slaps and Palm-Heel Strikes are the most effective.

KICKS

I personally know dozens of kicks. Many of these kicks are suitable for competition and for developing balance, conditioning and body awareness. But I have only ever used four (4), yes FOUR (and their variations) in real street combat situations. The Fabulous Four Kicks are:

Roundhouse: This also includes Cut Kicks and Shin Kicks
Front Kick: Lunging or Stationary
Side Kick: To the knee, body or back, as in a Mule Kick
Stomps: To the knee, shin or foot

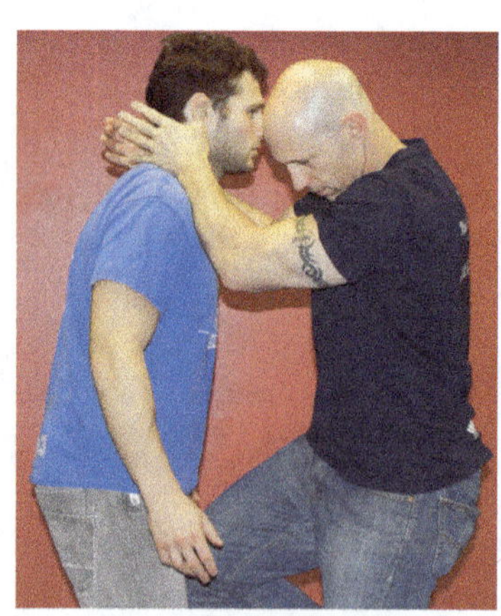

Knee drive & side head butt.

KNEE DRIVES AND ELBOWS

These are used at very close range when you are too close to kick or punch.

KNEE DRIVES

Straight knees delivered to the groin and bladder work best. Roundhouse Knees directed to the sciatic nerve, quads and hamstrings are extremely effective.

ELBOWS

Elbows can be delivered up, down, across, back and at angles. The top targets are the temple, jaw, groin, solar plexus, ribs and spine.

WHAT DO WE DO?

The most important component is your mindset and willingness to win; even more important is *your hatred of losing*. If you ever witnessed me win anything, I might smile but I never demonstrate much more excitement than that. Whether I'm in a competition or a "situation," I am supposed to win. That's what I'm there for. I EXPECT to win. When I win, I'm simply doing what I should.

In contrast, when I lose the reaction is much stronger. I hate to lose more than anything. Maybe you wouldn't be able to see that I was disappointed or mad, but I don't take losses lightly. Show me a "Good Loser" and I'll show you a loser.

Three weeks after I earned my Black Belt, I entered a professional karate tournament. My first fight was against the #3-ranked fighter in the world, Larry Kelly. I will tell you that he spanked me. I couldn't lay a glove on him. He didn't hurt me, but damn, he embarrassed the hell out of me! He avoided all of my attacks and simply hit me when I missed.

After the bout, I didn't speak with anyone. I was an amateur champion, and I had expected to win at my first pro event. When I got home that night, I ran five miles and then went into my basement and hit the heavy bag so long and hard that I was completely exhausted and both my hands were bleeding. I really didn't care; I was extremely pissed off at my performance. It was the last time I was ever embarrassed. I made sure it never happened again.

WHAT TO DO WHEN THE PROVERBIAL S**T HITS THE FAN?

Five-time UFC World Champion Frank Shamrock was once asked the question, "What's the best advice anyone has given you about fighting?" He stated that the best advice he was ever given was to "Keep your hands up."

That's some great advice. When you are in a fracas, get your hands up by your head, and don't let them drop for any reason. As I tell my students, you can do Push-Ups to strengthen your upper body, and you can do Sit-Ups to make your abdominals strong, but there is no such thing as "Face ups," So you had better protect your face and head by keeping your hands up!

I would also advise you to move. Simply start moving, but not backward. Move your head around and circle. Change directions. A moving target is much more difficult to hit than a stationary one, that's an eternal principle of fighting. *So, keep your hands up and move.*

WHAT'S A GOOD BASIC PHILOSOPHY TO ADOPT?

The *Element of Surprise* is especially beneficial to smaller and female practitioners. In most self-defense situations, the assailant is looking to impose their will on someone they believe they can subdue with minimal resistance. But you can surprise them by seizing the opportunity to launch an immediate counterattack.

Quick, repeated and powerful strikes in resistance are all that you may need to afford yourself the time to escape a conflict uninjured.

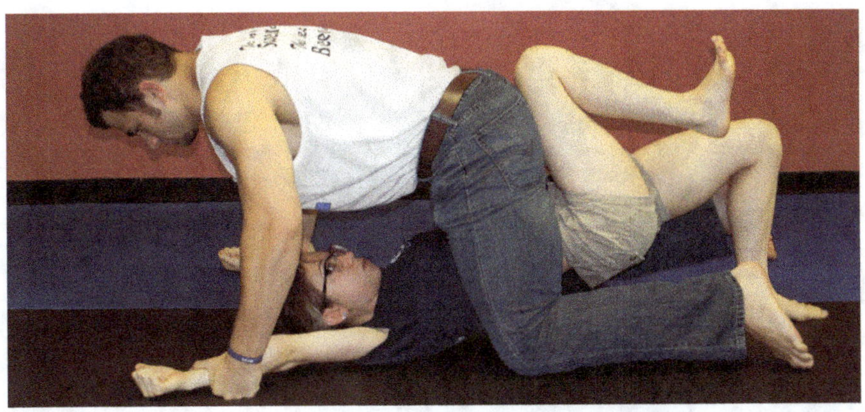

As far as actual movement and fighting strategies are concerned, a good premise to use as your base is what I refer to as the "X's and O's Principle." Think of it as the X's and O's in football, where the X's represent the defense and the O's represent the offense.

When defending, you should be doing X-shaped movements, and when attacking (or counter attacking), your movements should be O-shaped, in a pattern known as circle striking. There are many martial arts movements where the arms cross in front of the body, moving to another counter-offensive position. They make an X, in other words, and the X defense principle applies to ground fighting, stand-up battles and weapons.

The O's are for offensive circles of striking combinations. My preference for attacking and counter attacking is in a circle. An example of a Circle-or O-combination would be a Left Roundhouse Kick, Left Jab, Right Cross, and Right Cut Kick. You start low, move up, then across and down to the opposite side of where you started, thus making a complete circle. I will say that there are certain circumstances when I employ an X for striking, but as a general rule, I utilize a circle or an O.

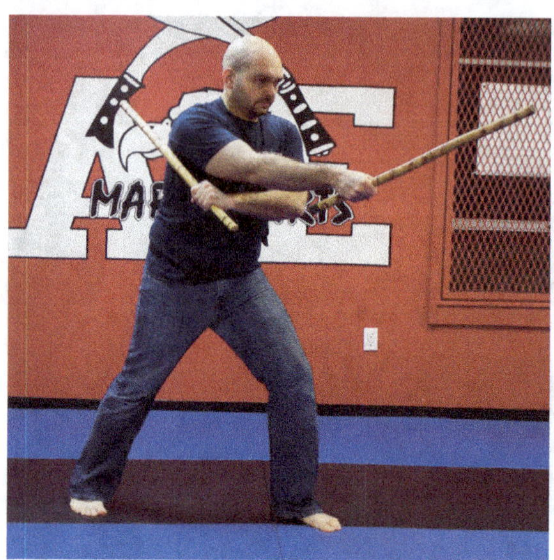 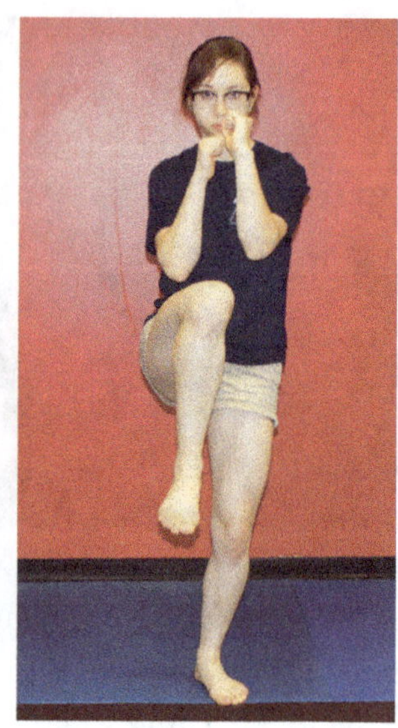

HOW SHOULD WE TRAIN?

There is a false opinion espoused by some so-called experts that all you need to do is to practice your self-defense and "death techniques" and everything will be alright (*chuckle*). Others claim that if you are used to "pulling" or controlling your strikes, you will do so in the street, so therefore you shouldn't do it while training.

In truth, both ideas are incorrect. If you didn't pull your techniques or exhibit control while sparring, everyone would be banged up and unable to compete, or train for that matter. There are plenty of knock-outs and submissions in competition, so that theory is out of the window.

When you are in a real-life situation, you should treat it like a training session where all restraint is abandoned. If you don't "roll" or spar live, you'll never be able to develop the kinesthetic awareness of movement with and against another human being. This is also why live drilling is also paramount for your training. You need to practice your real Sport Combat *and* your defensive tactics, plus strength and conditioning as well as your body toughening techniques. Don't neglect any of these areas, being complete in these aspects is what is required to be completely prepared for anything and everything.

I have never had an issue making the transition from my training in the studio to applying what I know in the street. Neither have any of my friends, students or training partners. When I've squared up with someone in the street, I've treated the situation like I was sparring - except with more emotion, adrenaline and knowing that I *didn't* have to hold back! It was GO TIME!

Those who disagree with this either never have had a fight or have been trained in an inferior system. The sparring and reaction to human movement, getting hit yourself and seeing how you react, plus practicing your defensive tactics, all of this training-related activity will prepare you for a street encounter.

You need to train so that your defensive maneuvers are purely reflexive. Once you reach this stage, "IT" takes over. You have now developed Instinctive Technique. The body and mind are in such sync with each other, and you are so attuned that you will respond properly to any circumstance that arises.

Here's an example of what I'm referring to. I had graduated college a year or so before, and I was in a bar in NYC with a group of friends. As we were making our way through the crowded, dark and very loud club, I felt someone grab me by my traps from behind. I immediately turned and captured both of the assailant's arms with one of mine and readied my fist to smash into his face. Luckily for him, I recognized him. He was a buddy from college. I pulled the punch before I hit him in the face and let go of him. I said, "Greg, what are you doing?!?" He said, "You are crazy!" I replied, "Me? You know me and ought to know better than to grab me from behind!" IT took over. IT responded. IT did what I had trained IT to do: protect me. IT did its job. As IT had many times before and would again many times after.

Listed below are specific responses to specific attacks. While it is impossible to train for every potential situation, the concepts behind these responses are universal and applicable to multiple attack scenarios. The attacks addressed are some of the more prevalent, and the defensive tactics employed are the most universal. This means that most people will be able to perform these movements against most assailants.

All self-defense techniques have three components (or ingredients as I often refer to them as): Distraction, Release and Finish. *The Distraction* is in the form of a stomp, smash or strike to the vital and semi-vital areas. *The Release* occurs when you free yourself from their grasp or hold. *The Finish* takes place once you are free and are able to temporarily (or permanently) disable the assailant while securing your safe escape. In the worst case, once you are grabbed or attacked - *immediately strike back.*

Listed below are over 50 highly recommended self-defense techniques. It would be an arduous, if not impossible, task to teach, train and practice every possible defensive tactic maneuver. Not to mention developing the muscle memory required to execute so many techniques under duress. Instead of focusing specifically on the techniques, we focus on the principles of responses to attacks.

So why do we even practice techniques? There are several reasons, a major one being that we need to know how to move with another person and how a body will react when both being attacked and attacking.

These are some well-known, prevalent attack scenarios. Preparing oneself for such instances is practicing due diligence. The main reason is to teach your body how to apply the principles of human movement, thus developing the "IT" or Instinctive Technique necessary to effectively protect yourself.

REAL-LIFE EXAMPLE

It was May 1984, and I had just finished finals at the University of Maryland. It was a long day of celebration and the night had wound down. It was around 2:00 AM and there was a group of us hanging out in my apartment eating pizza and snacks. Only the screen door was closed, and suddenly, there was a knock at the door. I got up to answer it, and there was a large guy there, approximately 6 feet tall and 210 pounds. He was covered in blood, said that he had experienced an accident, and asked if he could use the phone to call his brother. I said OK.

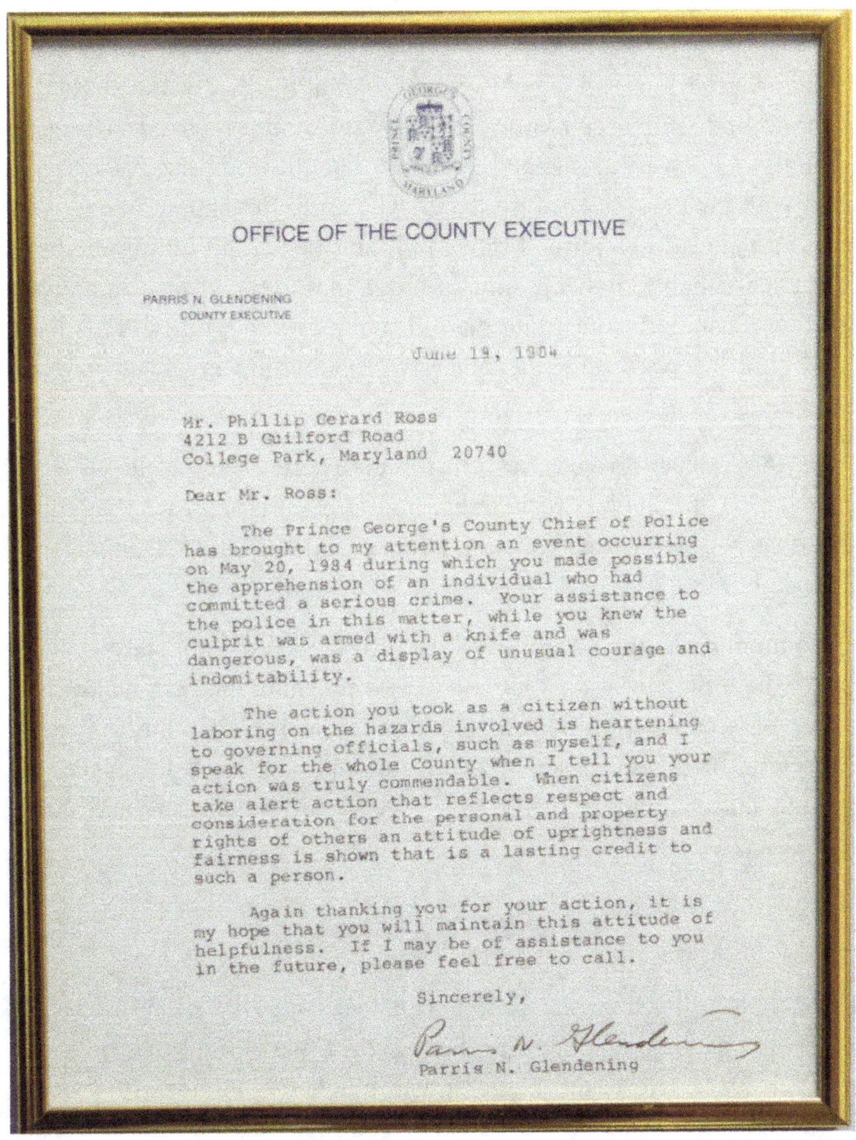

Well, as he was on the phone, I noticed something bulging under his shirt in the back. I was getting a strange feeling, so I followed him out of the door and looked around as he started walking off to the right. I looked to the left and saw a guy lying on the ground, bleeding about half of a block away. I yelled to the guy that had just left my house. He took off - GAME ON!

I took off after him and caught up with him at the end of the street. He spun around and faced me with the knife in his hand. Reacting instantly, I open-hand slapped his knife hand, hitting the back of his wrist with the palm heel of my hand. The knife flew about twenty feet or so and landed in a gully. I moved to the side and hit him in the back of his neck, then foot-swept him and took him to the ground in a prone position. Pushing his face into the dirt with one hand, I jacked his hand up behind his back with the other while jamming my knee into his tailbone.

Soon the police arrived in full force! There were a dozen cops surrounding the action, with lights and sirens blaring and their guns drawn on the two of us. Quickly, I looked up and said, "Don't worry, boys, I got him!"

By some miracle, the victim lived. He had survived eight stab wounds, one of them puncturing his lung. I wound up being the recipient of two letters of commendation from the Prince George's County Chief of Police and the County Executive. If you look at what I did, there was nothing fancy about it, just concise, powerful movements and quick action.

COMMON ATTACKS

The defenses listed to the following attacks may be performed with either side of the body. For simplicity's sake, we will discuss only one side per attack. However, be certain to practice both sides; you never know what circumstances will dictate. You may have an injury, or your dominant side may be otherwise occupied.

We describe initial responses to attacks. If executed with intensity, precision and power, the prescribed techniques will resolve the situation. However, things don't always go as planned, so you must be prepared to improvise. I call this "catch as catch can:" whatever comes up, hit it. Adhere to the principles of movement and you will tilt the scales in your favor.

There are many bonafide self-defense techniques. The responses listed are the ones I have found to work the best for the majority of people. I've performed most of these techniques personally in a real-life situation, or someone I trained with had performed them in similar circumstances. After years of practice, you may discover variations that better suit you. If so, perfect! Good for you, use them. We're simply giving you a point to start at or a different perspective to consider if you are already trained.

CHOKES

FRONT CHOKE, TWO HANDS

This is the "stereotypical" Front Choke attack when someone reaches out with both hands and attempts to strangle you with their hands. Bring your shoulders up with a shrugging motion as you bring your chin down, just as if you were a turtle going into its shell. As you are doing this, strike your opponent in the nose with a Palm-Heel Strike with your right hand. Next you will simultaneously step back with your right foot as your left hand comes over with a slap to the assailant's ear. These combined motions will free you from their grasp.

Plant your right foot firmly on the ground and deliver a Side Kick to the attacker's knee. On a side note, if you have fingernails that are long enough you can scratch their face with your open-hand slap and leave identifying marks.

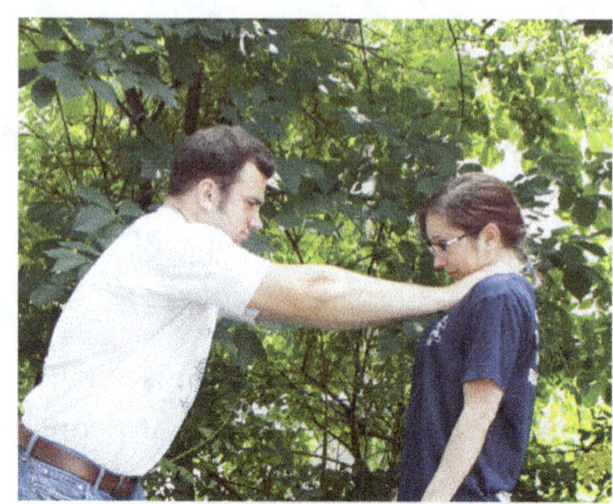
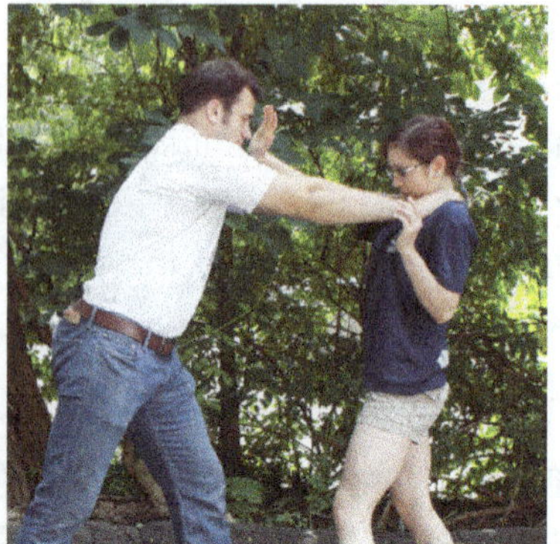
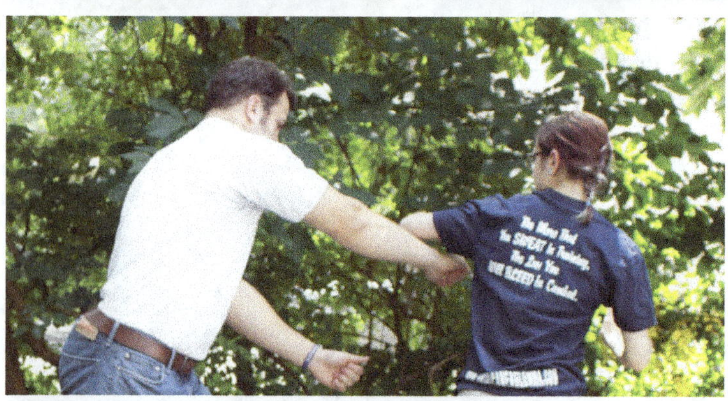
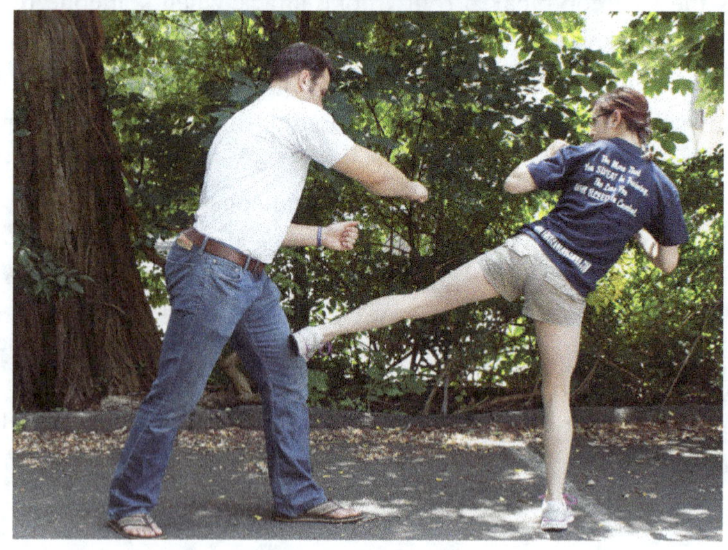

FRONT CHOKE, ONE HAND

There are two basic methods that you can use to defend yourself in this situation. One is to the inside, and the other to the outside. The latter is the preferable method, but you are not always afforded the luxury of a choice.

Outside: When you get attacked with one hand, the hand will most likely be used to punch you in the face. This is why moving to the outside of the opponent is preferable. If the assailant grabs you with their left hand, you grab their wrist with your left hand and place your elbow up so that it is covering your face. Step in with your right foot, making sure their left arm is straight as you deliver a Hammerfist Strike to the extended arm at the elbow. As you finish that blow, immediately strike their face with a Side Hammer Smash.

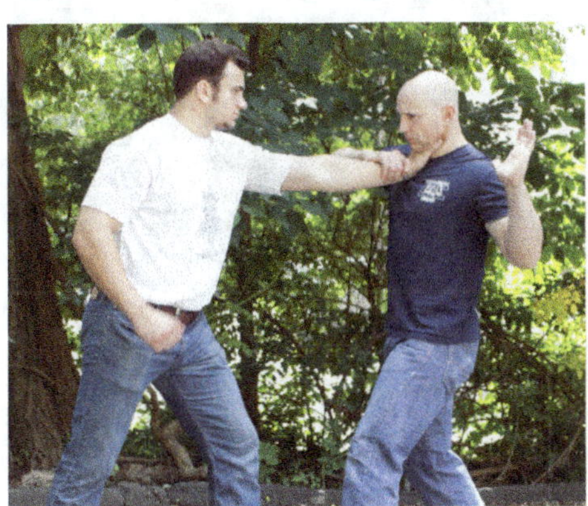
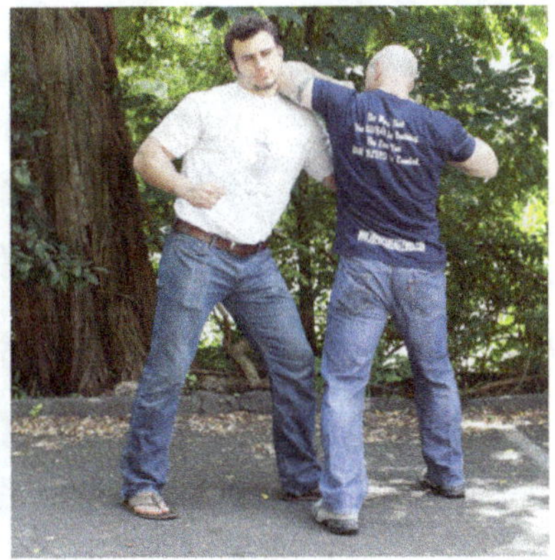

Inside: There may be an occasion where the outside path is unavailable, and you need to be aware that you could be stepping into a punch. If the perpetrator grabs your throat with their right hand, secure his wrist with your left as you step in, making certain that your right hand is up. We do this for two reasons: one, as a means to protect your face when you move in, and two, so that your hand is in position to deliver the Knife-Hand Chop to the bicep's insertion. This is located above the bend in the elbow. Bounce your strike from the biceps and drive an elbow into your assailant's face. Your fist will be clenched and your palm facing downward. Capture your opponent's neck with your right hand and deliver upward Knee Strikes to the groin, head or bladder.

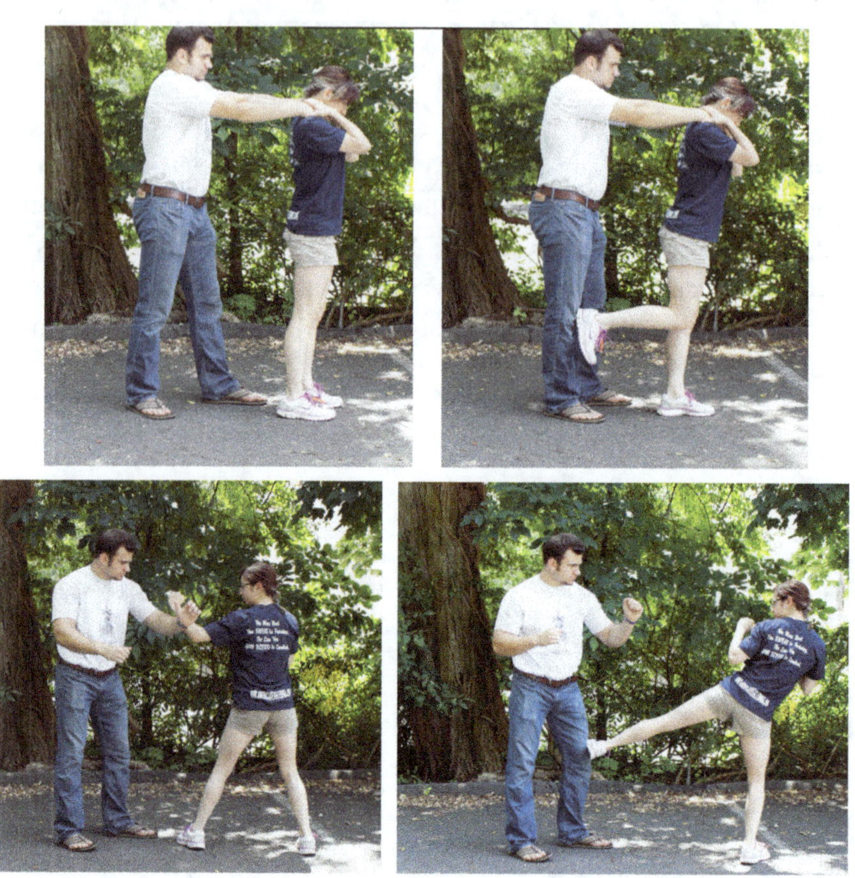

REAR CHOKES

There is a common thread with all choke defenses—you need to make space and act quickly. If the assailant knows what he's doing, you'll be unconscious in three seconds or less. When you have an arm around your neck, you'll need to bring your shoulder up, tuck your neck in, take your middle and ring fingers from one hand, insert them into the crook of the attacker's elbow and pull down. You will now need to turn so that your chin is placed in the crook of the elbow. You have now bought yourself some time to escape.

REAR CHOKE WITH ARMBAR

This is a very commonplace restraining attack. The assailant will wrap their right arm around your neck and force your left hand up high by grabbing your wrist and driving it up. Lower your weight, stomp their toes and kick their shins, drive your head backward into their face and then perform the sequence of movements described above.

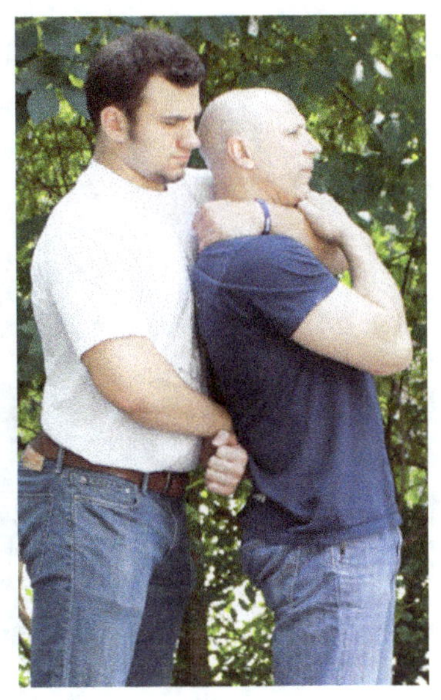

Once you have loosened the grip and executed your techniques for distraction, take your left foot and step behind your right foot as you bend your waist and duck out. This motion will free the arm they are jacking up your back. As you turn and move, hold your grip on the arm that was once around your neck with your right hand and your newly freed left hand. You will wind up at the side of your opponent. Drive your right shoulder into their arm as you side-step and drag your opponent by the arm in the direction of their hand.

REAR NAKED CHOKES

There are more people practicing martial arts nowadays than ever before. Most thugs get their techniques from television, and many of these guys watch MMA Fighters putting Rear Naked Chokes (RNCs) on their opponents in combat. It's only natural that they will try them on you. It's best to be cognizant of this fact and prepare yourselves.

Standing: If attacked in this manner, you should follow the same movement pattern as you would if attacked with the Rear Choke and Armbar. However, you may not be able to throw the backward Head Butt, as the lock may be too tight. You will, however, most likely be able to back into the attacker as you deliver a barrage of kicks and stomps to the feet and shins. Repeat the same steps used in the Rear Choke with the Armbar to complete your escape.

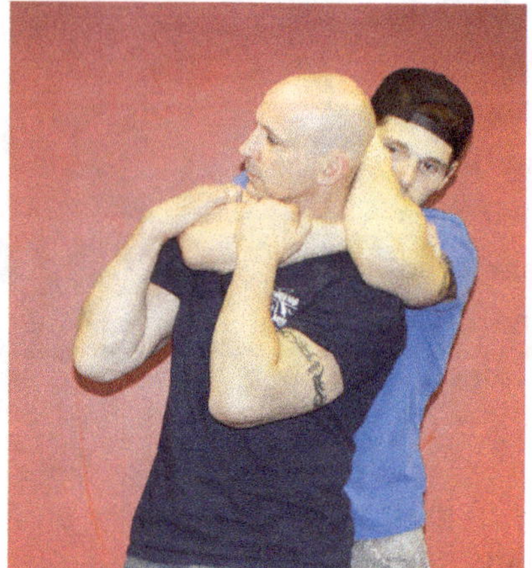
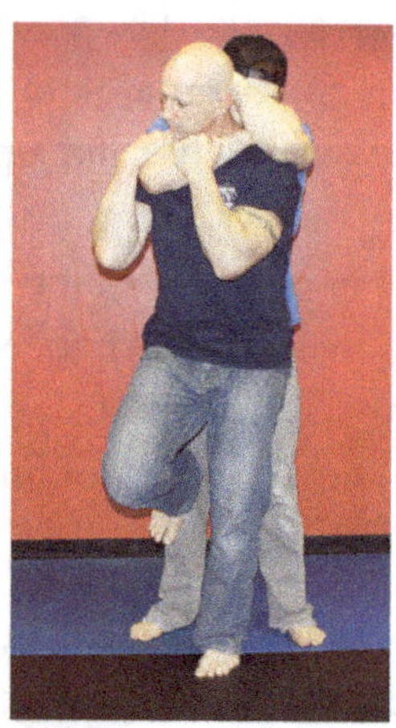

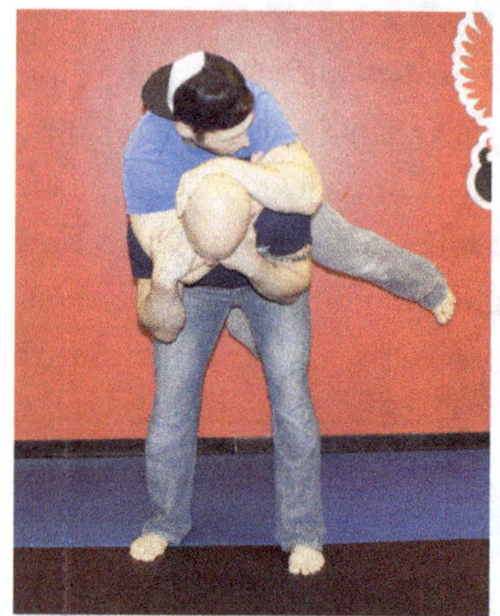
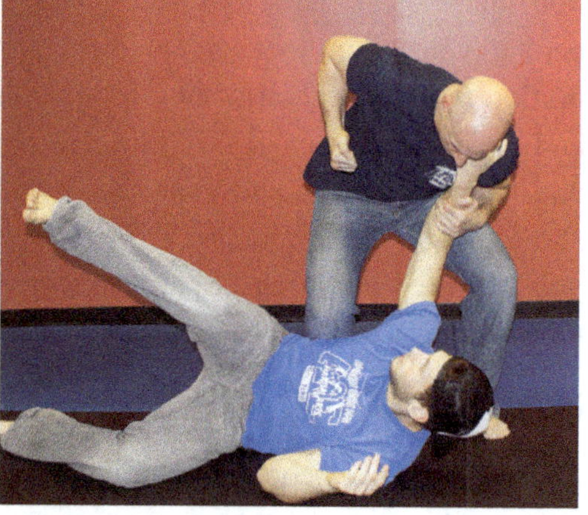

On the Ground: This position is a little more dangerous, unless you have friends with you to kick and stomp the attacker. Assuming you don't, he will most likely have his hooks in on both of your legs, pinning you down. Some people like to escape to the choking side arm, others like to get to the free arm side. You may not have a choice, so practice your escapes to both sides—but for now let's consider escaping to the choking arm side. Follow all of the steps to relieve the pressure on your throat as you slide your body down toward his feet as you put your butt on his thigh. Eventually you will slide downward far enough to get your butt on the outside of his leg. You will now be able to cut your hips and flip over so that you are belly down and can scramble around and launch your own counterattack.

WRIST GRABS

When someone grabs your wrist, at least one of their hands will be compromised. They are as tied up as you are, for the time being, anyway. You need to take advantage of this before they realize that they do not have the advantage. They are also vulnerable to strikes, having one-half of their defense compromised. It's important to keep in mind that you are most vulnerable while attacking. You will also always want to twist your wrist so the edge of the wrist on the side of your thumb is lined up where the thumb and finger come together.

There are many controlling techniques that you can use when your wrist gets grabbed, but they are reserved for situations that dictate control and non-lethal responses. We will not address these here. Controlling techniques are only recommended for those working in security or law enforcement. You have to be extremely proficient to subdue another human being without inflicting pain or damage.

ONE-ON-ONE (SINGLE) WRIST GRAB

Let us suppose that they've grabbed your left wrist. The attacker will not simply stand there holding your wrist. They are either going to pull you, try to punch you or a combination thereof. Moving rapidly, step into the assailant with your right foot as you deliver an Axehand with your right hand to their head. Now, as you twist your left wrist as described above, execute a Downward Chop to their wrist. Bounce that hand off of their wrist and strike them in the side of the neck as you grab that neck. Thread your left hand under their right arm and onto their back. Stomp the ground with your left foot and perform the Springboard Knee with your right knee, striking them in the groin, bladder or head. Repeat the strikes until they drop.

Whether you are attacked with the same side-wrist or the assailant grabs the cross-side wrist, the defense remains consistent.

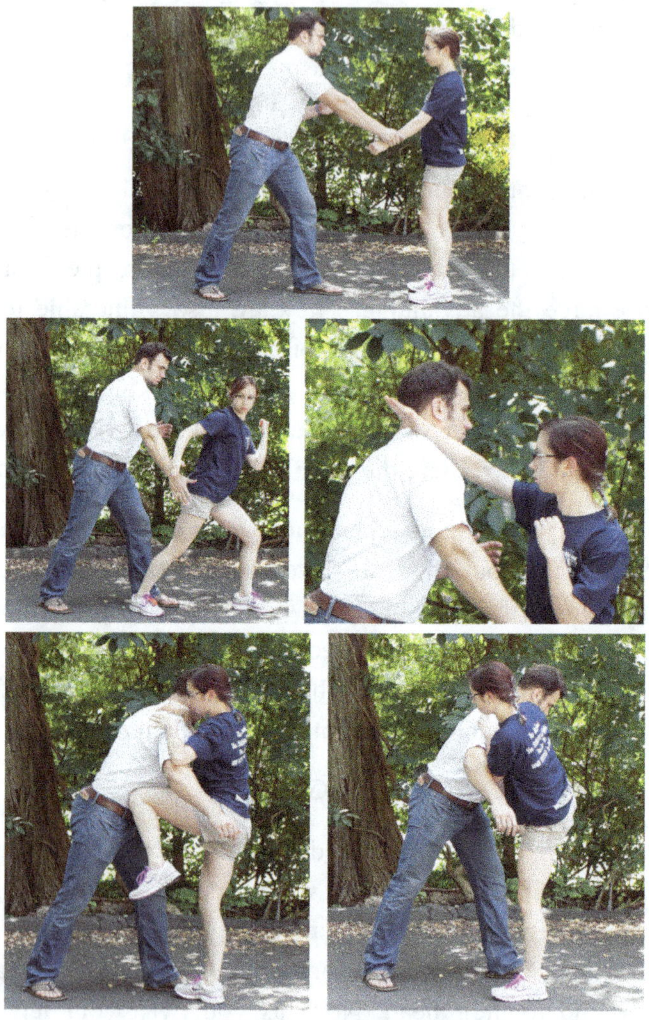

One-on-one (single) wrist grab.

TWO-ON-ONE WRIST GRAB

The assailant grabs your one wrist with two hands. You deliver a Palm-Heel Strike to their face, aiming for the nose. Reach between their arms and "shake hands" with yourself and step back with the opposite foot of the hand that is being grabbed. If your right hand was grabbed, step back with your left foot as you pull your hand free. If the opponent steps toward you, deliver a Side Elbow to their face. If they step away or remain stationary, administer a Sidekick to the knee.

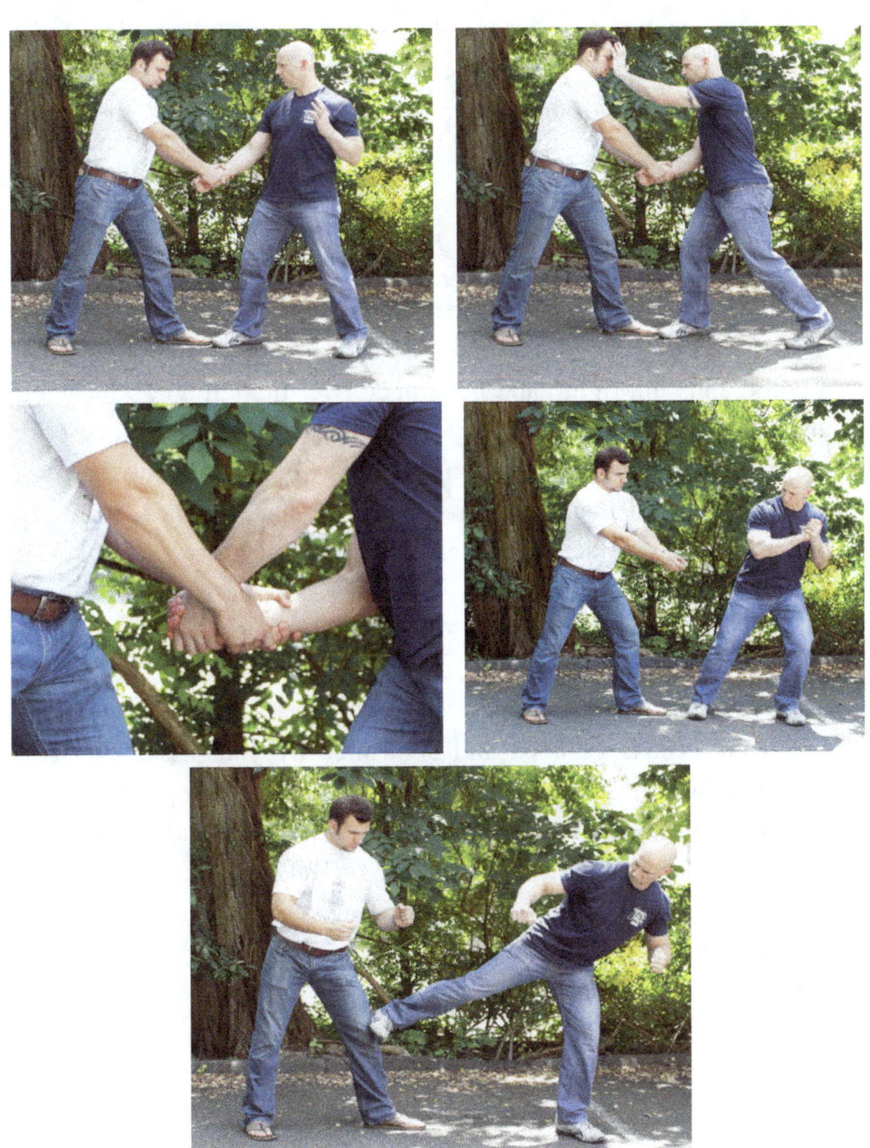

TWO-ON-TWO WRIST GRAB

One of the easiest and most effective ways to free yourself from a two-on-two wrist attack is to force your hands in and, as they pull your hands outward, to counter what you have done, deliver a Front Knee strike to the groin. Repeat this until they fall. If they don't pull your hands apart, punch your left hand downward and grab their right wrist with your right hand as you deliver a kick to their left shin with your right foot. Stomp the ground and move to your left and kick their right knee then step to your left and Side Kick their right knee as you free your hand.

TWO-ON-TWO WRIST GRAB, CONTROL

If the situation arises where you need to control an attacker, and both of your wrists are grabbed, first deliver a kick to their talus or shin. Next, turn both palms up, right hand positioned over the left. Grab their left hand with the fingers of your left hand on the thumb portion of their palm. Your thumb will be up as you pull your fingers toward you; push your thumb toward them as you shove their hand toward them and downward to the outside as you deliver a palm heel to the side of their head.

TWO HANDS ON ONE ARM FROM BEHIND (ARM BEHIND BACK)

If your right arm is grabbed and controlled by your assailant's two hands and your arm is placed behind your back, first stomp his feet and kick backward into his knees as a distraction. Next, bend at the waist and step across with your left foot and pivot 180 degrees. You will now be facing your attacker, but off to their right side. Free your hand either by creating a small circle with your wrist or by attacking with chops to his wrist. Employ a finishing technique.

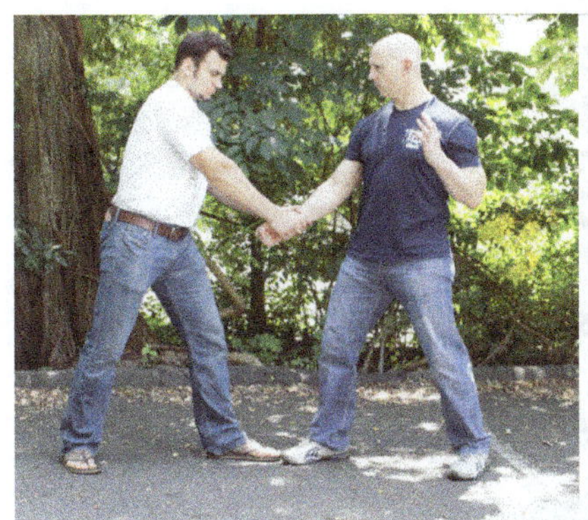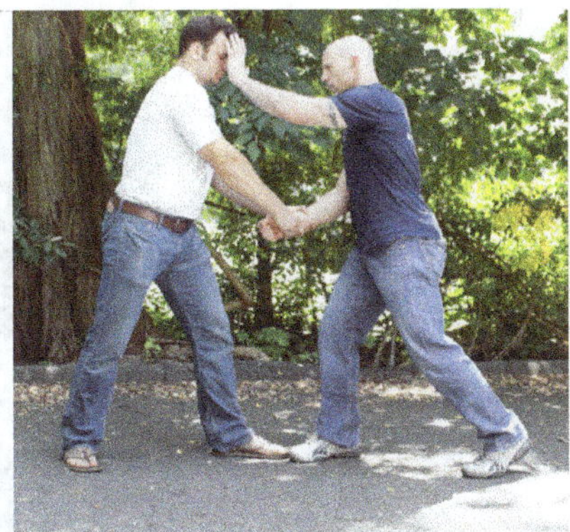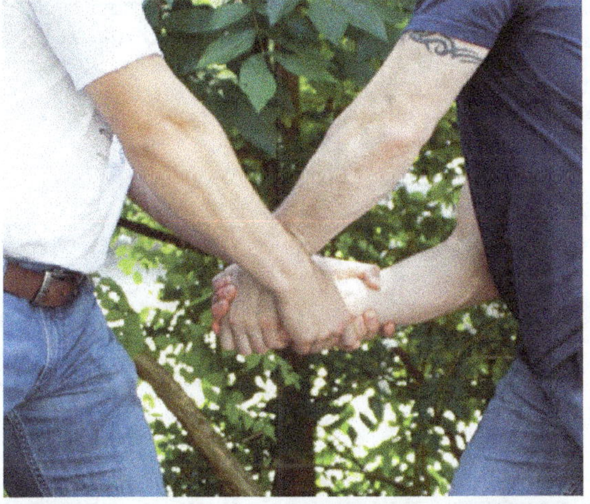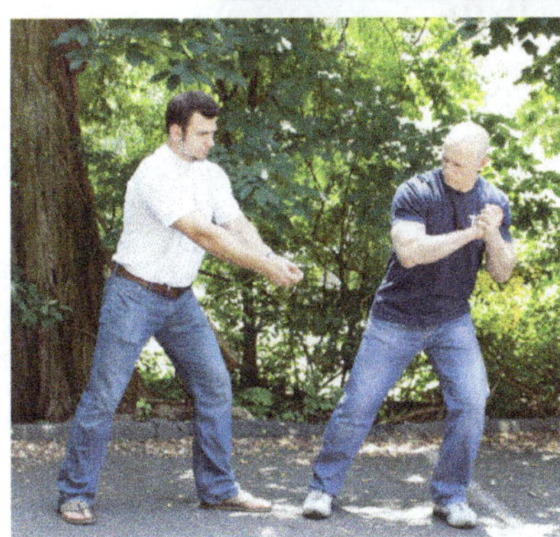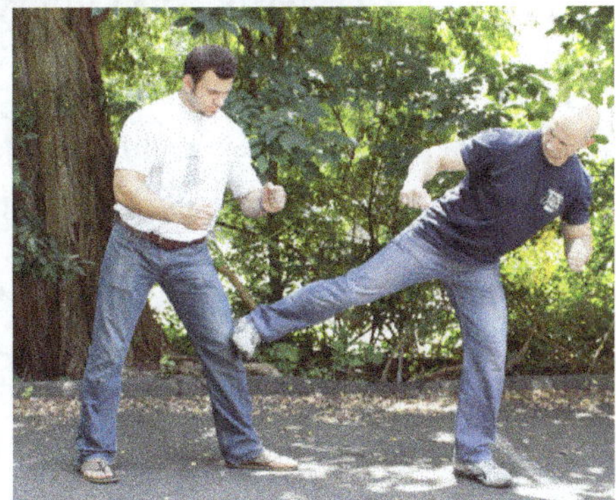

Two-on-two wrist grab, control.

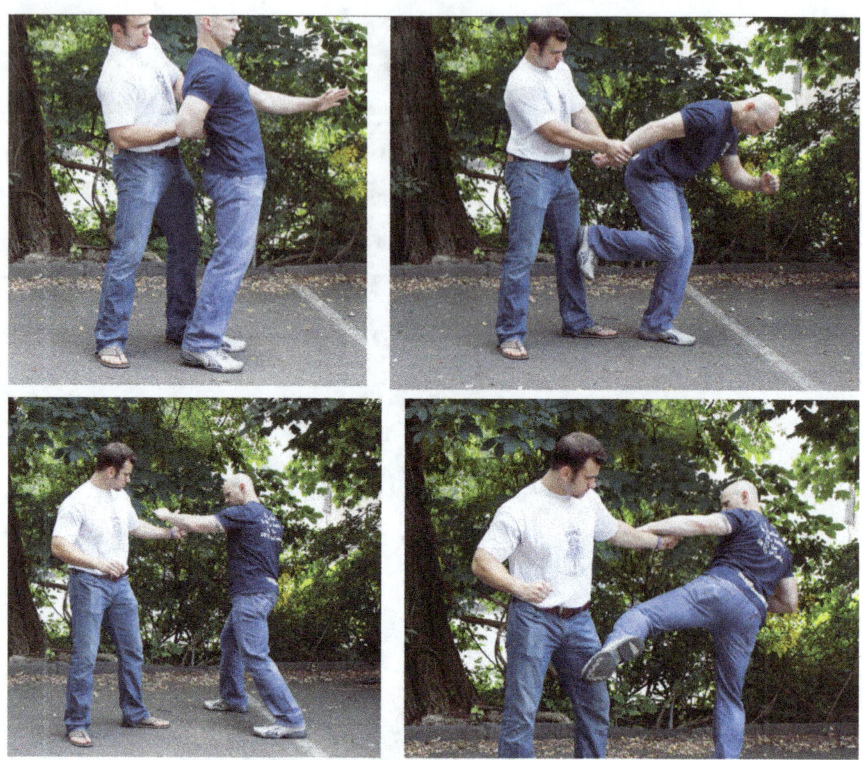

Two hands on one arm from behind (arm behind back).

TWO HANDS ON ONE ARM FROM BEHIND (AROUND WAIST)

Suppose you have been grabbed from behind and your attacker grabs your left wrist with their right hand and grabs your right forearm with their left hand. This is generally referred to as a Two-on-One Wrist Control position. If they position themselves properly, their face and groin will be obscured. You'll only be able to use Foot Stomps and Shin Kicks as distraction techniques.

To free yourself, take your right hand and thread it under their right hand as you grab their left wrist. Bring your right elbow up high as you "pop" his right hand off of your wrist and then drive your left hand straight downward. You will now be free to unleash your barrage of counterattacks.

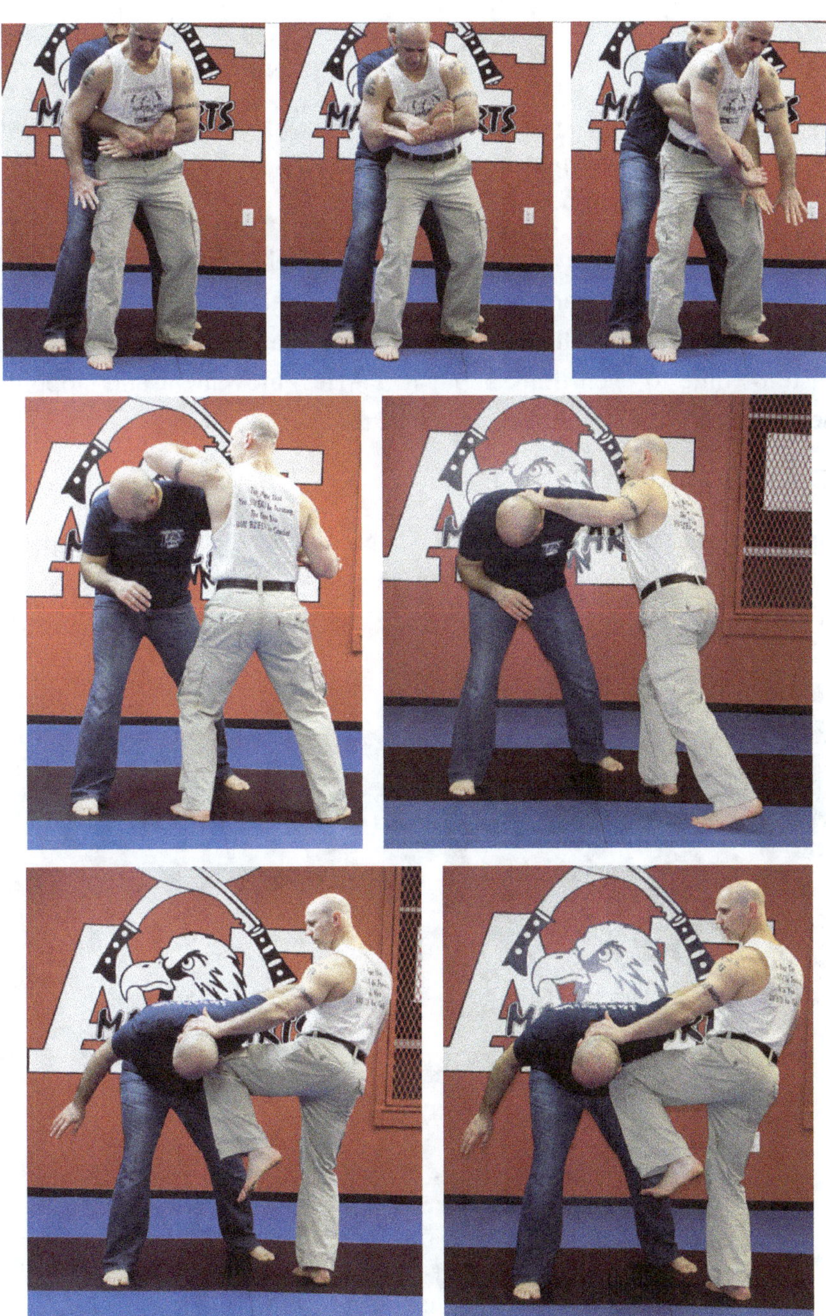

Two hands on one arm from behind (around waist).

PUNCHES

It's very humorous to watch movies and see these "action stars" catch someone's fist in mid-punch and then proceed to flip them through a wall. This will not happen in real life.

We need to concentrate on the fact that all punches begin at the hip and then come from the shoulder. Stopping the punch at its origin is the only chance that you'll have. You'll never catch their fist, so it's a waste of time to even think about it. Parries, movement and stopping the punch at its origin are the strategies that work best.

SINGLE STRAIGHT PUNCH

If you are attacked with a Straight Punch, the person throwing it probably has some idea of how to throw a good shot and most likely has had some training. This person is more dangerous and will leave fewer openings.

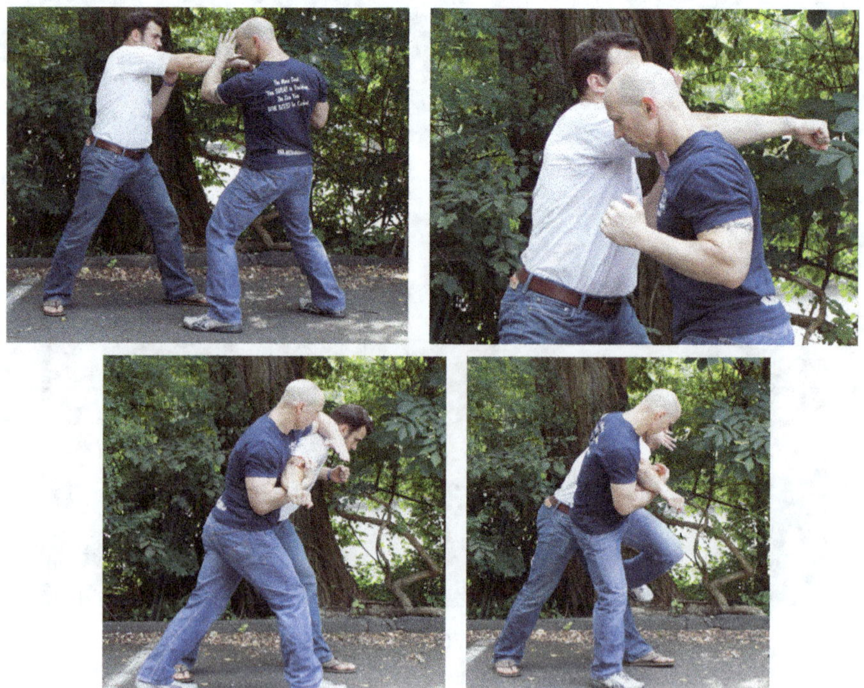

Let us assume that you have your hands up and that the attacker is throwing a straight right hand at you. Move to your left and toward them with a "6 Step" (Pie-Stepping in Chapter 10) and parry their strike with your left hand anywhere between their fist and elbow as you deliver a strike to their abdomen with your right hand. Next, slide your right hand up to capture their extended right arm and deliver an elbow strike with your left to their head.

TWO STRAIGHT PUNCHES

This defense is identical to the Single Straight Punch, except there are two parries due to the two punches. We'll finish with a Knee Drive to the groin and a Downward Elbow Smash to the back of the head of the doubled-over attacker.

GRAB AND PUNCH

If someone grabs your lapel, you can bet that there will be a punch sailing to your head shortly thereafter. If they grab you with their left hand, cover it with your right and immediately direct a Palm-Heel Strike to their right shoulder with your left hand. We strike the shoulder because every punch, whether a Straight, Hook or Uppercut, emanates from the shoulder. Stop the punch at its source.

Back to the defensive maneuver: keep their left hand secured to your chest, and after you have struck their shoulder with your right, execute a Chin Jab, then an Elbow Strike across their chin from right to left. Next, perform an Axehand Strike from left to right and then grasp their neck with your right hand as you slide your left hand under their arm and across their back. Now you deliver Knee Strikes to the groin, solar plexus and bladder until you determine its time to implement your redirect throw.

DOUBLE PUNCH (HAYMAKER)

This defense is against an attacker throwing haymaker punches at you. As the looping punch comes in, deliver hard chops to the biceps of the assailant. Once you have blocked, immediately counterattack with a

Knifehand Chop to the neck, grabbing behind his head with the same hand and then delivering an Elbow Smash to the face. Now repeat the position and the finishing as we had done in the Grab and Punch attack.

We use this finish on many attacks.

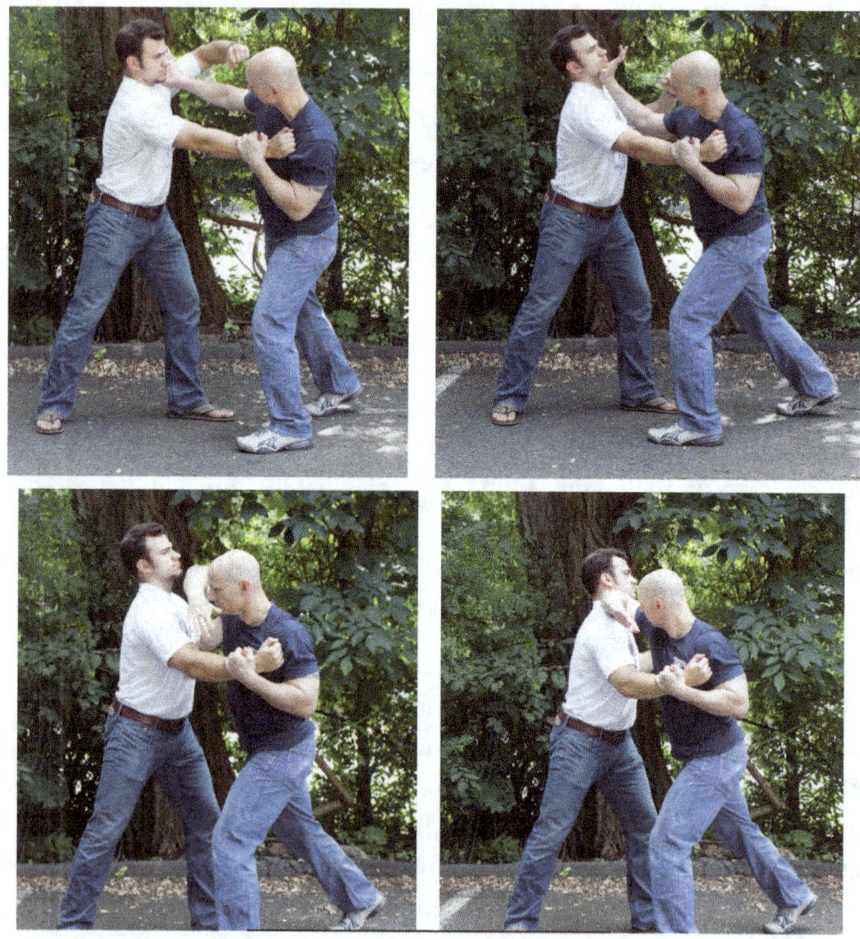

Grab and punch.

BEAR-HUGS

Let's consider who will be attacking you. The chances are that you will be attacked in this manner by a larger, stronger individual who feels that they can overpower you. Just think about it, if you are 6' 2" and 225 pounds it's highly unlikely that a 5'1", 123-pound assailant will attack you in this fashion.

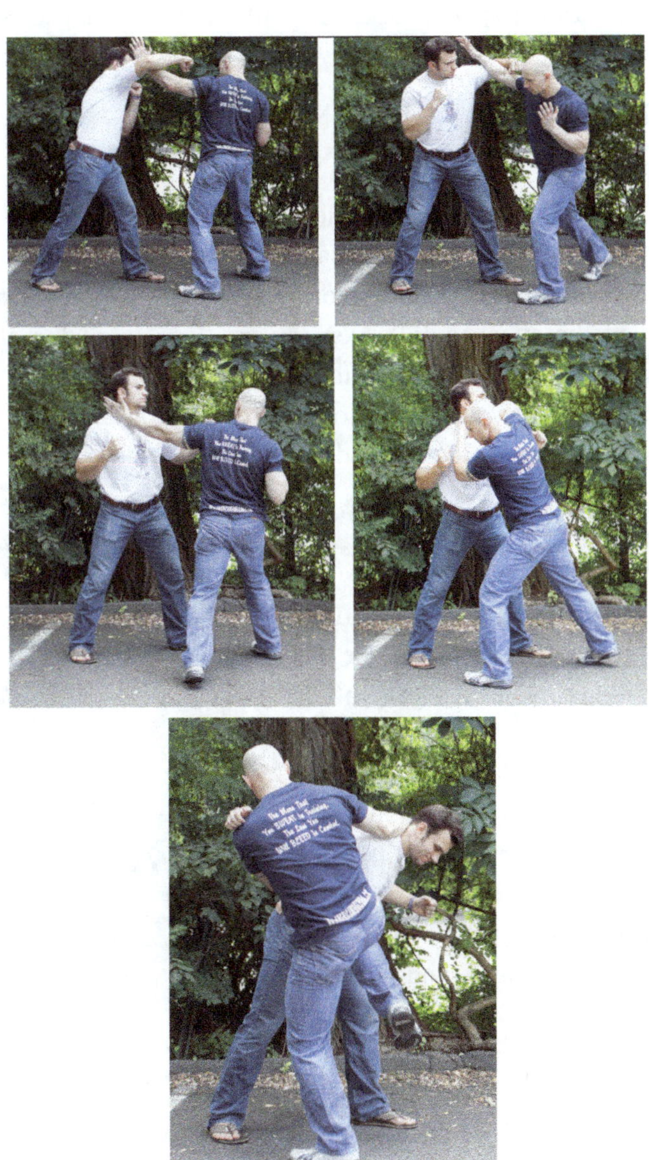

Double haymaker.

FRONT BEAR-HUG

There are three different scenarios with the Front Bear- Hug attack: entering with arms trapped, locked in with the arms trapped, and arms free.

ENTERING, WITH ARMS TRAPPED

An assailant steps in to grab you and wrap their arms around you. Step back into a front stance with one leg straight and locked out and the other knee bent as you drive your palms into their hips. Make sure that your thumbs are pressed against your hand so your hands form "flippers." When the attacker pulls you toward them more forcefully, go with it and deliver Knee Drives to their and/or bladder until you are able to free yourself or they fall to the ground. You may now execute kicks or a Parachute Stomp to the downed perpetrator.

FRONT BEAR-HUG, ARMS FREE

Both of your hands and your arms are free. You have most likely been lifted off of the ground, so you can't use the ground to aid you in generating power. No worries, you won't need that to administer a Head- Butt and then cup your hands, clap their ears, and gouge their eyes with your thumbs. As we explained before, take your thumbs, start at the bridge of the nose, dig your thumbs in, and scoop to the outside.

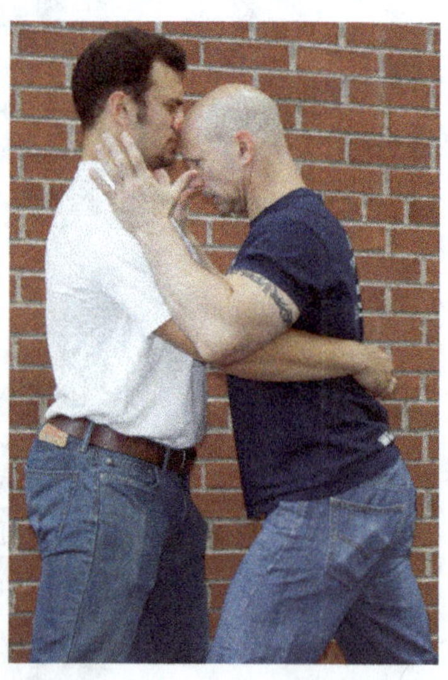

FRONT BEAR-HUG, ARMS TRAPPED AND TIGHT TO YOU

You may have been caught completely off-guard, and your assailant has secured a tight Bear-Hug over the arms and is crushing you. Begin with a Head-Butt to the nose as you make your hands into fists and press them together, lower your weight, pull your hips back and drive your thumbs into their bladder or groin. If the attacker is a male, grab, twist and pull the groin. If they are a female, strike to the groin and then gain enough space to deliver Knee Drives.

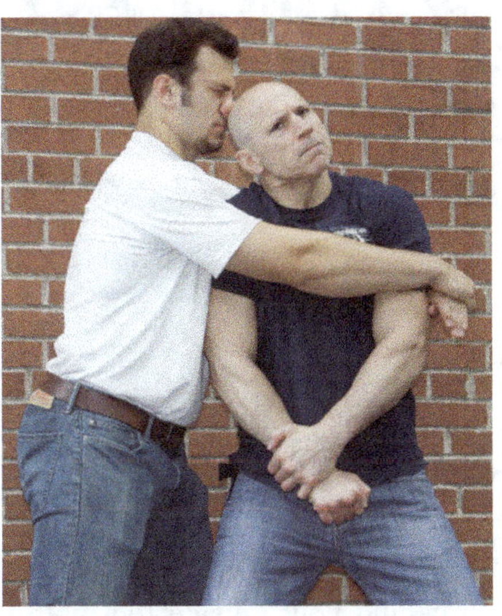

Side bear hug.

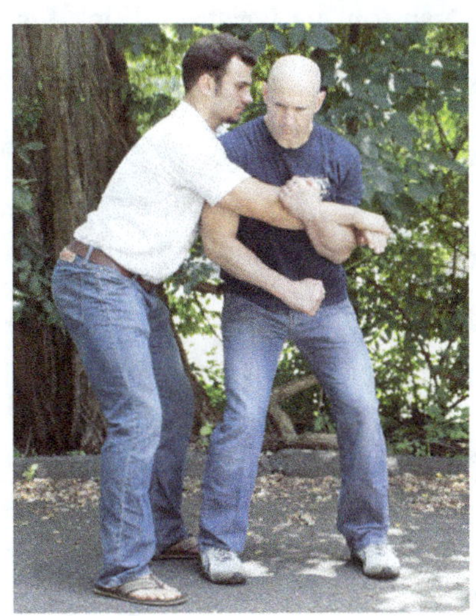
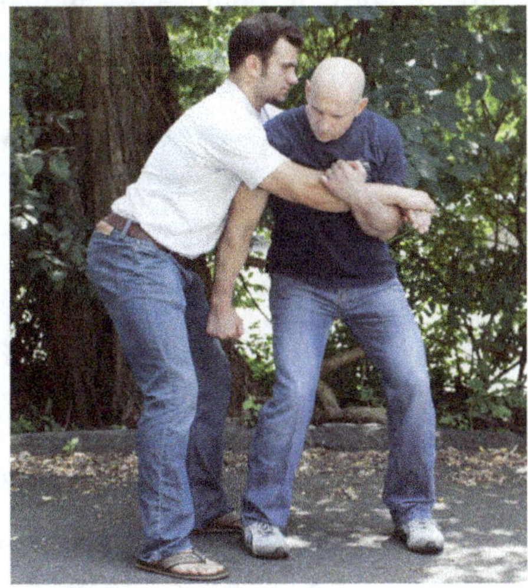

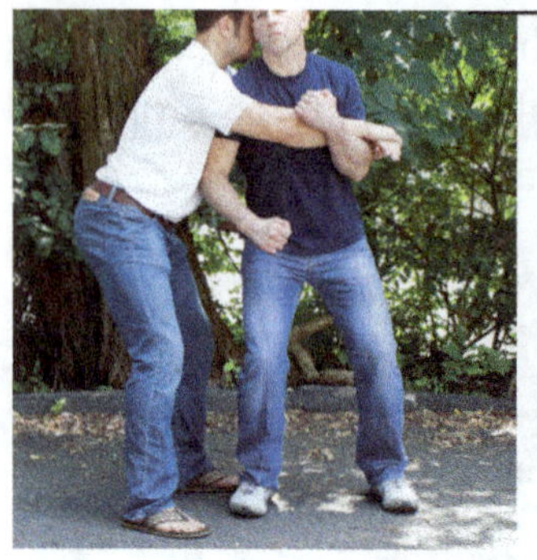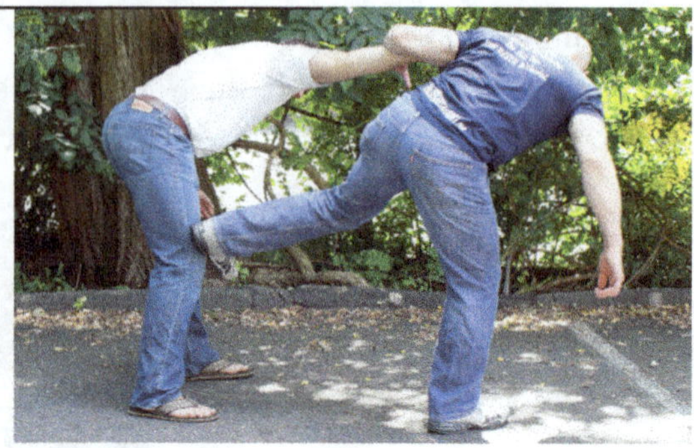

Side bear hug.

SIDE BEAR-HUG

You've been attacked from the side and your arms are trapped. Lower your weight by bending your knees and keeping your back straight. Capture their hands with your hands and stomp their foot, do a Side Head-Butt, and then a Hammerfist Strike to their groin with the hand closest to him. Step behind your outside foot with the foot closest to him and drive your outside arm up into the air as you make a 180-degree pivot with your feet. Maintain a grip on his wrist and kick his knee with a Lead-Leg Side Kick.

REAR BEAR-HUG

You will either be attacked with your arms trapped or free. With arms free is an easier attack to defend.

REAR BEAR-HUG, ARMS TRAPPED

The defense for this attack is virtually identical to what you do in a Side Bear-Hug attack, except you add a "Butt-Butt" into their groin as part of the loosening-up sequence. The Butt-Butt technique is exactly as it sounds. You drive your Butt into their groin.

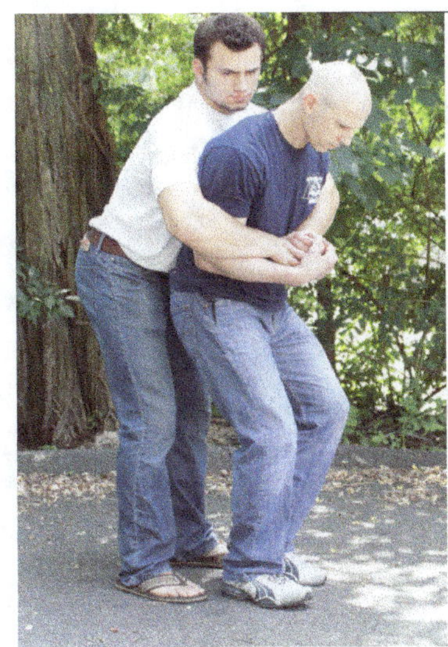
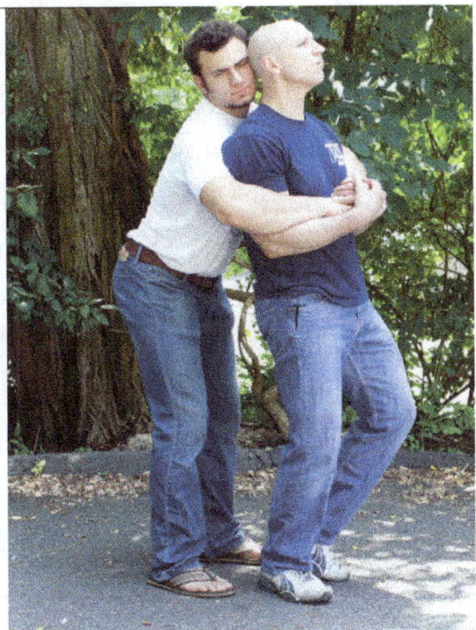

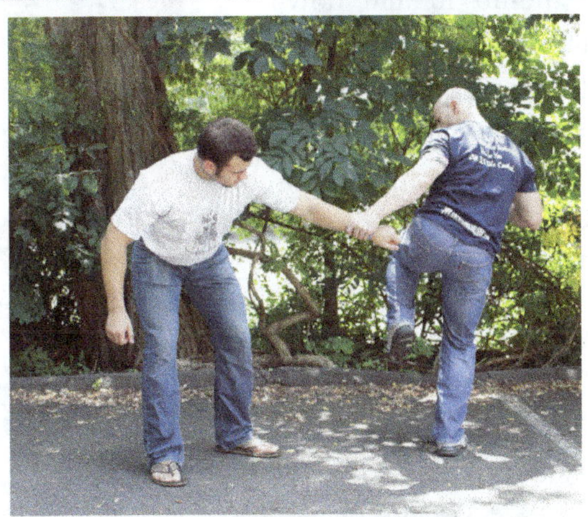

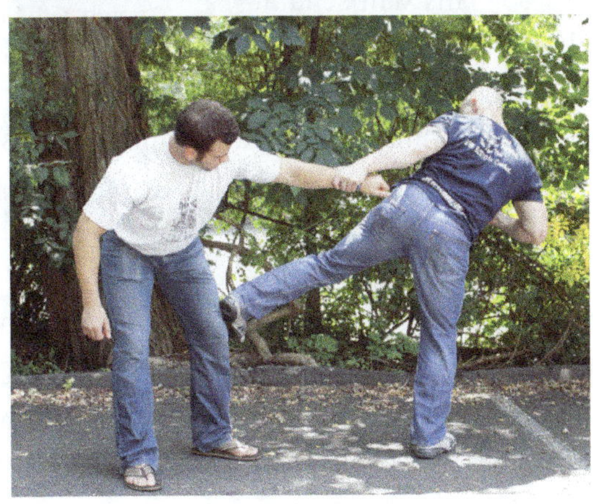

REAR BEAR-HUG, ARMS FREE

When your arms are free, drop one leg back and deliver a double ear slap, cupping your hands as you force the air into their ear canal. Then move to an eye gouge, knees to the groin or any of the many other finishing techniques. Alternatively, when grabbed you may attack their Episternal notch, the little "hole" at the base of the throat above the collar-bone. I like to brace with one hand behind their neck and drive my thumb in and downward. If you simply go straight in, you will not shift the throat cartilage to the side, thus enabling your thumb (or fingers) to get at the sensitive throat. If you have smaller hands, use two fingers to jab the area.

My favorite move here is the Thumbs to the carotid. Grab their neck and place your two thumbs on their carotid artery and jam them into the area with great force. This will send a "shock" through the assailant's body and enable you to deliver Kicks, Knees or other Strikes to finish them off, enabling your escape.

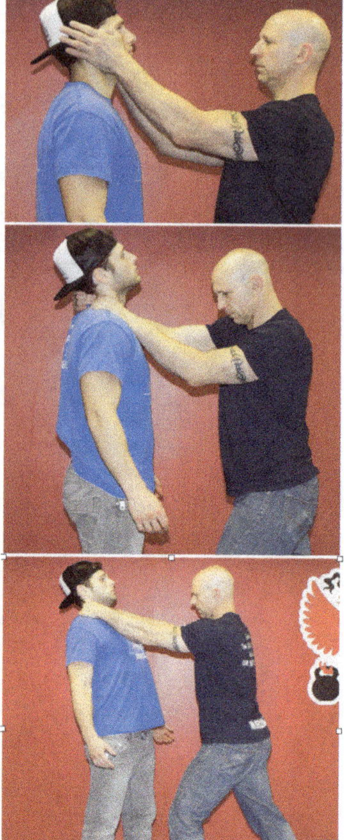

Double ear slap | Episternal notch with brace | Thumbs to the carotid.

KICKS

If you are being attacked with kicks by someone who throws them with proficiency, the attacker has probably had some training. Also, a kick, even from an untrained person, is more powerful than a punch. Your legs are much stronger than your arms. This is a fact. Also remember that your movement and blocking drills will come in handy when facing a kick attack.

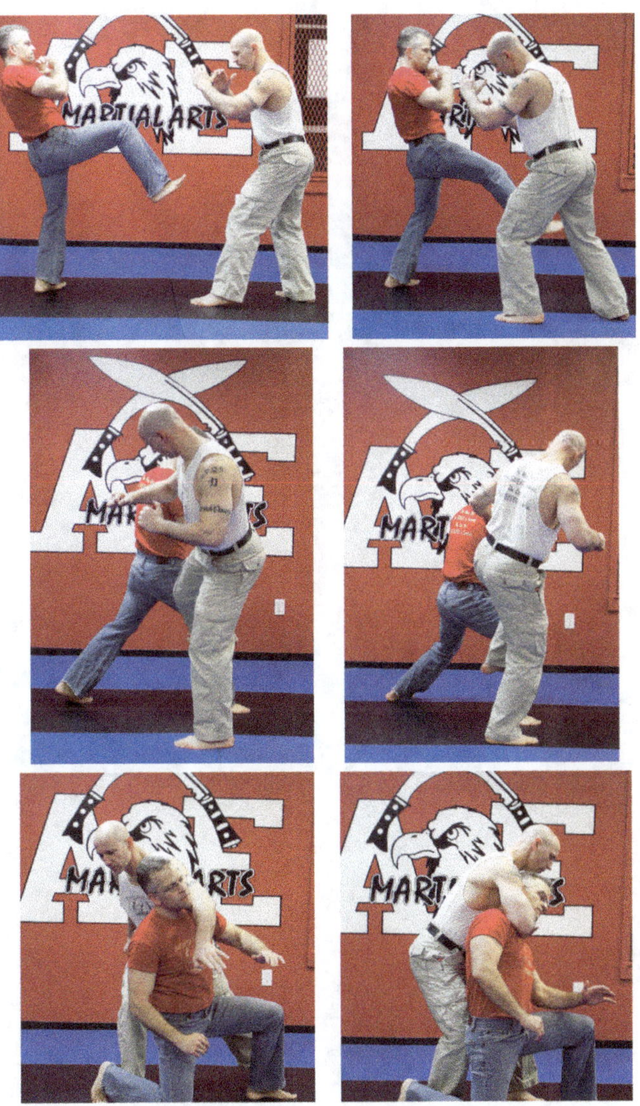

Front kick, a lot of room.

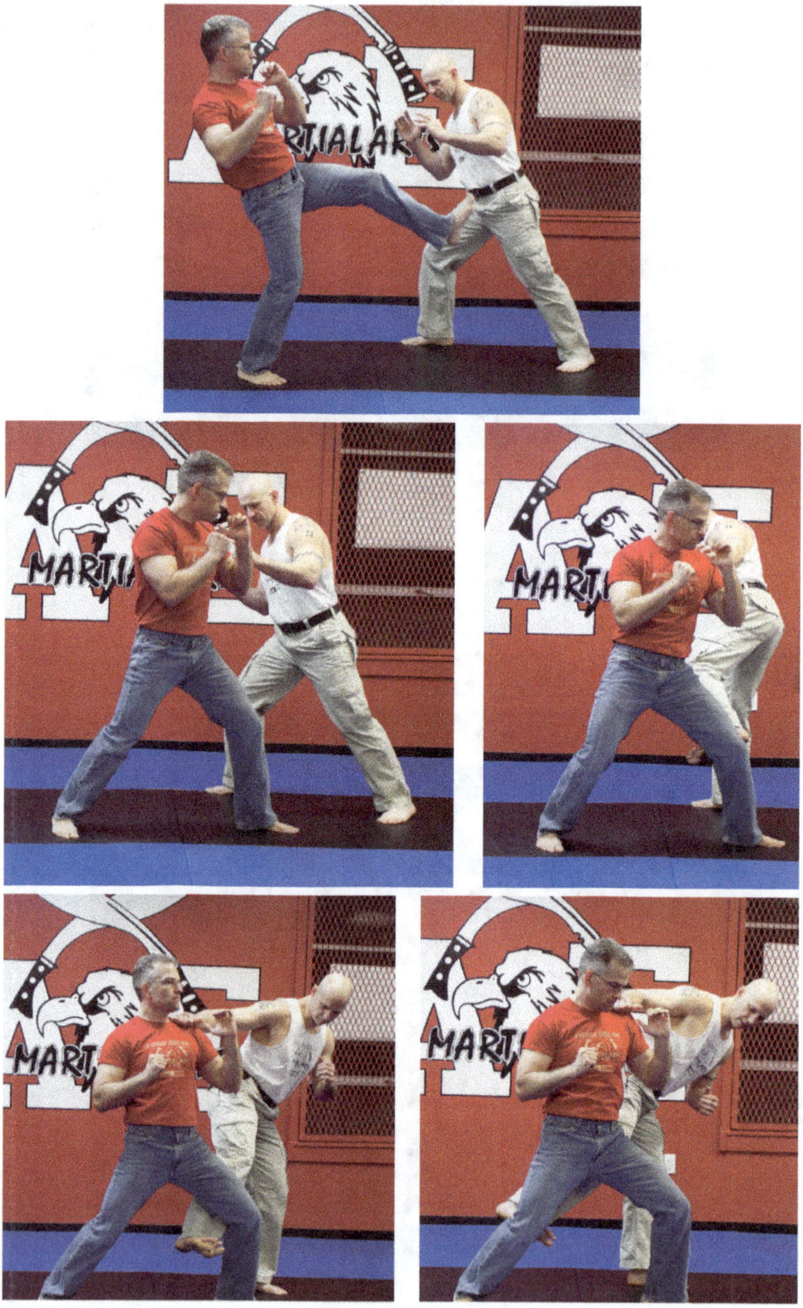

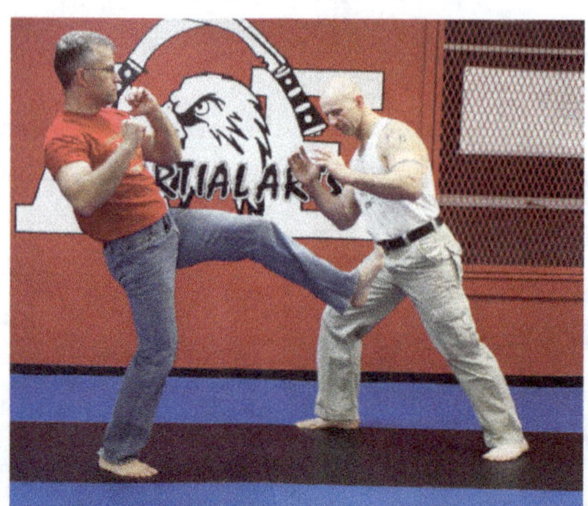

Front kick, a lot of room (opposite side).

FRONT KICK ATTACK

If you are attacked with a Front Kick, you will either have a lot of room or very little. For example, a lot of room would be in a mostly empty parking lot, while a little room would be in a parking lot between two cars.

FRONT KICK, A LOT OF ROOM

Use your Box Step and deliver a Side Kick to the back of their knee with your right foot and then Cut Kick their same leg with your left. Next, send a Side Kick into their other leg with your left foot before putting it down. Now, either deliver Elbow Strikes to their head or apply a Standing Rear Naked Choke.

FRONT KICK, NO ROOM

You will need to parry their foot to the side with your hands. We normally don't drop our hands this far down, but in some instances, you will need to take chances to neutralize an imminent attack. All else is identical to the aforementioned defense, minus the first kick.

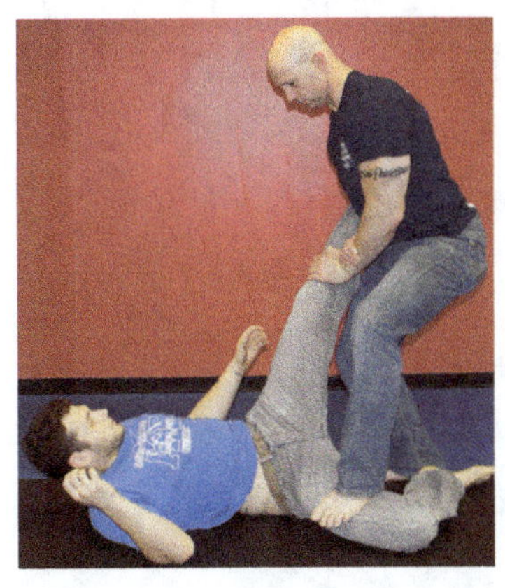

ROUNDHOUSE KICK ATTACK

The most dangerous part of this kick is the foot. A well-placed Roundhouse Kick is like a powerful whip. If you get hit in the head, groin or ribs, the results can be devastating. It's important to get inside the kick and cut the power off at the knee. Step in with your hands up, elbows directed into their leg as you perform a combination block/ strike. Next you will grab their leg and secure the Python Lock (Figure-4) on their leg, kick them in the groin, and take them down by lifting the captured leg and sweeping the remaining leg. Maintaining your hold on their leg, it's now time to employ the Italian Gas Pedal. What this means is that while your opponent is supine and you are standing above them with one of their legs in a Python (Figure 4) Grip, take the foot closest to their groin and stomp down on it as you pull up on their leg.

CUT KICK ATTACK

As we are aware from our training, a Cut Kick is a particularly devastating blow. The following are some of the most effective methods to defend yourself from this powerful weapon.

KICK STOP

If you are being attacked by someone's right leg, pick up your left foot and Push Kick the attacker anywhere between the knee and the hip.

QUICK KICK

Once their attack is launched with the right leg, quickly switch your hips, bringing your left leg to the back. Immediately "bounce" your foot off of the floor and deliver a counter kick to the back of their leg.

LEG CHECK

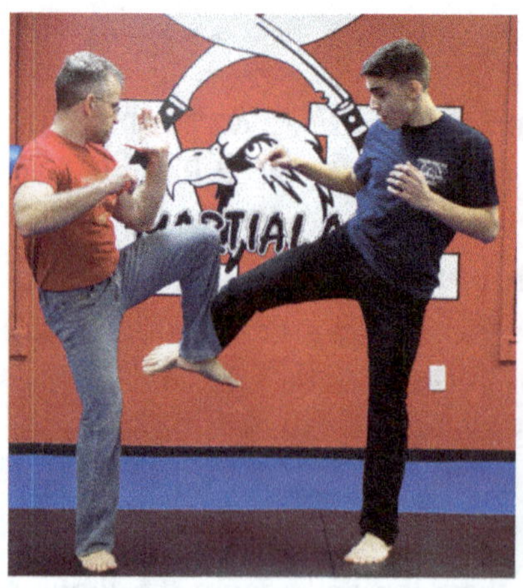 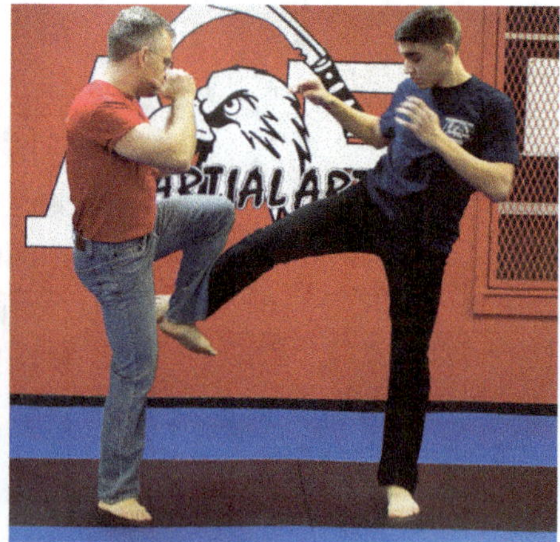

As the right-leg kick comes at you, lift your lead leg and angle your knee or upper shin toward the oncoming kick. You'll want to have your knee slightly pointed toward the outside of your foot at approximately a 15-20-degree angle. Step to the inside and implement your counter-attack.

KICK STOP AT THE HIP

Since we know that all techniques start at the hip, we will focus our attack here. If the opponent starts to throw a kick or if you believe that they are about to, bring your corresponding leg up quickly with your leg straight and "shove" your foot into any spot from the top of their knee to their hip. You will be stopping the kick at its origin. Then move forward with your counter-attack.

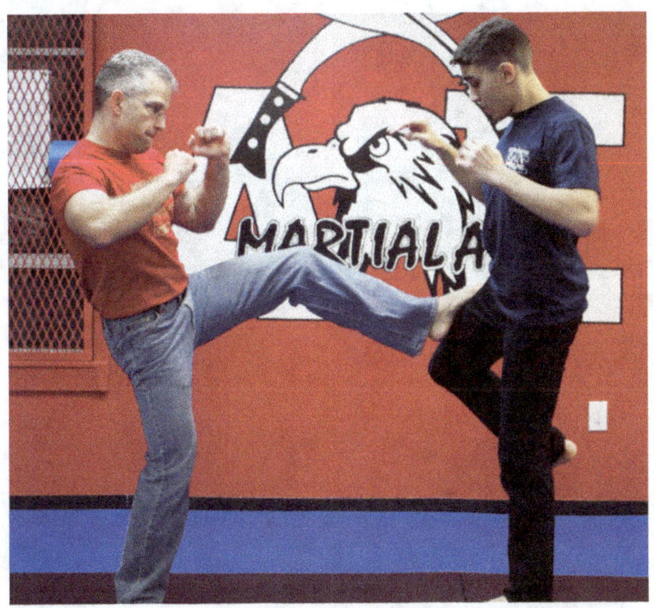

GRABBED LEG

You now have become an accomplished kicker and you train to throw your kicks in a confrontation. Fine, but what do you do if your leg gets grabbed? Sprawling is one excellent option, but what if your leg is up too high? What can we do first?

If your leg gets grabbed, your opponent's hands will be occupied, leaving his face and head open for a counter attack. Instead of moving away from them, launch yourself toward him and grab the back of their neck with one hand while delivering Elbow Strikes to their face and head. Once you have loosened them up, drive your knees into their groin and bladder until you are free or they are incapacitated.

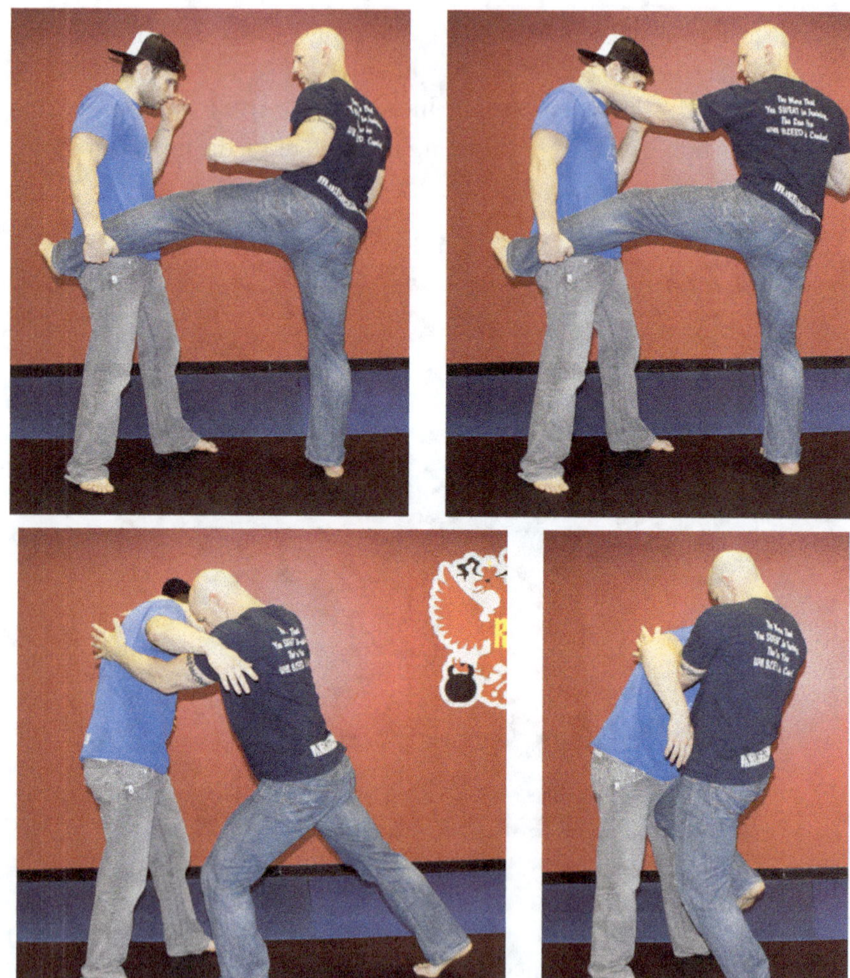

Grabbed leg.

GROUND PINS

Before we discuss Ground Techniques, you must consider how you got there. Were you taken down or knocked down? Were you hit with a strike that caused you to fall? Were you simply lying there and got caught by surprise? You may need some recovery time to gather your wits. This may entail hugging the attacker until your head clears.

We will focus on the worst of the scenarios: your assailant has you in a Full Mount with either your arms pinned or they are choking you.

ARMS PINNED

You are in the Full Mount and your assailant has your wrists both pinned against the floor. There are several movements that must be done simultaneously to make a successful escape. Shoot your hands off to the side,

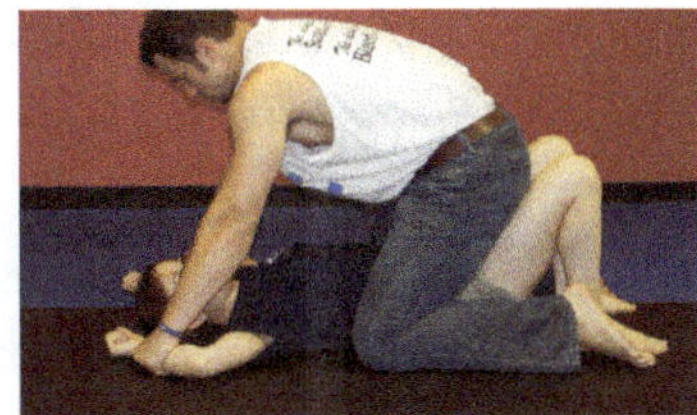
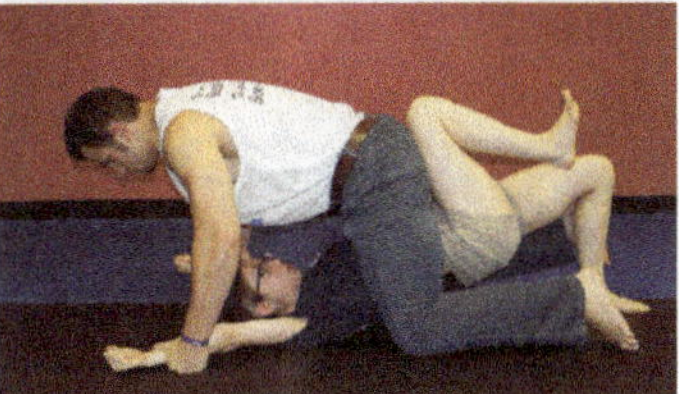
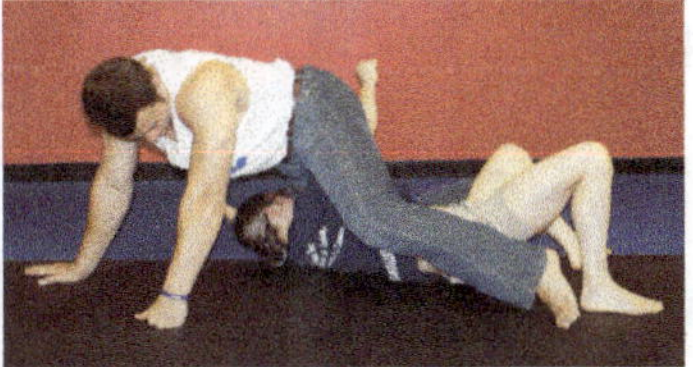
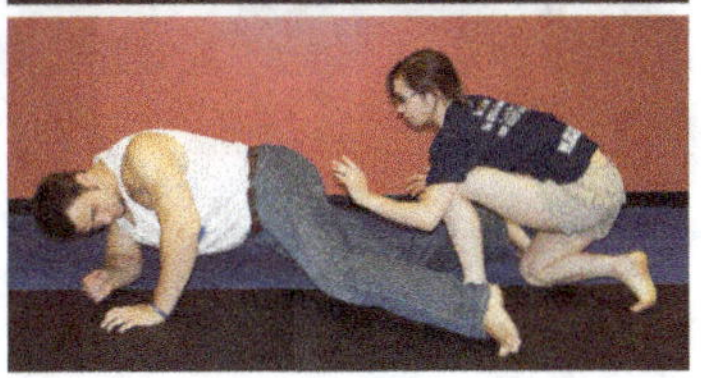

Arms pinned.

Bridge toward the ceiling, and drive your right knee into their coccyx bone. Trap their left arm with your right, Bridge again, and roll to your right while pushing on their ribs with your left hand to add power to your move. It will then be time to finish the maneuver. You will be in their guard, or at least between their legs and on top of them. Place your forearms on their abdomen and levy punches to their chin and elbows to their thighs until their legs open. Now you smash the groin.

CHOKING

You are in the same position as you were in the previous move, except the attacker is choking you while sitting on your chest. You do not have much time. Your first action will be to punch your attacker's ribs and then Finger-Jab them in the eyes. This is followed by a double Knife-Hand Chop directed to the assailant's elbow pits. After the Chop, clamp their left hand to your chest with your right hand. Strike them in the throat with a left-hand Scissor Punch as you perform a Bridge Pop and roll to your right. Do the same finish technique as you did for the Arms Pinned defense.

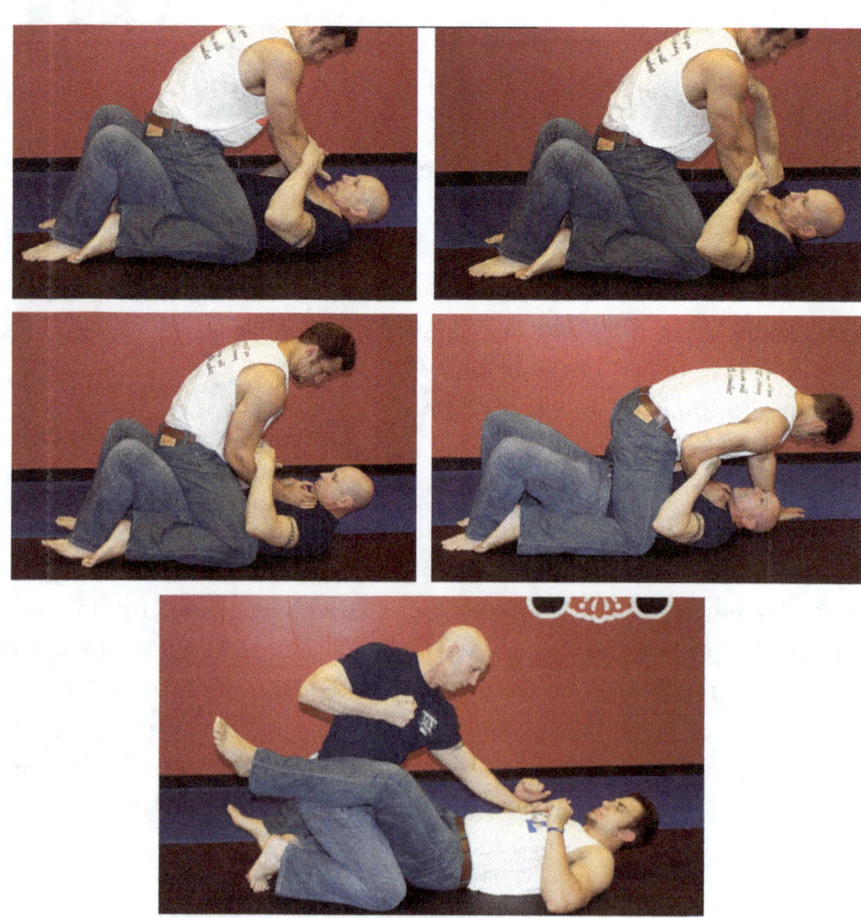

Choking.

HAIR GRAB

I personally have the world's best defense for the Hair Grab: my head is completely shaved. So, unless you are sporting the same hairstyle, you'll need to learn a defense for this attack. Another important tidbit to note, men who plan to assault women love ponytails, which they can use as handles to grab and control their intended victims.

FRONT HAIR GRAB

The assailant facing you grabs a fistful of hair with their left hand. They will tend to grab and twist, tightening their grip, and then pull you forward and down.

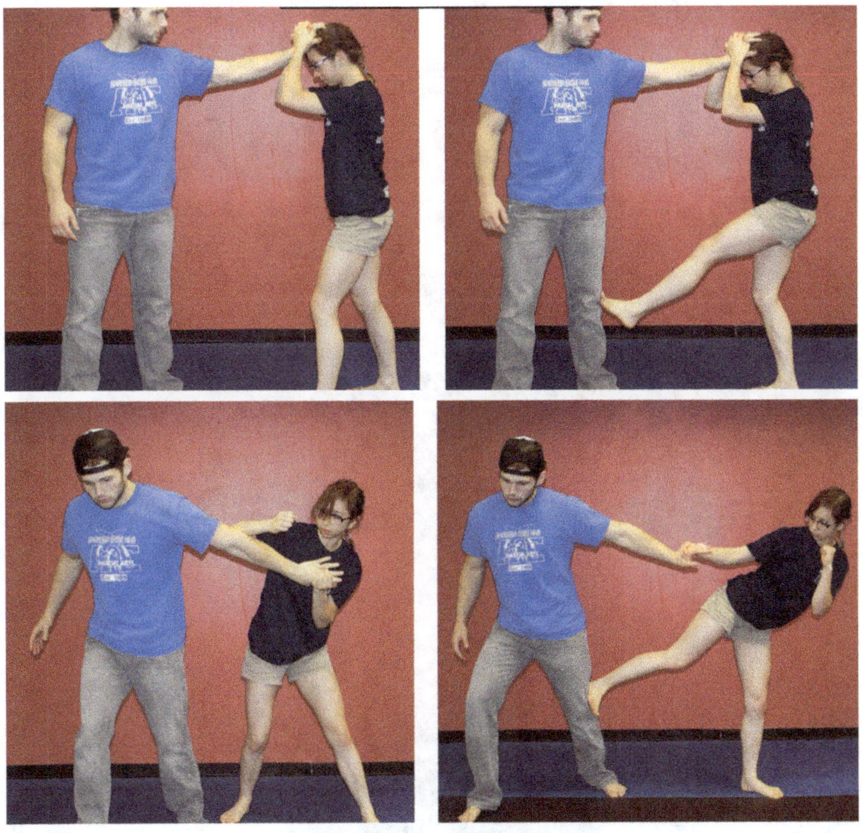

Front hair grab.

Place both of your hands on top of their left hand and step into them. As you step in with your left foot, deliver a Knife-Hand Chop to their bicep insertion with your left hand while maintaining the grip on the hand on your head with your right. After the Chop, smash them in the face with your elbow as you pull their hand in the opposite direction. Think of the movement as if you were yawning and stretching, making your chest big, only doing this very quickly. Grab them by the back of the neck, thread your hand under their arm and give them Knee Drives until they drop, just as we have done to finish several other defensive tactics.

REAR HAIR GRAB

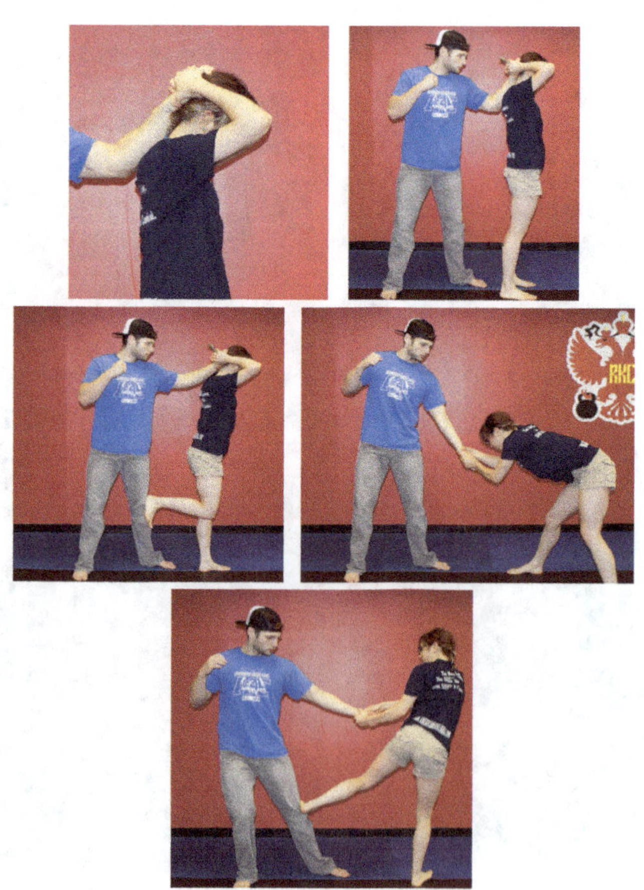

When you are attacked from behind with a Hair Grab, place both of your hands on the grabbing hand and move backward quickly into them as they pull. They will be expecting you to pull away, so this will disrupt their balance and buy you some time. As you are moving backward, Kick and Stomp their shins and feet, which may free you. If not, and they have grabbed you with their right hand, step backward with your left foot and bend at the waist as you snap their hand down. Once they are bent over, pretend as if it is Fourth and Long and deliver a punt to their face. For the non-football fans, simply kick them in the face with an upward Front Snap Kick.

DOUBLE LAPEL GRAB

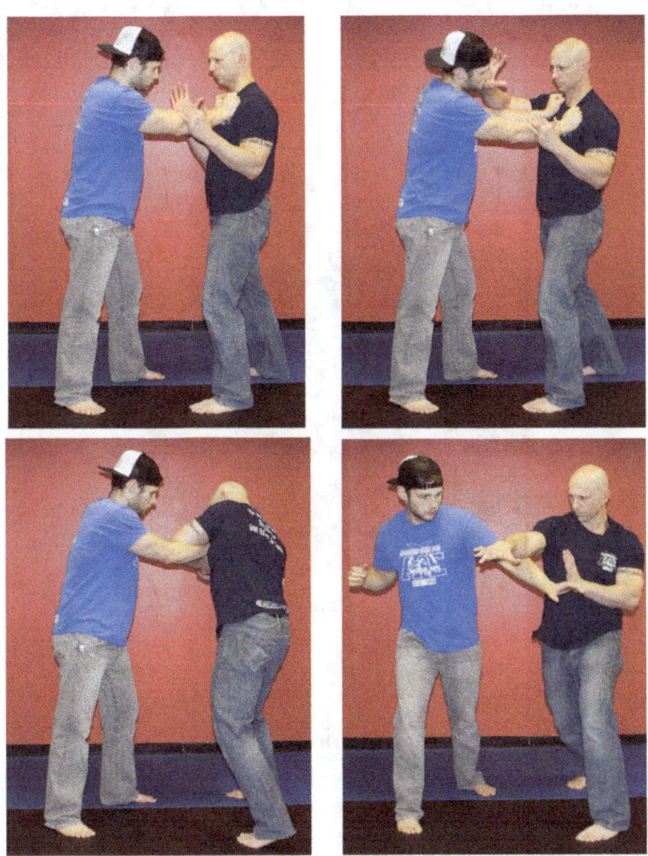

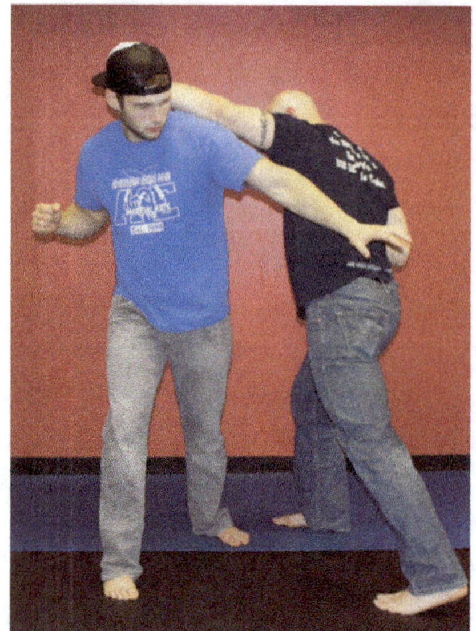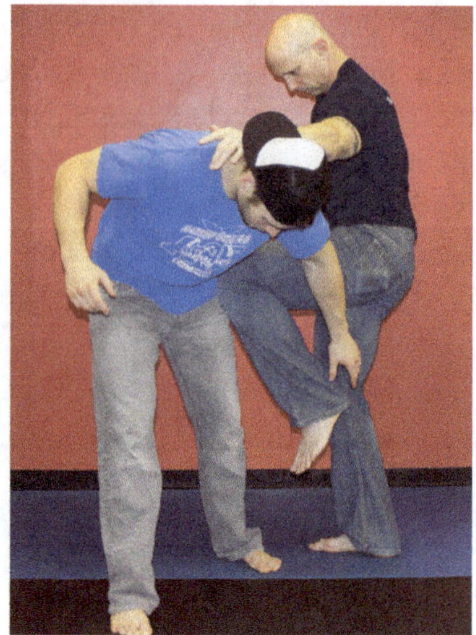

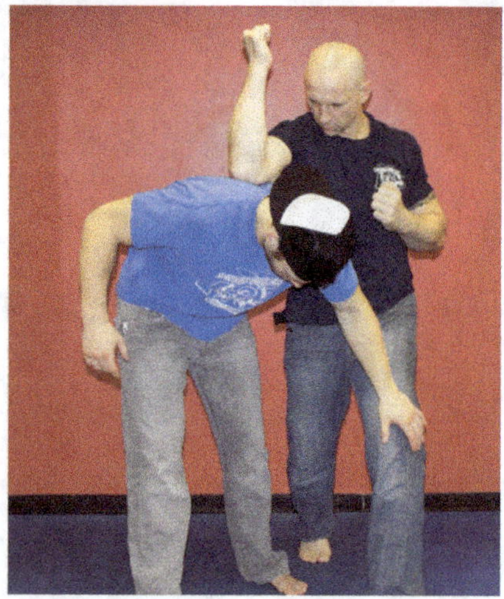

Double lapel grab.

In this attack, it's important to note that both of your attacker's hands are compromised. He probably thinks that you won't resist, and he wants something from you. This is an advantage for you.

A disadvantage in this situation is if there are multiple attackers, one grabbing you and the other committing some other sort of act against you. We'll address the single-attacker defenses here and the multiple attackers at the end of this chapter.

CHOP DEFENSE

Once your lapels have been grabbed, Palm-Heel Strike the assailant in the nose, double clap their ears, rise up on your toes and drop your weight as you do a double Knife-Hand Chop downward on the bend in their elbows. Finish them with a Head-Butt to the nose and Knee Drives to their groin and bladder. Push them away and Front Kick them in the nearest, most vulnerable available target.

THREAD DEFENSE

Begin your defense again with a Palm-Heel Strike to the nose. If you Strike with your right hand, thread your left under their wrist. Apply pressure downward on their right wrist with your left elbow and position your left hand so that your fingers are facing upward and the back of your hand is against their left wrist. Twist your hips from right to left while keeping your arms locked. Trap both of their arms with one hand. This position is transitory, so start to strike immediately, directing your blows to their temple, floating ribs and peroneal nerve.

TACKLE

A Tackle is generally a Rage Attack, and the attacker will be filled with fury as they rush you. The negative for you is they are committed to the move and they are coming at you hard.

This is also to your advantage, however, since they are unable to change directions easily when attacking in this fashion. In this situation there are three basic options for defense: the Front Kick, the Knee Drive or a Redirect.

FRONT KICK

You need to be very confident and possess a very powerful and quick Front Kick to pull this one off. As they charge, stand your ground and time your Full Front Kick (off of the back leg) to land as they get into range. It's risky, but if you're good at the Front Kick your results will be favorable and the damage that you cause will be debilitating.

KNEE DRIVE WITH SIDE STEP

When they are charging at you, wait until the last possible second and hop to the side and deliver a Round Knee to their midsection and a Knife-Hand Chop to their neck.

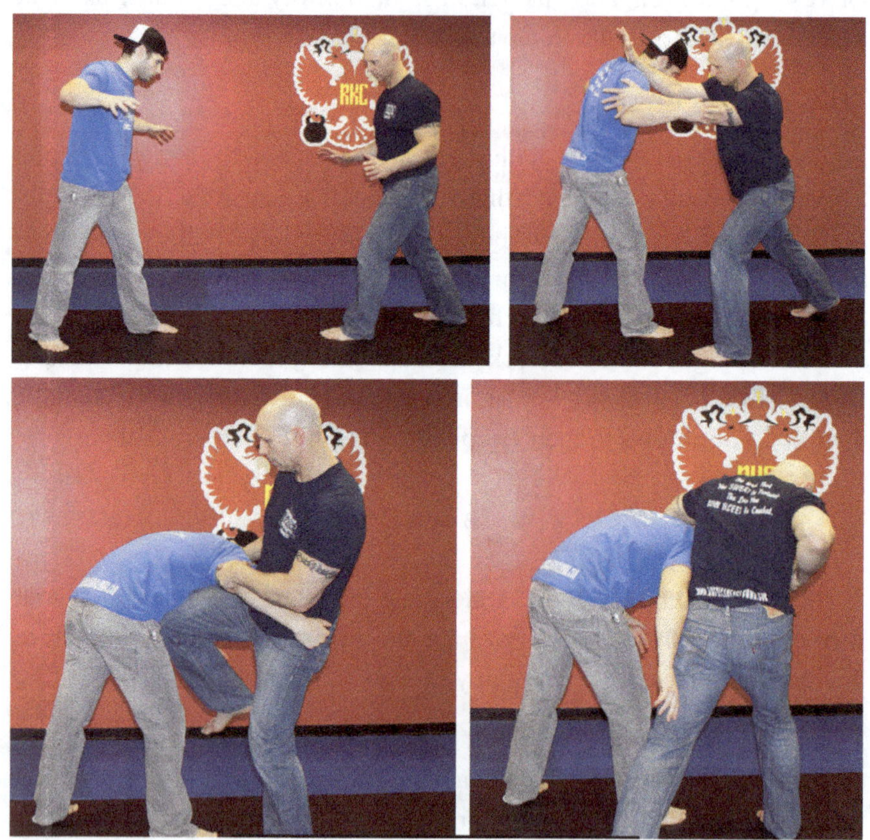

Knee drive with side step.

REDIRECT

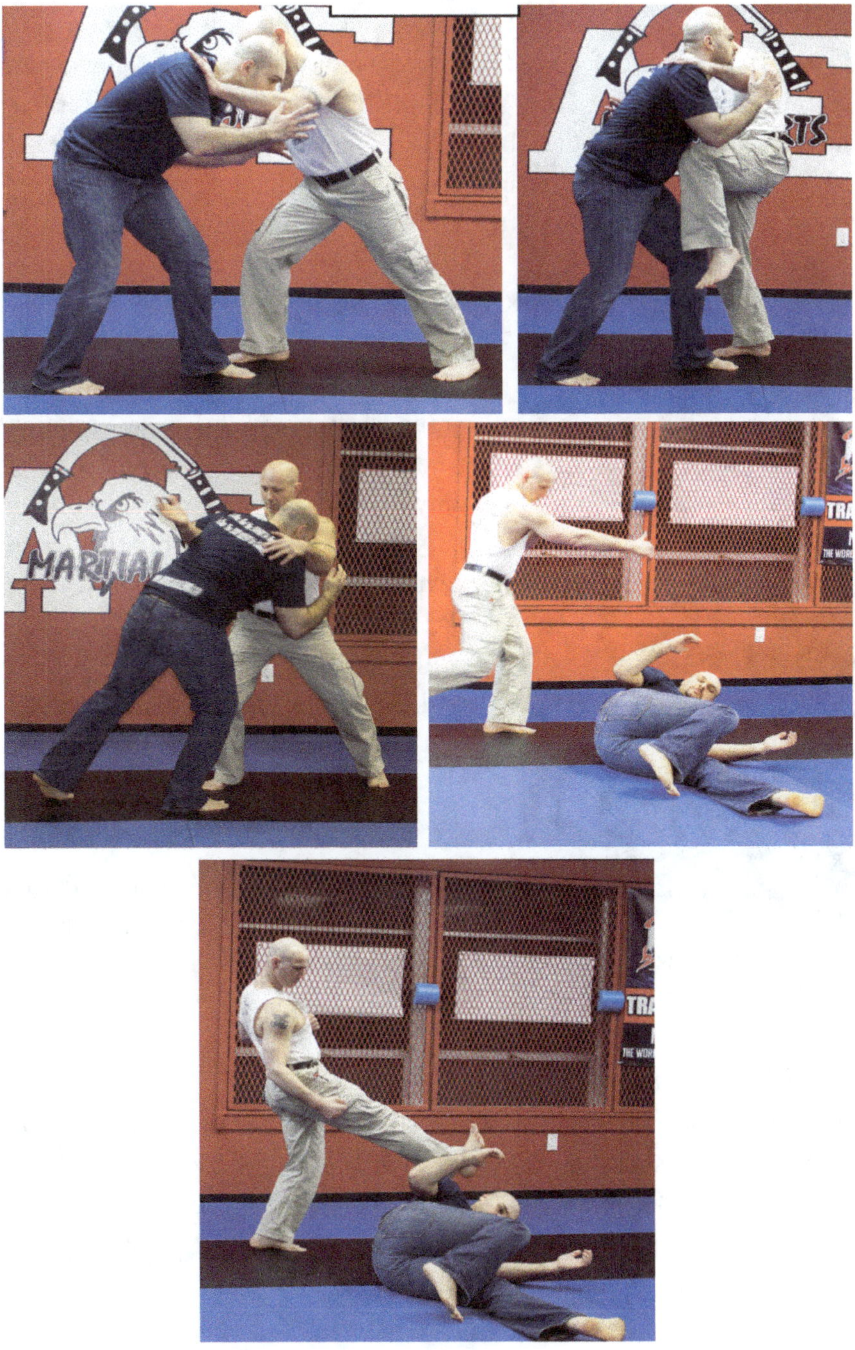

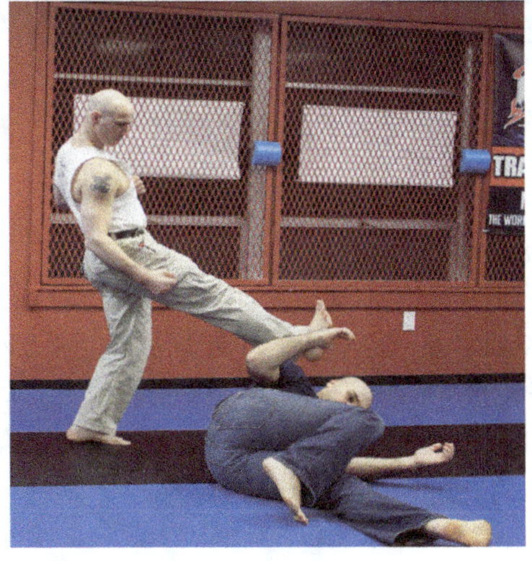

This is another timing-based defense. Just before they reach you, hit them with an Axehand Strike to the side of the neck or head with your right hand and thread under their outstretched left arm. Perform a 180-degree step with your right foot as you redirect their head downward and toward their right knee as you lift up your left arm, thus turning them so they fall onto their back where you were previously standing. Do what is necessary to finish them. Throw kicks their head and body, or use your Parachute Stomp to end it.

FROM THE GROUND (KNOCKED DOWN)

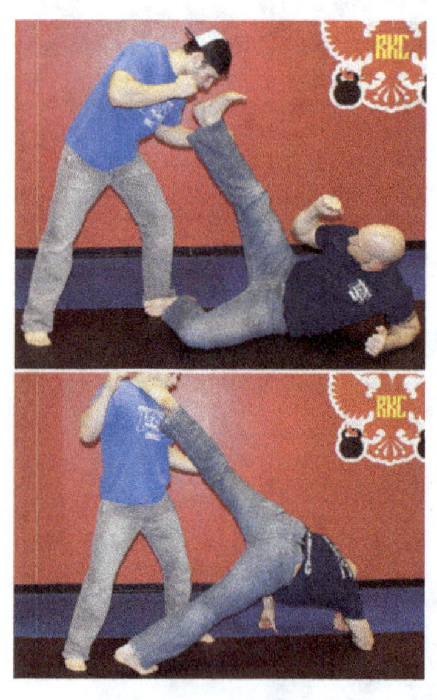

Up-kick heel | Up-kick roundhouse.

If you fall or get knocked to the ground, assume the side position where you are up on your elbow with only one side on the ground, not lying on your back. This position has great advantages for fighting, other than the fact that you are on the ground and could easily sustain an injury from broken glass, nails, sticks, etc. if you're in a littered area. However, if you are here, you need to be able to defend and move from this position.

I generally mix the following defenses together, changing from one type to another. I change sides and circle to throw off the attacker.

UP-KICKS

This is seen a great deal in MMA. I would not rely on this for the street, though, as your groin is open. In MMA, the groin is an illegal target area. In the street, there is no such thing. Knowing this, Up-Kicks are still acceptable to mix into your defenses, provided you deliver a Side Kick to the perpetrator's face as you rise up on the non-kicking foot and balance yourself on your elbow and the hand of the side of the kicking foot.

CIRCLE AND KICK

While propped up on your elbow and on your side, rotate and follow your attacker as they try to circle to your back. You may also flip to your other side by changing which hip is on the ground. As you implement a barrage of kicks to their knees, move into them and "chase" them down, kicking and launching yourself aggressively at them.

CIRCLE AND SCISSORS SWEEP TAKEDOWN

You are on the ground and on your side, you're kicking away at his legs, and either he manages to step in, or you close the distance. If his left leg is forward, place your right foot on top of his left and your left foot behind his left knee. Use your hips, not your legs, to turn toward him, rotating 180 degrees. This will knock him to the ground face-first. To keep things simple, roll on top of him and take his back or stand up and kick his ribs and head.

MULTIPLE ATTACKERS

There are an infinite number of possible multiple attacker scenarios that can arise. It would be virtually impossible to even attempt to address them all. As with all of the other described maneuvers, focus on the principles and apply them to the situation at hand.

ONE IN THE FRONT AND THE OTHER ON THE SIDE

If you are confronted with one assailant grabbing you in a Double Lapel attack and another assailant on your right, grabbing the back of your shoulder and chest from the side, here's what to do: direct a Side Elbow with your right arm to the face of the attacker on the side. With the same hand, smash the other opponent in the face and then strike them with your right knee to the groin, and without placing your foot down, direct a Stomp to the side attacker's inside knee with the same foot. It's catch as catch can at this point. Move and do whatever is necessary to secure your escape.

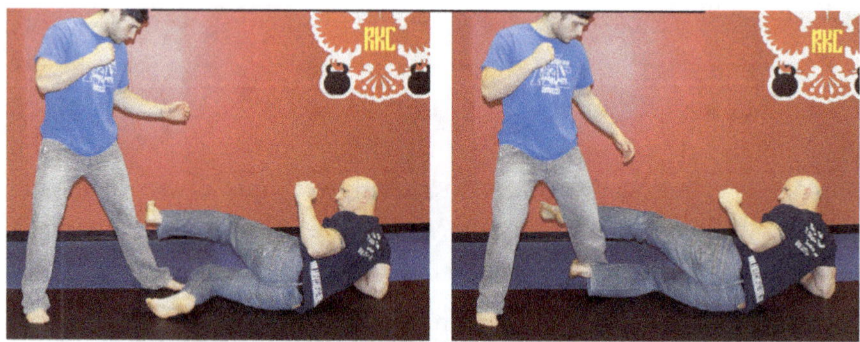

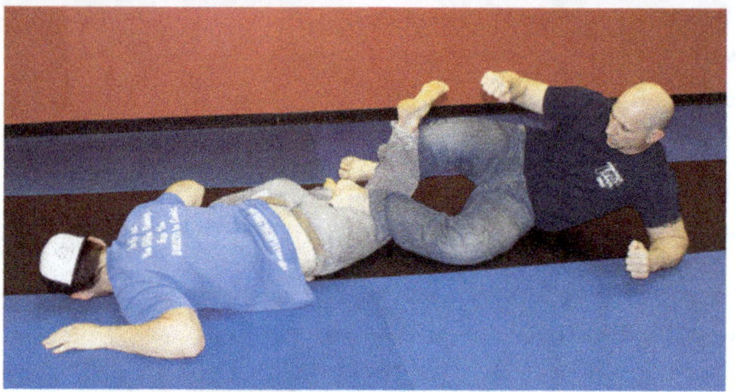

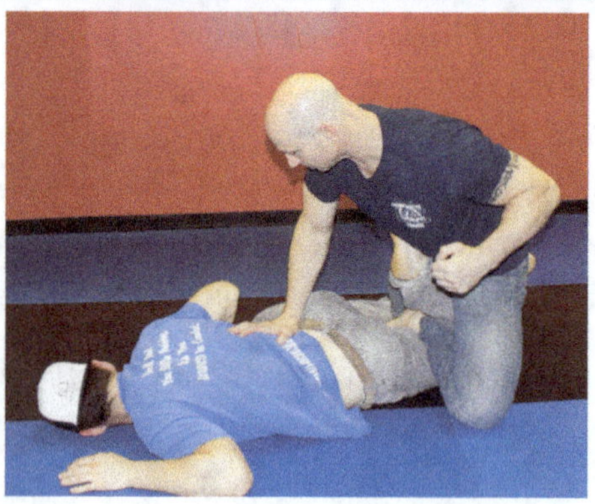

Circle and scissor sweep takedown.

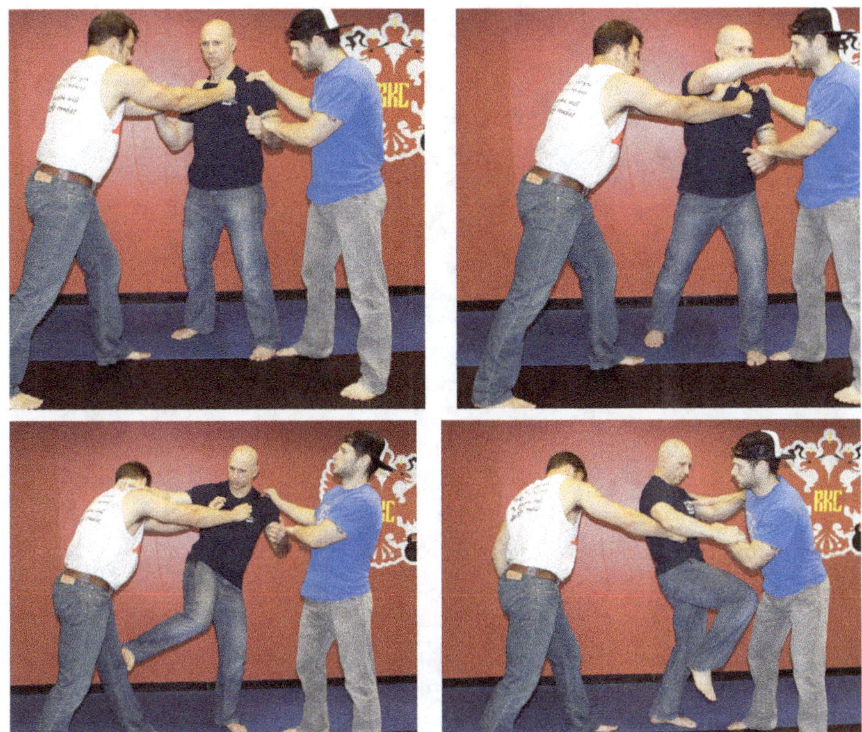

One in front, one on side.

ONE ASSAILANT ON EITHER SIDE

Two guys grab you, one on each arm, and they are trying to take you someplace against your will. Resist first for a short time and then go with it, but run ahead of them. As they strive to catch up to you, jam on the brakes and stop dead in your tracks, and you punch both fists straight down. This will break their grips and they will release you. It's now time to unleash a hellish onslaught of Kicks, Stomps and Strikes to make your escape.

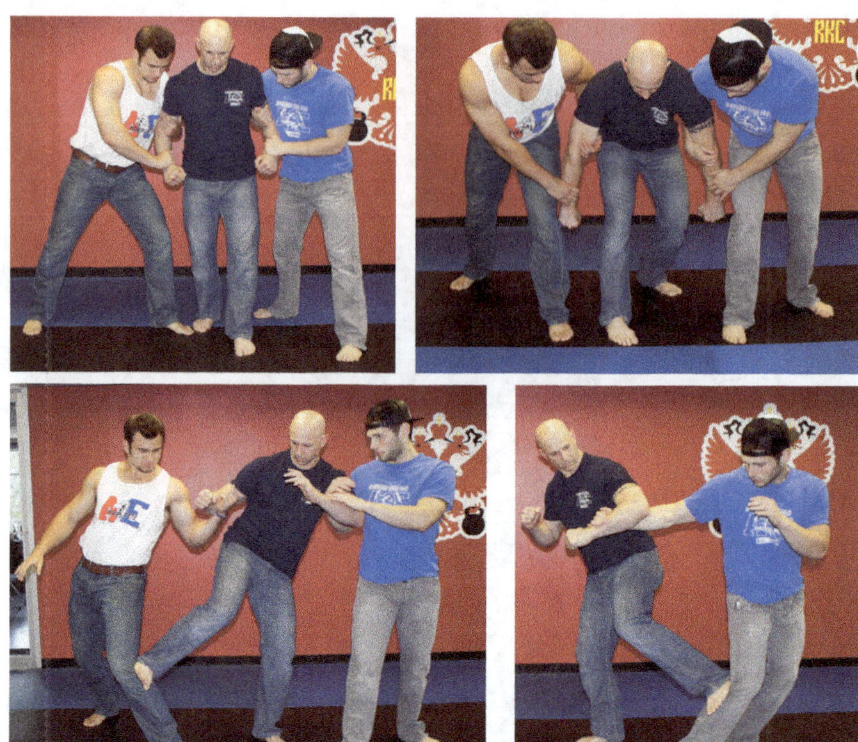

One on either side.

BASEBALL BAT AND CLUB

Blunt, accessible and extremely lethal, the ends of a bat or club are the business parts of the weapon. There are techniques using other sections of these weapons, but for the most part, you will be faced with an instrument being swung at you, even if the assailant has been trained.

Back in the 1980s and 1990s, police were issued and trained in the use of the PR24, which is essentially a tonfa. This was a club with a handle on it that was supposed to revolutionize policing and crowd control. All of the departments were issued the PR24 (Tonfas), their Billy clubs discarded, and they were trained for hours on end in how to swing and block with them. Well, after a few years, it was discovered that the Police were simply flipping the PR24 over and either using the handle like you would a hammer head or using it like a regular club. The bottom line: no more PR24s. Man, I wish I had that contract for the furnishing of the PR24s and the administration of the training; I'd already be retired!

The point that I'm trying to get across is that, under stress, people will only rely on gross motor movements. Swinging a bat or a club is a gross motor movement. Fancy movements are not. As a general rule, you will be attacked with either a Side-to-Side swing, an Overhead (downward) strike, or from somewhere in between.

SIDE TO SIDE

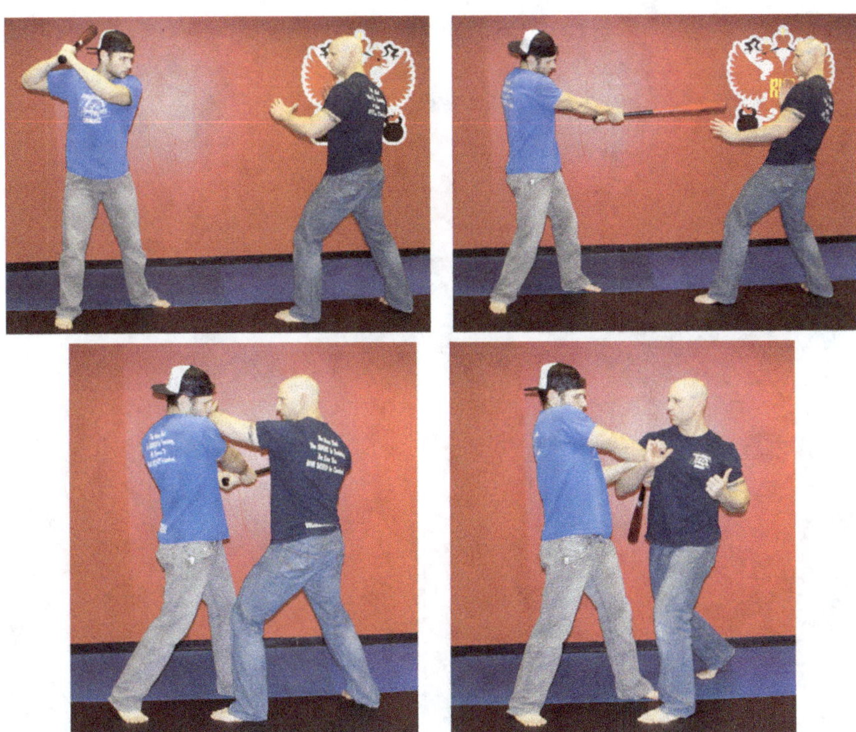

If the attacker swings a bat with two hands like Mike Trout, you need to avoid the business end of the bat at all costs. If you get hit with any part of the bat from the sweet spot (middle section) to the end of the barrel, you will sustain damage. You have two choices here: either move in quickly with a Lunge Step as the bat is drawn back, or fade back out of the way and lunge in after the barrel has passed the center of your body. Once it has passed, you'll be out of danger until the perpetrator comes at you with a backswing. To stop this do an aggressive Step-In Defense, lunging at the opponent with both hands up at a 90-degree angle with your fingertips facing up. Smash into him with both of your arms and grab the bat by looping one arm over it as you Axehand his head with the other and execute Knee Drives. For the Fade Back and then Attack, do as described above, and once the tip of the barrel is past your midline, lunge at him and perform the same finishing technique as before.

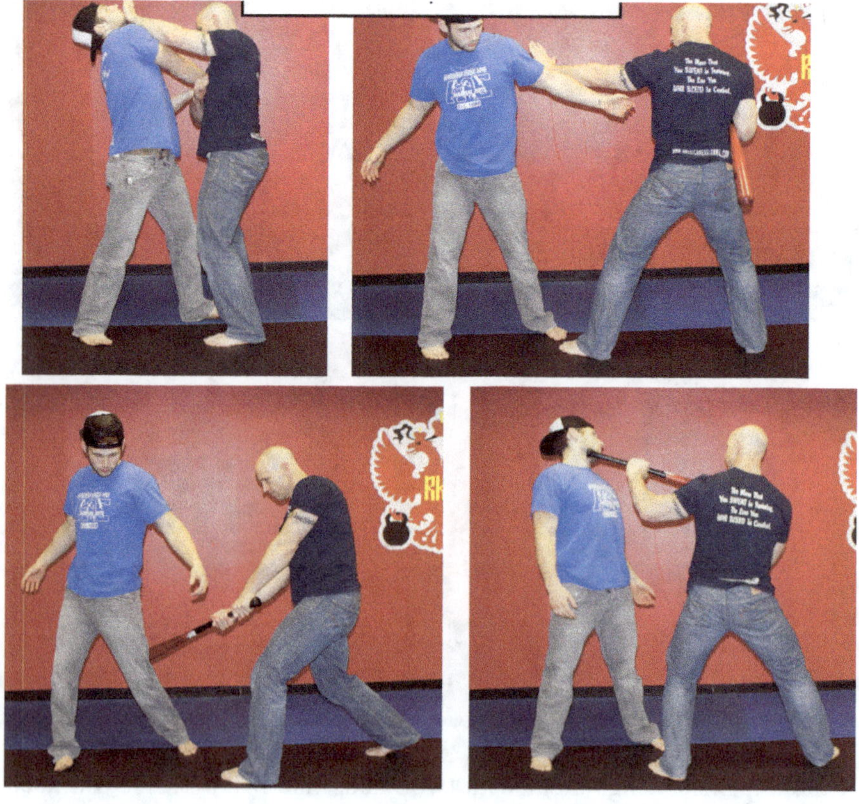

Baseball bat, side to side.

OVERHEAD

Pick a side and use lateral movement, and parry with the inside hand as you step. Take that same hand and wrap your arm around both of his as you Palm-Heel Strike him in the face with the other hand. Kick, Knee and Stomp, and deliver more Palm-Heel Strikes until you are able to secure the weapon and incapacitate the attacker. If you are being attacked from an angle, step to the side the attack is coming from, not to where it's going.

If it's a one-armed attack with a club, either move to the outside or the inside. As a general rule it's always better to move to the outside, it gives you a better position and your opponent fewer options for counterattack. However, you will not always be afforded that luxury and you may be forced to step inside due to the environment or maybe because a person you are with is in the way.

OUTSIDE STEP

If you are confronted with a right overhead or angled downward attack, step inward at a 45-degree angle with your left foot, and perform a High Block with your right hand with your wrist meeting theirs. Take your left hand and do a Downward Chop (thumb first) at the bend in the assailant's elbow. Shoot your left hand across, locking your left hand onto your right forearm, thus creating a Figure-Four Lock. Continue the step inward with your right foot and bow in a semi-circle to your left. This will put a great deal of stress on their shoulder and elbow and cause them to fall to the ground. Disarm them and render them helpless with kicks and stomps.

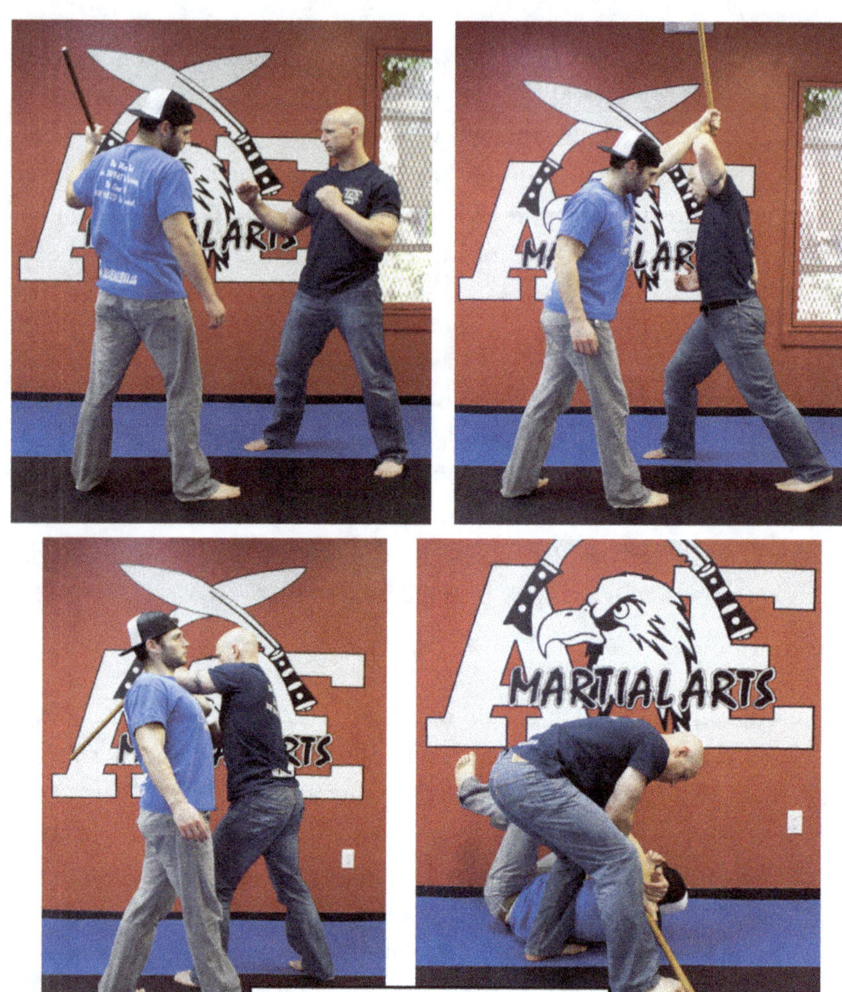

Club, outside step.

INSIDE STEP

If the attack is with the right-hand, step in with your left foot and execute a left High Block. Do a Thumb down Knife-Hand Chop with your right hand and thread your right hand through to your left fore-arm, locking in a Figure-Four. Step with your right foot and pivot toward your left, bowing in that same direction, taking them to the ground. Finish them as detailed above.

KNIFE

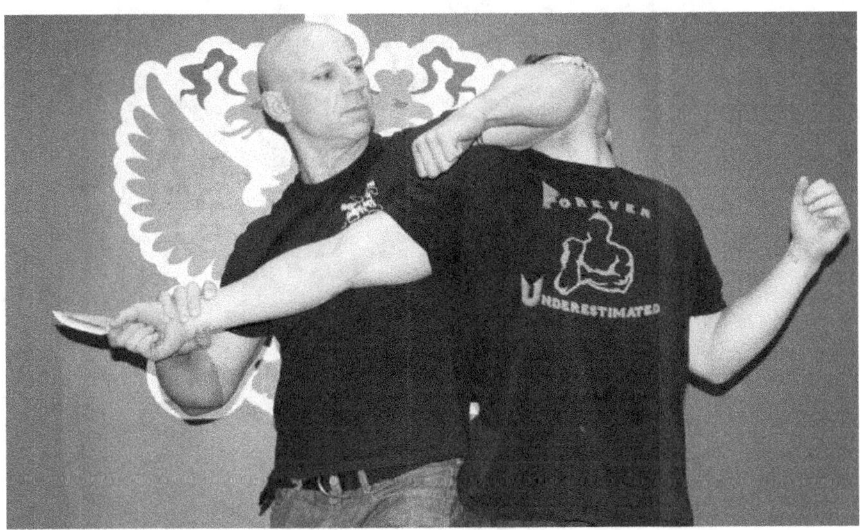

Know this, if you are attacked with a knife, you will be cut. Bearing this in mind, it is important to note that if the opportunity to run away affords itself, TAKE IT, and save yourself. Knives are very accessible, so everyone has them. Heck, you used to get a free set of steak knives when you filled your tank with gas back in the day. Statistics demonstrate that the percentages of people who die when stabbed is higher than the percentages for people who are shot. Imagine that! You have a better chance of surviving a gun attack than you do a knife attack. So, not only are knives more accessible than guns, but they are more lethal. If self-defense is your intent, you had better know your way around a knife.

THROAT

If you find yourself with a knife to your throat, consider yourself dead and every second that you are breathing is extra time on earth. On the good side, if they wanted you dead you would be dead already. Lucky for you, they want something from you first. Once they have that, though, you are done, so you had better act quickly.

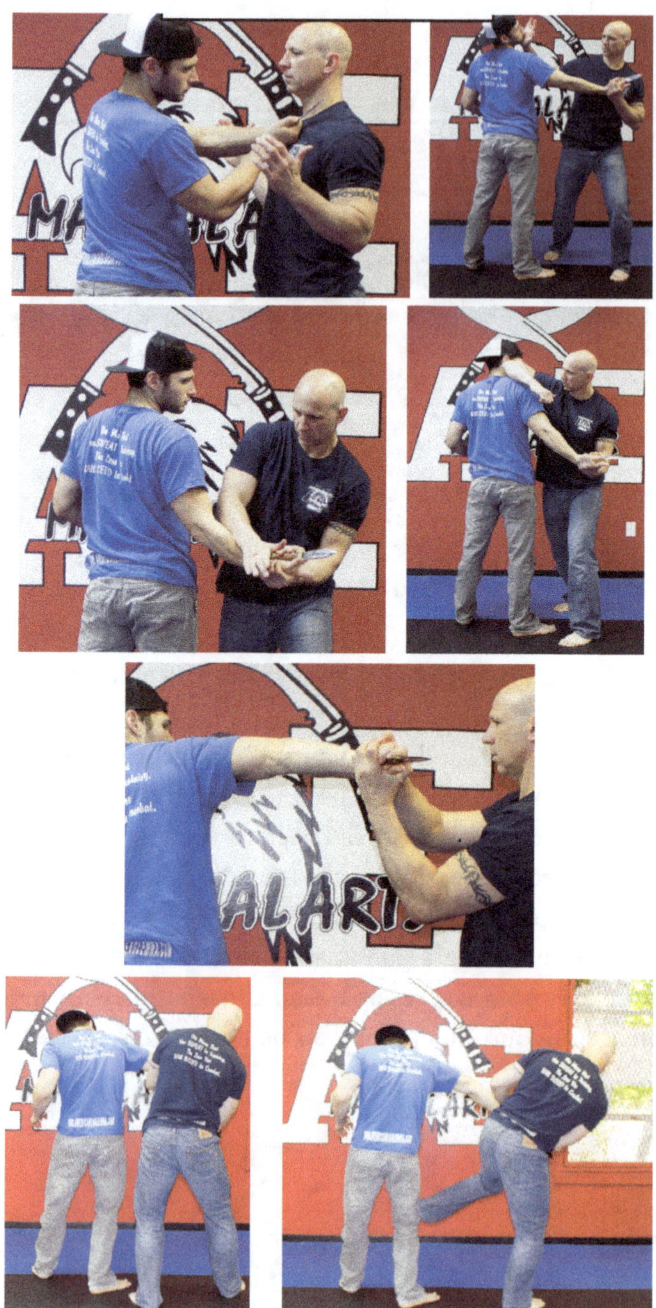

Knife, front of the throat.

To have a chance you'll have to create space between your throat and the blade. This may entail sustaining a cut on your hand, but that's quite a bit better than having your throat cut!

FRONT OF THE THROAT

Let's presume that the attacker has the knife up against your throat and the knife is in their right hand, with the knife point facing toward your left. Put your hands up in the air, placing your right hand slightly higher, and shake it. This will draw their attention to the right hand and away from the left. This is important because you will grab his knife hand with your left. This is the gutsy part; you don't pull away from the blade on your throat. It's against all of your natural instincts, but if you shy away from the blade, you'll rob yourself of much-needed room when you need to execute your defense. You need to perform several motions simultaneously. Rip your head backward and turn your right shoulder forward, and you grab his blade hand with your left hand.

You may have to grab the knife, not just the hand. As you do these movements, slap the assailant with your right hand and then smash them with a Back Hammerfist to the face. Take control of their knife hand with both of your hands, placing your thumbs on the back of the hand and grabbing their hand with your fingers, thus placing them in a Wrist Lock. Step forward with your right foot and snap their arm to the left over your right hip and target their knee with a Mule Kick. Secure the weapon and finish them with any of the variety of methods you've learned.

KNIFE ON THE THROAT FROM BEHIND

You have a knife to your throat with an attacker behind you. Let's make it even more interesting; they have your arm jacked up behind you. The knife is in their right hand, and their left hand is controlling your left. Rip your head backward as hard and as fast as you are able as you grab the knife hand with your right. Step behind your right foot with your left and direct his knife into his chest or abdomen. Do what is necessary to secure your escape.

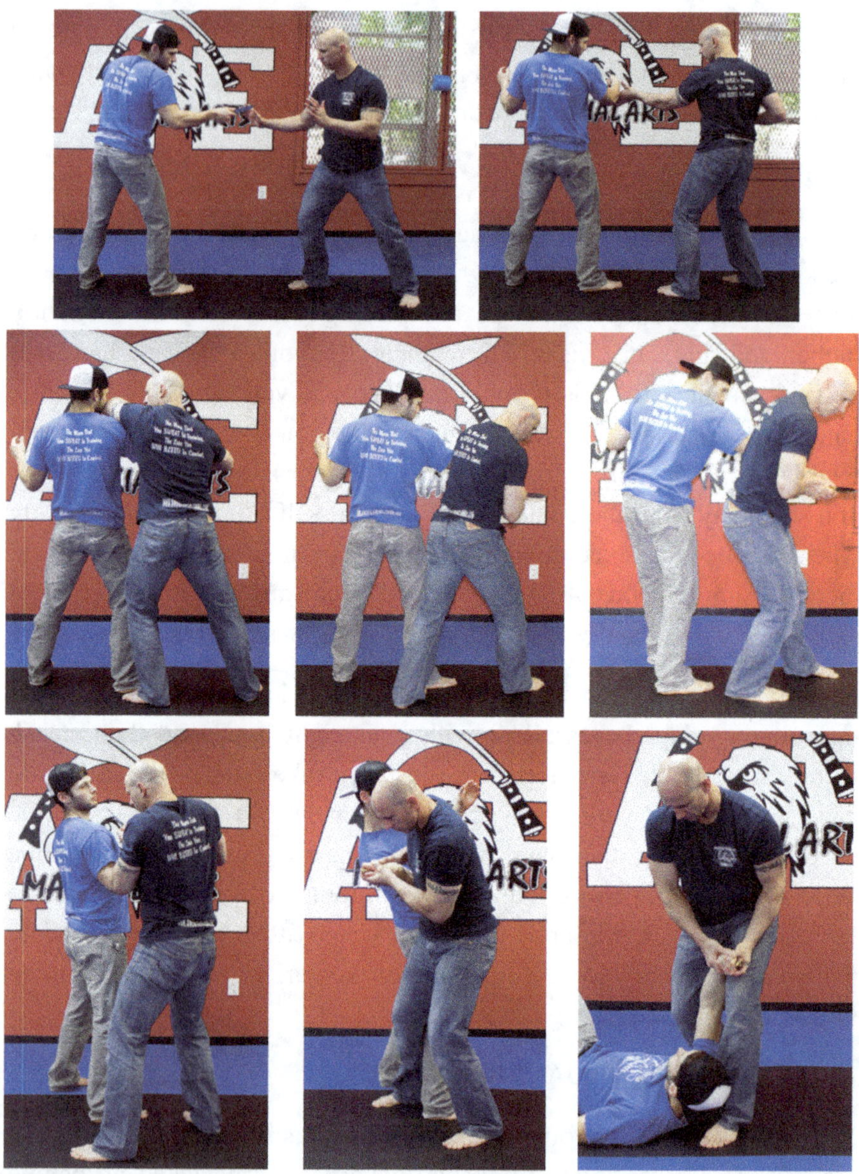

MENACING

If you are approached by a knife-wielding attacker, it will be in one of two manners. They will either be moving a little or moving a lot. It makes no difference what the attack is, and Overhead, a Thrust, a

Slash; it simply doesn't matter; only the movement matters. Look, this is NOT a movie. You are not going to simply grab the knife, flip the guy around, and throw him through a wall. It won't happen like that.

In the real world, the rule of thumb is if they move a little, you move a lot. If they move a lot, you move a little. Abide by this axiom, and you will prevail. When it comes to fighting an attacker with a knife, Boot him. Read on to see how.

MOVING A LITTLE

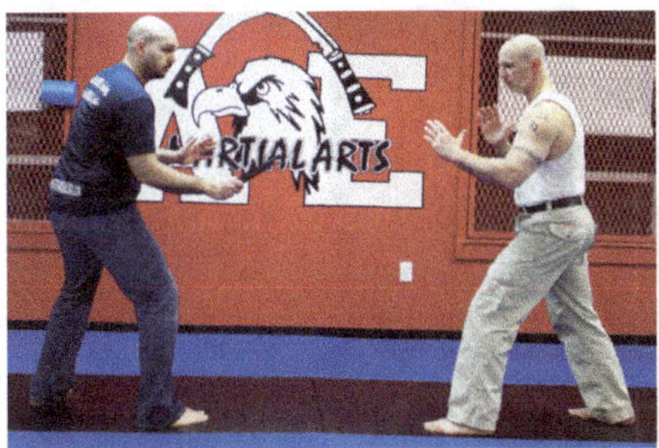
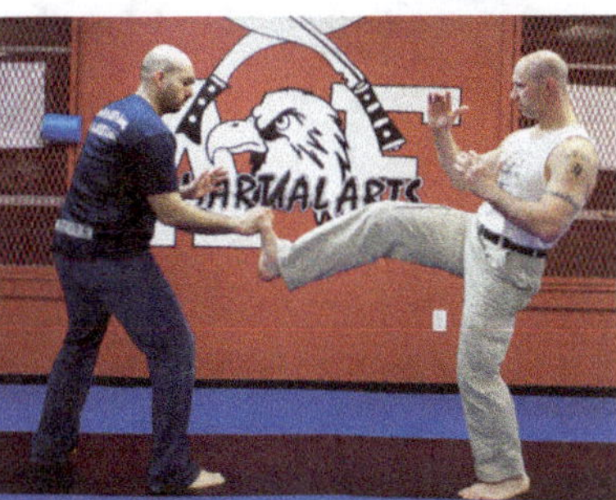

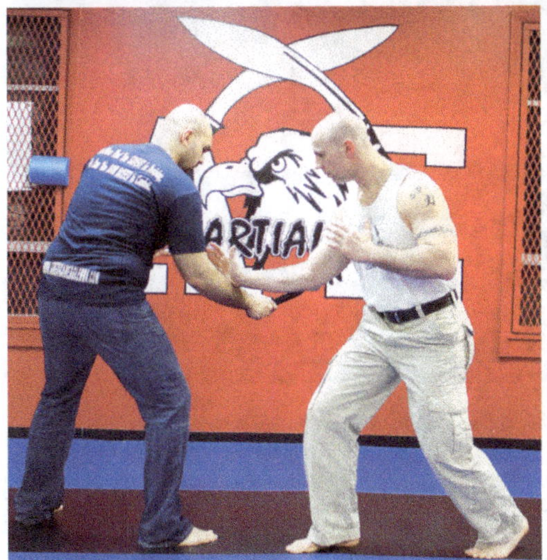
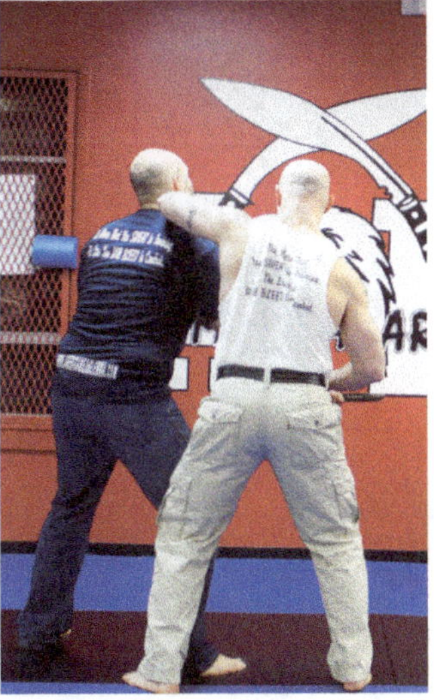

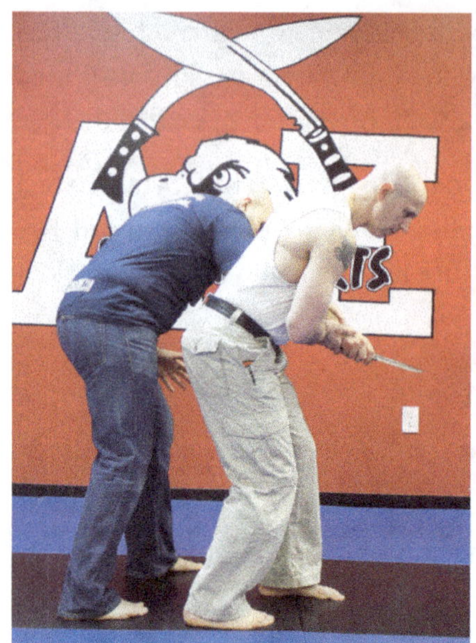

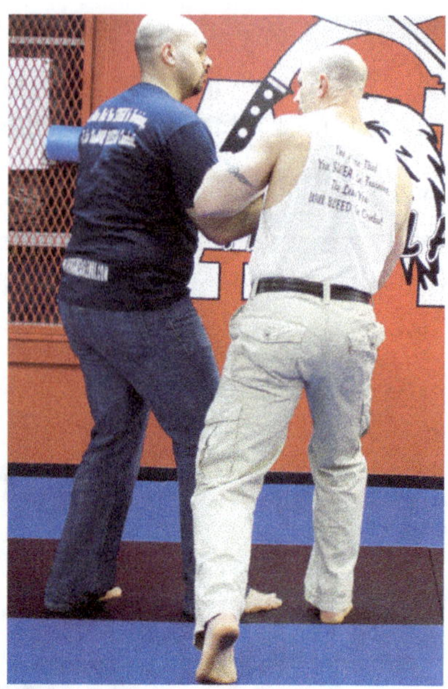

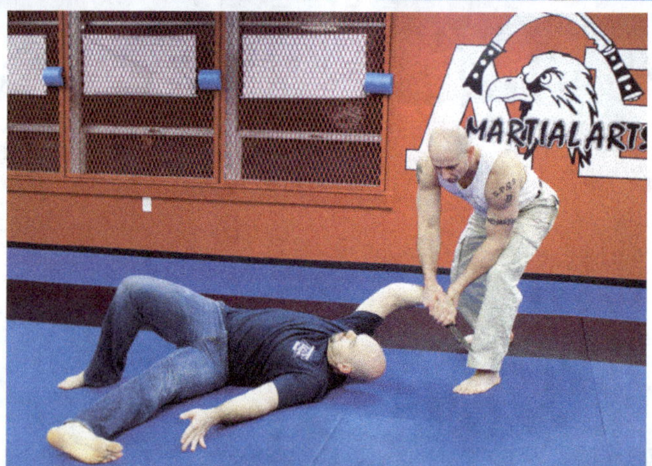

Knife, moving a little.

Suppose your attacker is only moving a little. Meaning they are standing between you and your escape, menacing and preventing you from leaving. As the rule goes, you need to move a lot. So, launch your attack with the Big Boot (Lunging Front Kick) directed toward their center mass. Generally, they will be holding the knife out in front and somewhere in the center of their body. The chances are good that if your kick is directed to the center, you will kick the knife. Whether or not you kick the knife is inconsequential, because you will drive them back and levy Axehand Chops to the arm and wrist of their knife hand. You will next secure the knife hand and deliver an Elbow Smash to their face as you pull on the knife arm extending them and adding additional power to your strike. If the weapon hasn't flown out of their hand by this point, it's now time to secure the knife and administer any of a number of finishing sequences.

MOVING A LOT

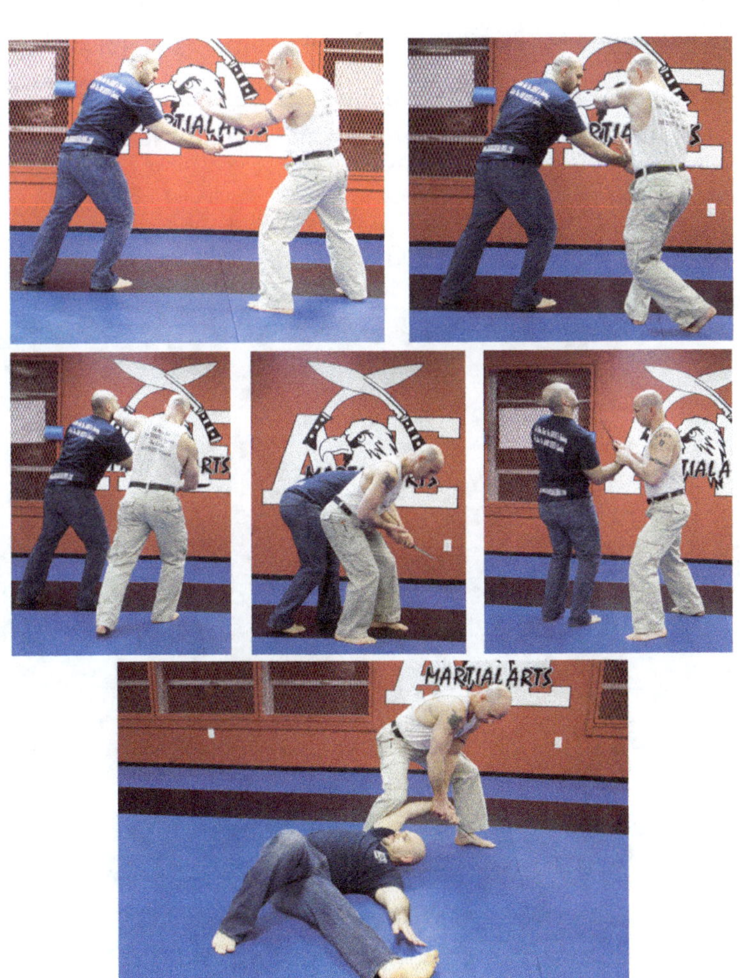

You are faced with an aggressive assailant who is coming at you fast, and thus moving a lot. To counter you will need to move very little and employ impeccable timing. The type of attack with the knife does not matter; overhead, thrusting, slashing or flicking. When you are charged, jump to the side at the last possible moment and deliver a Side Kick to their knee, driving it to the floor and forcing them to collapse to the ground. Follow this move by hacking their knife arm with down-ward Axehand Chops. If these movements do not cause the knife to be dropped, grab the knife hand and perform any of a number of Wrist Locks, securing the weapon and incapacitating the attacker. Finish with Kicks, Stomps and/or the Parachute Stomp.

It's important not to stop until you are sure the enemy is incapacitated. They may have another weapon on them, so don't leave anything to chance.

GUN

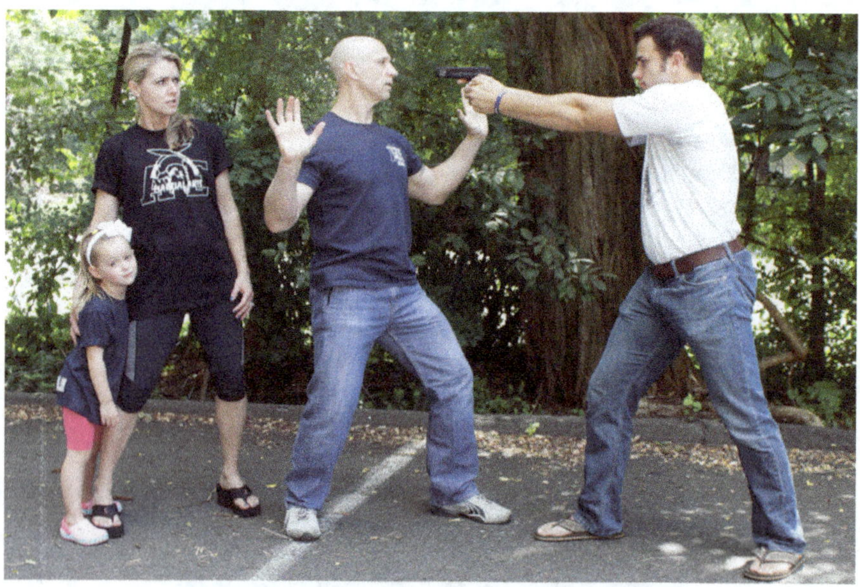

There are many things to consider when being on the wrong end of a gun. Both a fool and a coward can pull a trigger, so there is not much skill needed at point-blank range, just a willingness to do harm. If an assailant is five to 10 feet away from you with their gun pointed at you, it's a tough call; you'll be better suited to get them to come closer to you. As with the knife, consider yourself dead and living on borrowed time when staring down the barrel of a gun.

You have to understand the mindset of the gun-wielding assailant; they feel in control and are empowered by having this gun in their hand. They are in charge. They are the aggressor.

To draw them in, put your hands up and take small steps backward. Many times, this will prompt them to move toward you, generally with larger, more aggressive steps. This will bring them closer to you and within better striking range. If none of this works, you will need to move. Move to the side and in toward them. If you have to take a chance, so be it. Many times, you can get them to miss or their gun may misfire. Many guns aren't in good working condition because they haven't been taken care of properly. Most thugs don't spend the time to clean their guns or make sure their weapon is in good condition.

Remember who you are dealing with; they are most likely not going to be a professional hit man. If they are, you did something to someone that you shouldn't have. If a true professional wants you dead, you never know what hit you.

If you are attacked by a sideways-facing, gun-toting moron, they have no idea what they are doing and have learned their gunmanship from TV. If you hold an autoloader (semi-automatic) gun sideways and fire it, the chances of it jamming are very good.

Below some of the more realistic attack scenarios are listed. There are others, but the principles that you apply here will translate to other situations you may encounter.

GUN TO THE HEAD

A gun-brandishing attacker will generally come at you from the front or the back. Most thugs do not want to be seen, so they will generally be close to you. The good news is that if they wanted you dead, they would have fired already. They want something from you first. The bad news is that once they have gotten what they want, there is no guarantee they will let you live. But while you are alive, you can act. Use your opportunity while it's still there.

Here's how you can respond:

FRONT OF THE HEAD

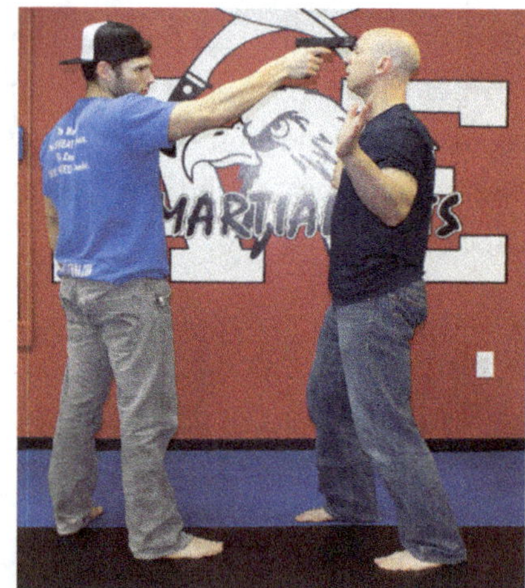
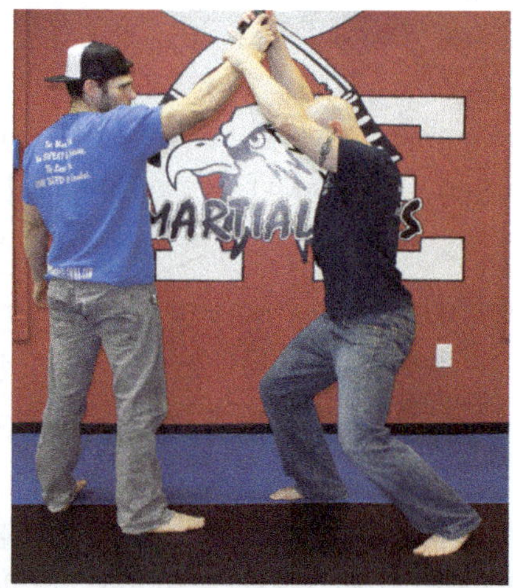
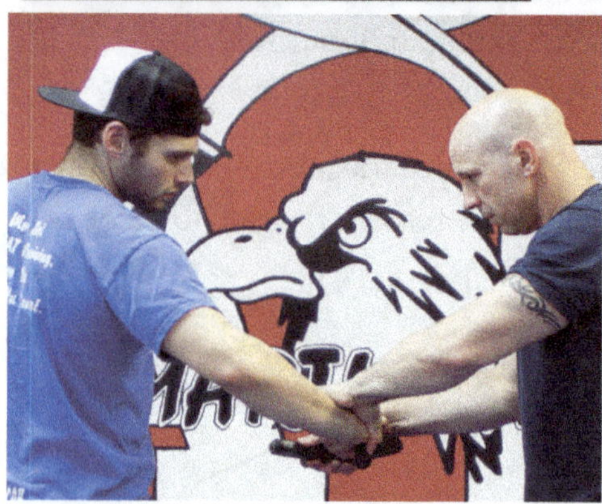
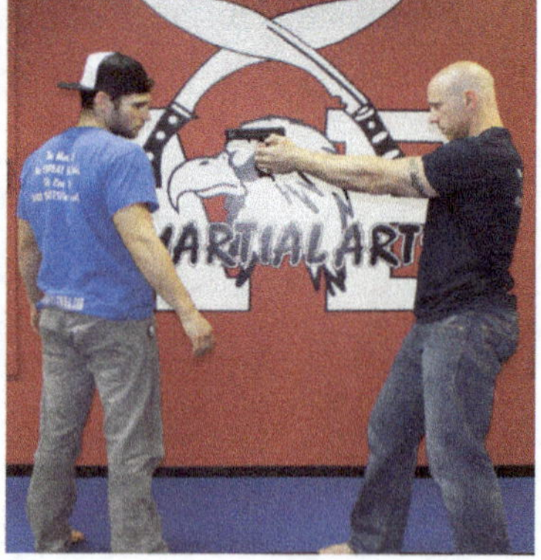

If you have a gun to your head, put your hands up as you did during the knife-to-the-throat attack. Drop straight down by bending your knees and drive your hands directly upward, forming your thumbs into a "V" as you pop the barrel of the gun first upward and then grab the gun with both hands. Snap the gun downward while pointing the barrel upward and toward the attacker. Straighten your knees and resume the standing position, pointing the gun at the assailant. Do whatever you deem necessary to escape with your life.

BACK OF THE HEAD

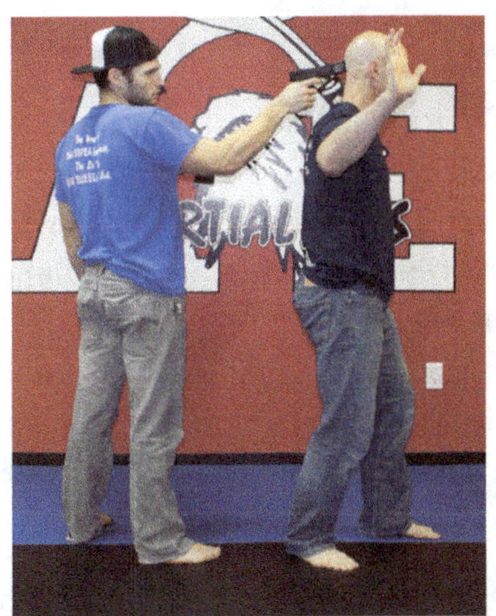
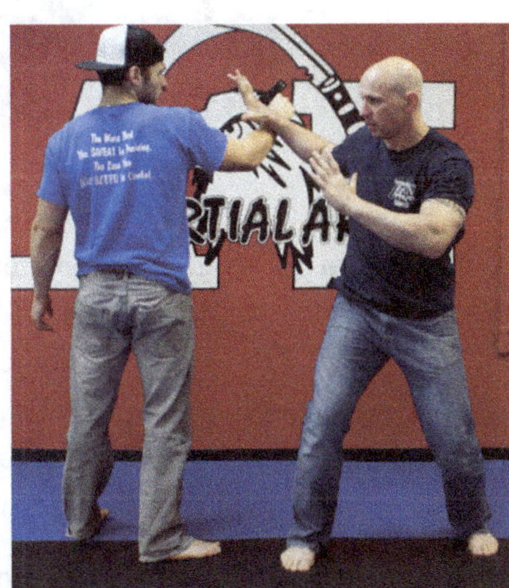
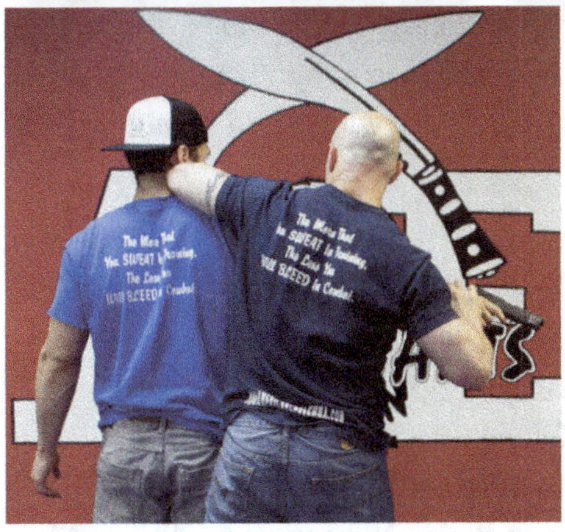
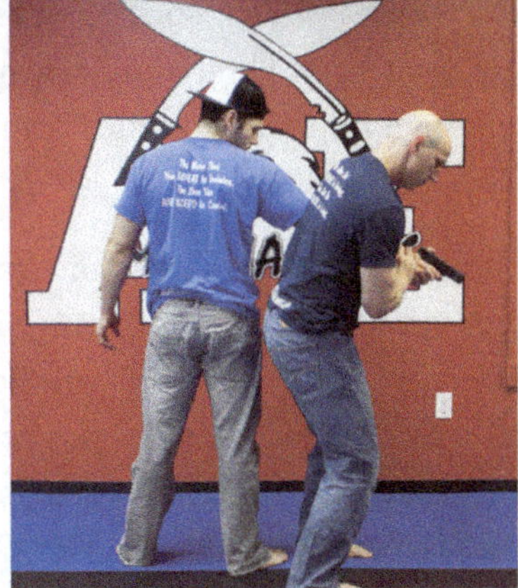

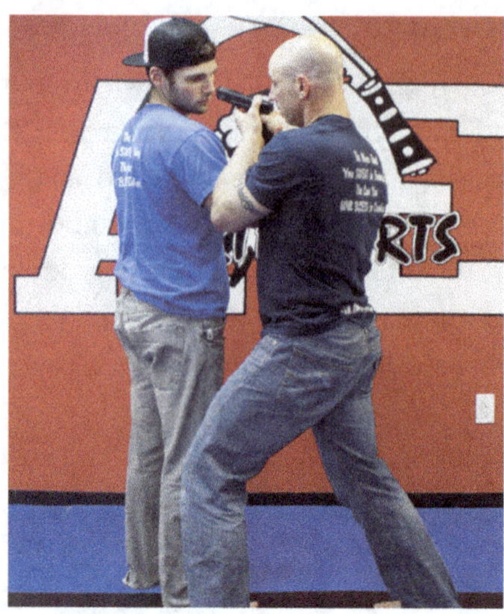

A gun to the back of the head poses several problems. First, you have a gun pointed at the back of your head, which is never a good thing. Second, you don't know which hand the perpetrator has the gun in. It is always preferable to work toward the outside of the gun hand. If, while you have your hands in the air, you are able to determine which hand he has the gun in, great; work to the outside. If not, no worries; the initial movements will be the same, just the finishing will be different.

Let us assume the attacker has the gun in their right hand. You will step with your left foot so it crosses your right as your hands hit their arm. Let your right hand slide down their arm, secure the hand at the wrist, and then hit their extended arm at the elbow with a Left Hammerfist as you pull on the arm.

Suppose we launch or counterattack only to discover that the gun is in the attacker's opposite hand. Since you are moving, keep going in that direction. Your left hand will go along the inside of their arm and make its way to their right hand, securing a grip at the spot where the wrist and the hand meet. As this is happening, your right will deliver an Elbow Smash to the attacker's face. Next, perform a Knee to the groin and then place both of your hands on their gun hand and deliver a Mule Kick to their right knee.

EXECUTION STYLE

If you find yourself on your knees with the attacker standing in front of you with a gun shoved in your face, here's what you do: put your hands up and start begging for your life. But then suddenly shift your head to the left, and drop your head down and to the left as you grab the gun with both hands. Your right hand will have your thumb facing upward, and your left hand will come over the back end of the gun. Push with your right and pull with your left and swivel your hips as you land on the ground, putting you on your right hip. You will now be pointing the gun at your attacker with the newly secured weapon on your left hip. Finish the encounter in whatever way seems appropriate.

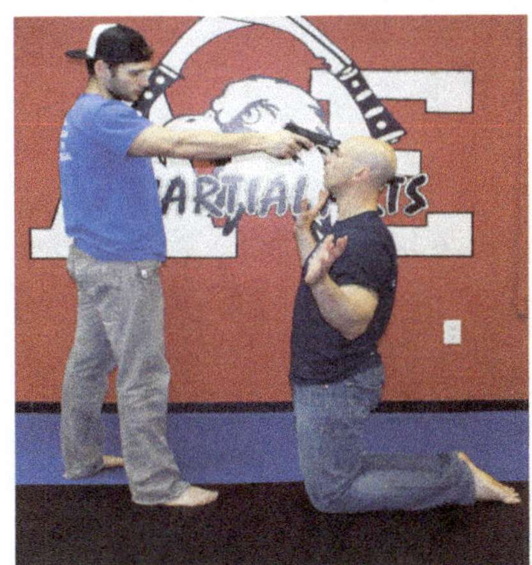

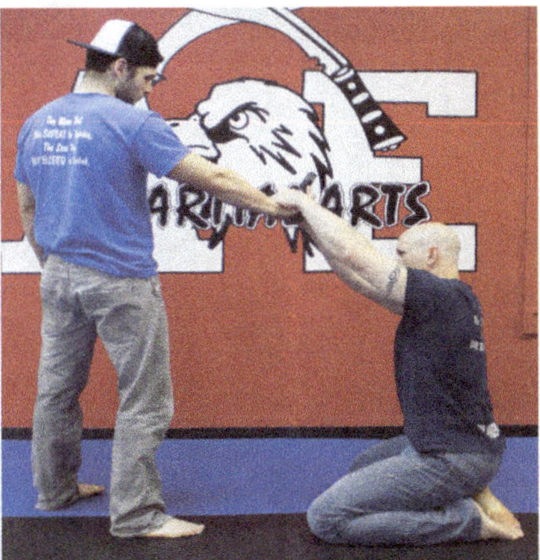

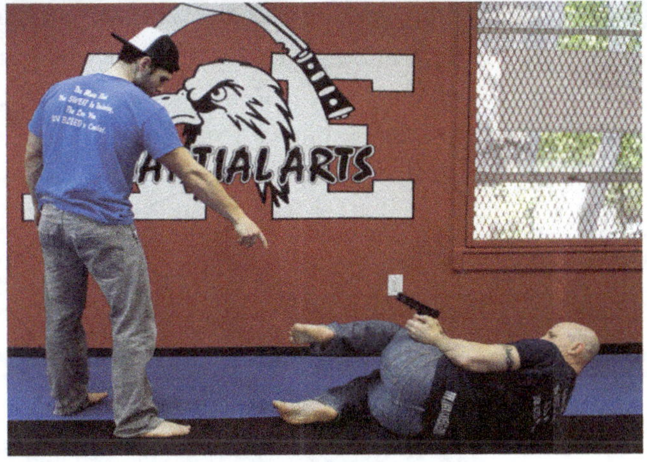

BACK

We addressed the gun to the back of the head, and the defense for a Gun to the Back is not much different. After you put your hands up, step with your left foot crossing in front of your right. This will put you off-line from the barrel of the gun. Turn and as your arms come in contact with theirs and slide your right hand, fingers up, down to their wrist and implement a left Elbow Strike to their head. Pivot your right hand on theirs so that your thumb is now upward and slide your left hand down, placing both hands on their gun hand. Step forward with your left foot and snap their elbow against your hip by driving your hip into their extended elbow, then yank their hand to the right using your hip as a fulcrum. Deliver Mule Kicks to their right knee and terminate the encounter.

STOMACH

Again, we will operate on the assumption that the gun is in the perp's right hand. However, be certain to practice being attacked with either hand holding the gun. If your hands are down and you find yourself with a gun pressed into your stomach, turn quickly toward your right and Smash the back of your left forearm into their right hand. As the barrel of the gun moves away from you and is past your body, slide your right hand, thumb facing upward, down to the wrist and hand of the assailant's gun hand. As you extend their arm, strike their head with a Side Elbow Strike and then secure the gun with both of your hands. As you do so, direct a Side Kick/Stomp toward their right knee with your left foot, causing them to collapse to the floor. Turn the gun back toward them as you bend their wrist inward and remove the gun. Finish the encounter as you deem most prudent.

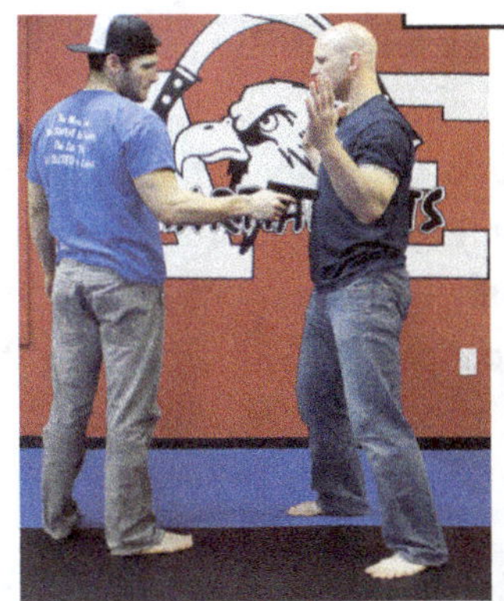
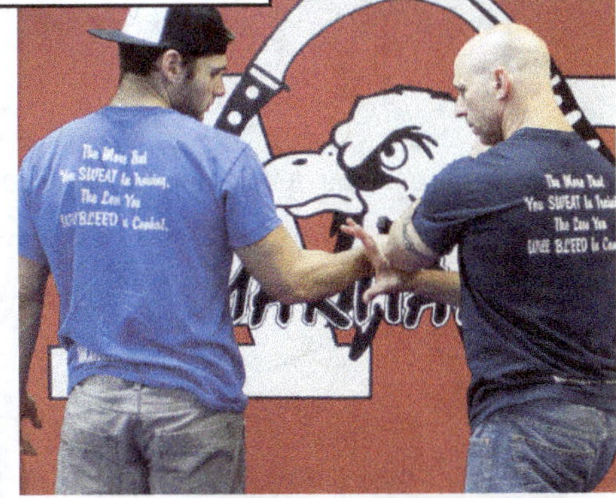
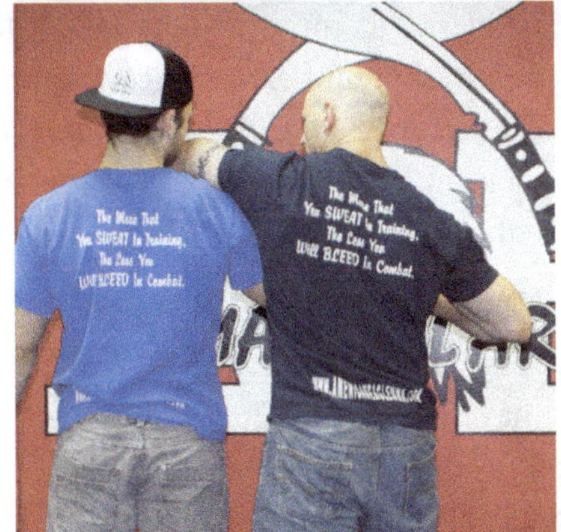
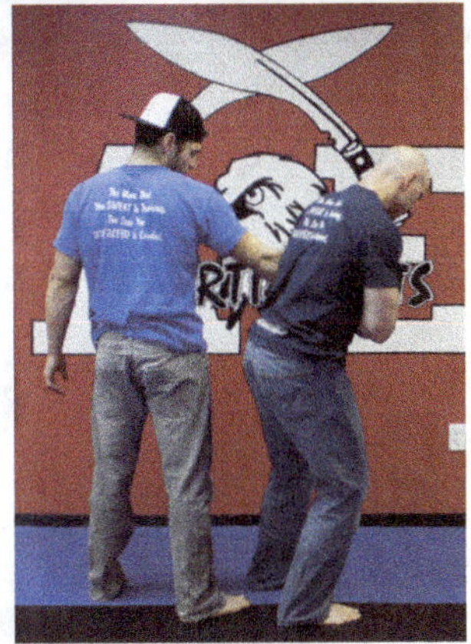
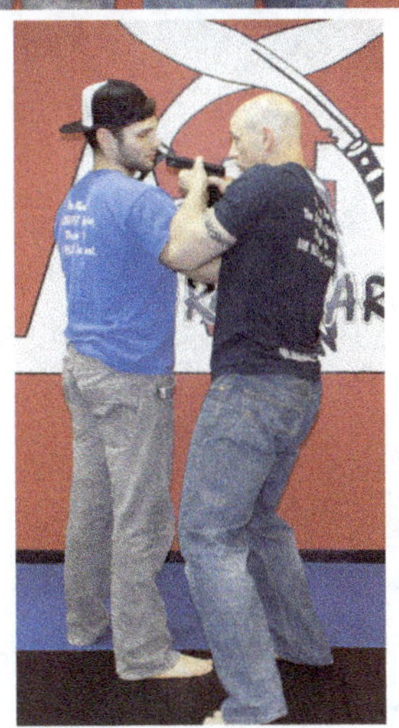
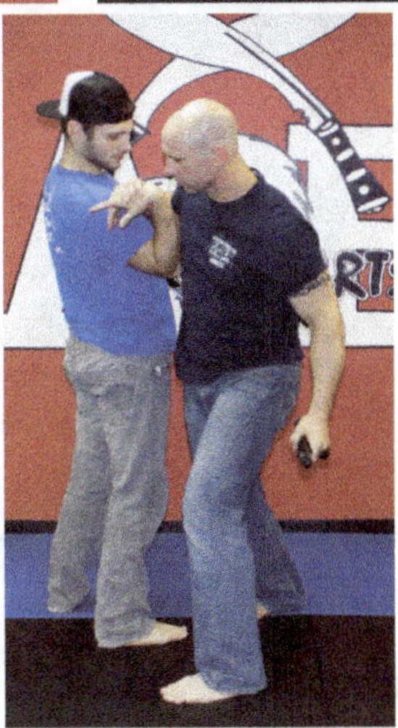

Gun to stomach.

LAST-RESORT MEASURES

We live in a different world now. Any of us, at any time, may find ourselves in dire circumstances facing seemingly insurmountable odds. We could get caught up in a hostage situation or terrorist attack, find ourselves in the line of fire of a psychotic shooter, or become the victim of a kidnapping.

Before we delve into such contingencies, we must be prepared to adhere to the tenets that we have espoused throughout this book: the belief that cooler heads prevail, and our commitment to the "all or nothing" principle. If we find ourselves outnumbered and on the wrong end of a weapon, every second we are alive is a gift, and we need to make the best of it. If there's a possibility of escape, no matter how small the chance, we have to seize the opportunity.

Now, it's a virtual impossibility to anticipate every single potential situation. But we don't have to, because the principles of self-protection are universal. Make sure that you have developed situational awareness and have put S.I.P.D.E. (Scan, Identify, Predict, Decide, Execute) into play. Don't bring attention to yourself. When the time comes to move, act swiftly and decisively.

Let's imagine a situation that could arise …

You're in a crowded area. This could be a restaurant, a concert hall, a stadium, a shopping mall, a park, a college campus, or just about any other place where large groups of people congregate. Suddenly, shots ring out, and they're not coming from far away.

Do not immediately flee. Hit the deck and do a visual surveillance of the area, before making an educated move. KEEP YOUR COOL! The perpetrators are counting on you to panic. They want to inspire mass hysteria, and you may run from the frying pan right into the fire if you run without thinking. Stick with the protocol. Remember that you can't count on anyone else. You have to have the mindset of "do something or perish."

Yes, there is an element of bravery involved here. But you are absolutely capable of rising to the challenge. You may recall an incident involving three Americans on the train in France. While others ran and hid from a terrorist rampage, they attacked and subdued him and saved countless lives. The lesson here is that when God gives you one shot, you take it. A second chance may never come.

In the event you are too far away to mount a counter-offensive, stay low and keep calm. If you see a clear path toward an escape route, take it. If not, you may have to "play dead" or wait until help comes. Try to become as invisible as possible. The good thing for you is that not everyone will buy this book, so a great number of those surrounding you will be panicking, thus drawing attention toward them and away from you.

If you are fortunate enough to have a legal carry permit, you might be armed and in a position to take action. This being the case, your best bet is to drop to the ground and find some cover. Assess how many assailants are involved. This may or may not be 100-percent apparent at first, but you have limited time to react, so you have to do your best to make an accurate estimate of the situation.

We will assume that you are very familiar with your weapon and have developed your shooting abilities. The chances of the criminal having a bullet-proof vest are pretty high, so a head shot would be best. If you are not an expert marksman, it would be best to aim your first shot relatively high on the chest and take your other shots moving up the body and toward the head.

Before anything actually happens, I recommend that you get some professional shooting instruction. There are many components to becoming a great shooter, and they must be addressed if you are to be successful in a stressful situation. There are tactical shooting instructors that have skills superior to mine. I know what works best for me, but I strongly recommend that you get the training you require to make you a confident and proficient shooter.

We will be discussing several self-defense responses. The tactics introduced are effective when you are unarmed or equipped with a knife. I do recommend that you carry a knife with you at all times, whenever possible. An assailant will either be drawing their weapon or reloading it, and you will be positioned either in front of them or behind them. There will also be times when they are simply looking around for more targets. If you are too far from them and have no escape route, it may be best to "play dead" until you see an opening to attack.

The most important physical aspect of this training is how quickly you are able to cover any particular distance. How far away can you be from the assailant and still reach him (or her) without being shot? How can you make them miss? What obstacles are in your way? What is available in the environment as an unconventional weapon? Are there chairs, tables or garbage cans within reach? Can you throw a salt-shaker or can of beans at them, aided by the element of surprise?

Here's what you can do when your attacker is:

DRAWING A WEAPON

If you are faced with someone and you observe them drawing a weapon, and you are within your practiced distance, rush them! Attack the weapon with your thumb up and fingers down as you shove the weapon into them and downward. With your free hand, strike them to the face or neck and then place your full attention on the weapon. Secure the weapon with both hands as you stomp and kick the assailant's feet and shins as you disarm them. Always keep the barrel of the gun pointed away from you and toward them, if possible. Place one hand on the barrel and the other on the pistol grip for a handgun and barrel and the stock of a longarm. If your left hand is on the barrel, step with your left foot in the direction of the barrel and pull in on the grip (or stock). You'll be bringing it toward you so that your hip becomes a fulcrum, with their arm on your hip as you apply force against the elbow joint with the goal of snapping it against your hip.

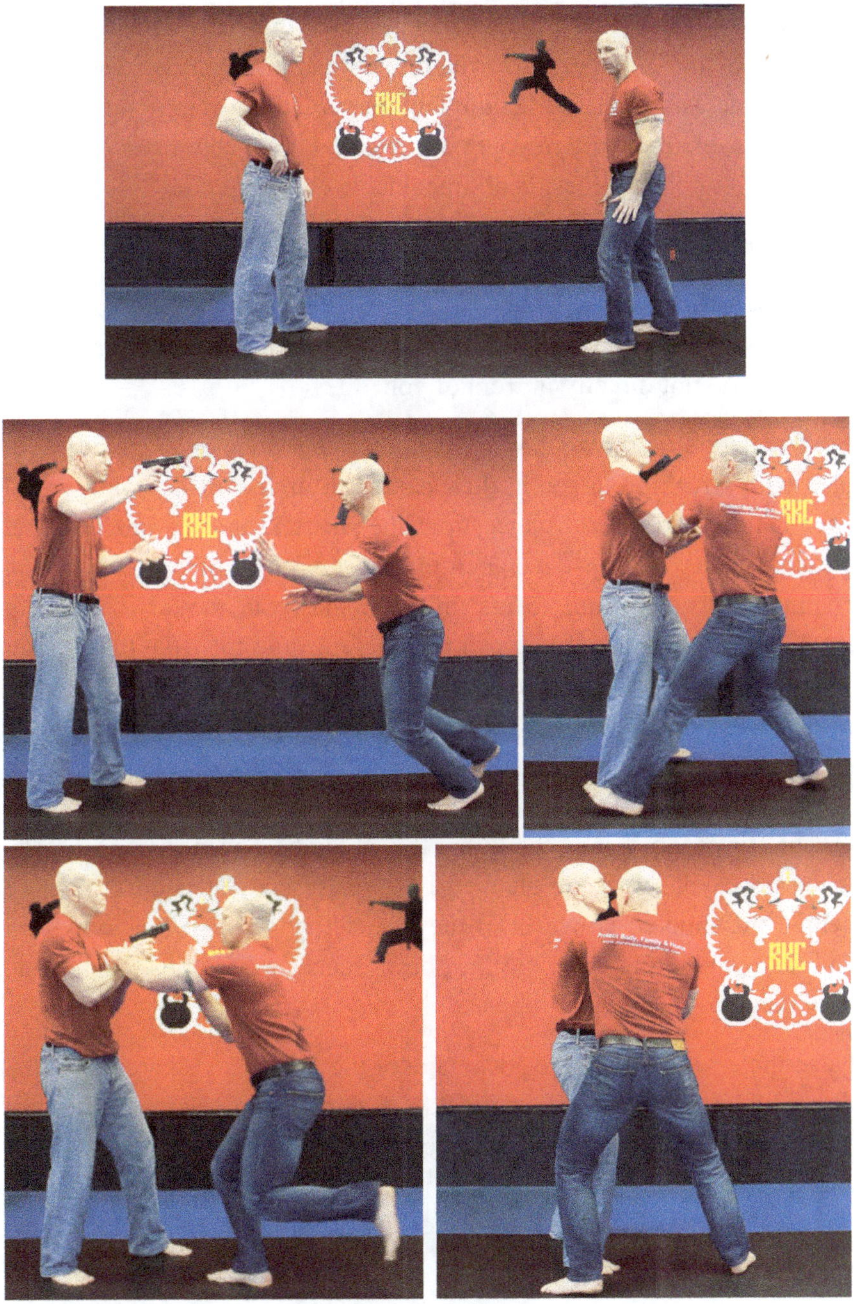

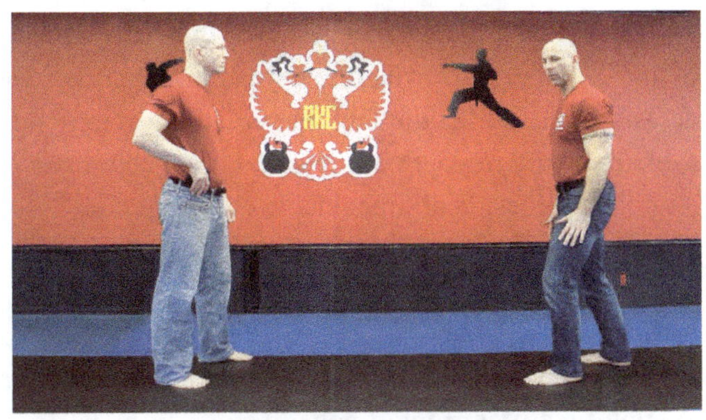

Drawing a weapon.

As mentioned previously, know the distance that you will be able to cover while the gunman is drawing their weapon. Practice these tactics with obstacles as well, for example with something lying on the floor, or with a table or chairs in your path that you must negotiate. You have to know your capabilities, in all imaginable circumstances.

RELOADING A WEAPON

The shooter is vulnerable for a brief time when they are reloading. If there are multiple shooters, you'll have to bear in mind your proximity to the one(s) not directly in front of you.

Let us operate on the assumption that the other shooter(s) are preoccupied with wreaking havoc in their particular area. At this point, you'll have determined your distance from the shooter, and it's one that you are confident you can cover before they are able to reload, aim and commence firing again; so it's time to make your move! If there's a small table or chair that you can pick up en route to strike the shooter with, do so. If you are unable, utilize the same tactics to disarm the assailant as you would do if they were drawing a weapon.

IN FRONT OF YOU WITH THEIR BACK TURNED

On the surface, one may think that this is the best scenario to be faced with, since you have the element of surprise on your side if you are behind the shooter. However, if they are actively firing, they may turn and face you at any time and the "best" scenario becomes the "worst" very quickly.

Nevertheless, you can take advantage of the fact that you are not in the direct line of sight and move quickly. Again, use your environment: if there is an object to strike with, pick it up. It may also act as a shield and help to deflect an attempted shot. If you are completely unarmed and void of any unconventional weapons, there are a few tactics that work best.

If you are reasonably big (at least larger than the shooter), tackle them. This will knock them to the ground and stop them from shooting others. Immediately secure a grip on the gun and shove the barrel into the shooter. If the gun goes off, they will shoot himself. If you are smaller, the tackle may still work, but you will need to generate enough force to knock them down. If you have any hesitation or aren't confident that you will be able to knock them off their feet, you will need to kick them in the back of the knee and deliver strikes to the back of the neck, occipital region and trapezius. Next, secure the weapon. It won't be pretty, but it will be nonetheless effective.

FACING YOU AND FIRING

The worst possible scenario is to be directly in front of a shooter while they are firing at you. It is an obvious understatement to say that you need to act extremely quickly, since outside of Superman no one can outrun an approaching bullet. You have to be a moving target and make yourself as small as possible.

There are three basic tactics to employ. Distance and environment will help you decide which of these methods to use.

Tactic #1: Execute a forward roll so that you end up rolling right into their legs. If possible, kick them in the groin on your way in. Immediately work your way up the body and gain control of the weapon. Unleash hell, reigning elbows down upon their head as you secure the weapon. Neutralize the threat, commandeer the weapon and either search for other assailants or exit the area quickly.

Tactic #2: Drop low and quickly "bear crawl" toward the shooter. Drive your shoulder into their knees as you cup the back of their heels with your hands. As you drive your shoulders into their knees, pull their heels toward you with all of your strength. As with Tactic #1, work your way up the body and finish the process.

Tactic #3 Move to the side prior to heading toward the assailant. If the perpetrator has the weapon in their right hand, move to your right. The attacker will have to bring their weapon across their body, thus causing the pectoral muscles to contract and making it more difficult to hit the intended target – in this instance, you! As always, move with purpose and conviction. Once the gap has closed, employ the "catch as catch can"philosophy and remove the weapon and neutralize the threat with any of the weapon neutralization tactics that we have covered – or by whatever means necessary.

With each of these tactics, you should practice with an airsoft gun and see which works best for you.

Again, folks, these are last-resort measures. Your dedication to the practice of the movements, conditioning of your body and willingness to perform these acts under duress will determine your success. When facing a weapon, death is always imminent. Every breath that you have is on borrowed time, and every second that you are alive is a gift. Use them wisely and do anything you can to save your life and the lives of others.

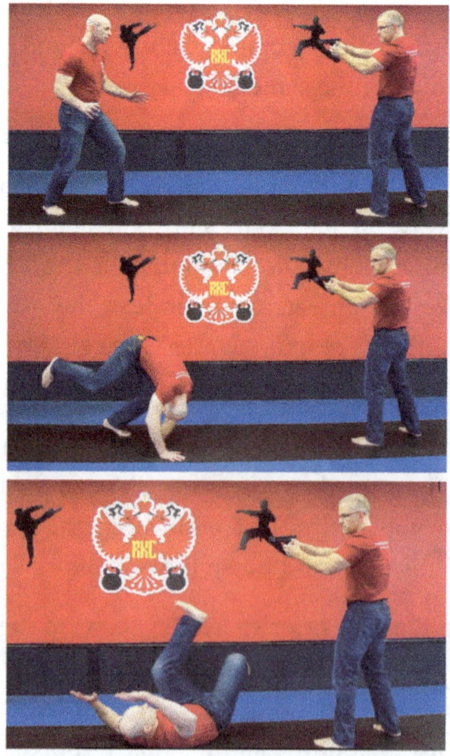

Gun from the front, tactic #1.

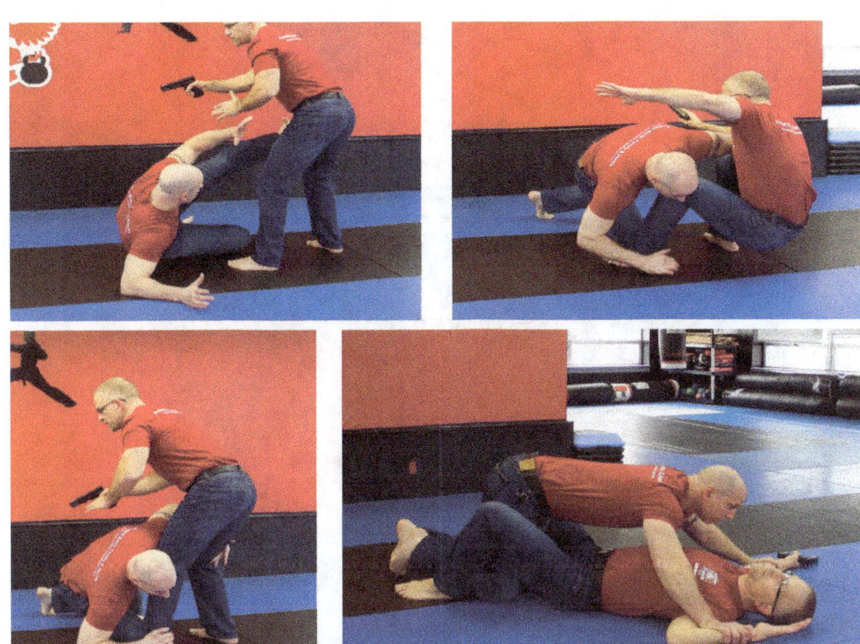

Gun from the front, tactic #1.

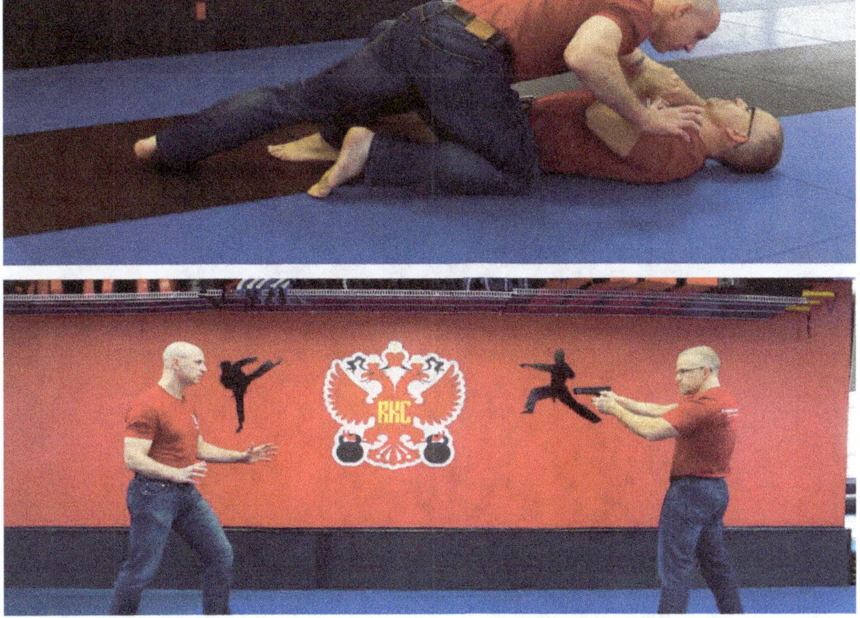

Gun from the front, tactic #2

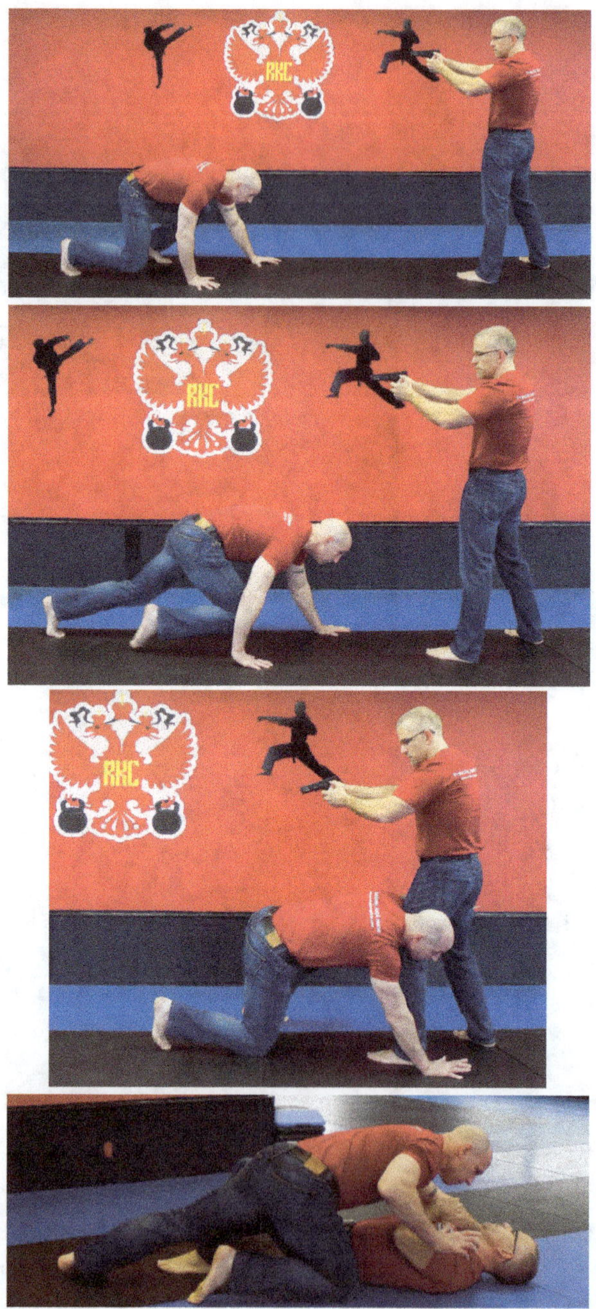

Gun from the front, tactic #2

Chapter 14
Practice and Training

MAN-TO-MAN STRENGTH

While strength of all types is vital, man-to-man strength is absolutely imperative in fights. There is a dynamic and chaotic nature to grappling, boxing and kickboxing that is impossible to perfectly prepare for without actually fighting or grappling. Therefore, it is important to not only improve your overall strength through proper training, but to also make sure that you spend some time with a bonafide "opponent."

Below is a collection of drills to help you develop strength, balance and quicker reactions to aid you in fighting. These drills should be incorporated as part of your regular practice.

MAN-TO-MAN DRILLS

1. **Push-Pull:** Stand facing your partner with both having the same foot forward. Press the outside of your foot against your partner's and lock arms, hand to forearm. Push and pull each other in an attempt to disrupt each other's balance. Practice this with both feet forward.

2. **Pummeling:** Stand chest to chest with your partner, and each of you should have one arm under and the other over. One person moves

forward as the other goes back, continually switching the Underhooks and Overhooks, smashing your posterior deltoids into each other as you move. Once you get to the end of the mat, go back in the other direction so that you have switched who is moving forward and who is moving back.

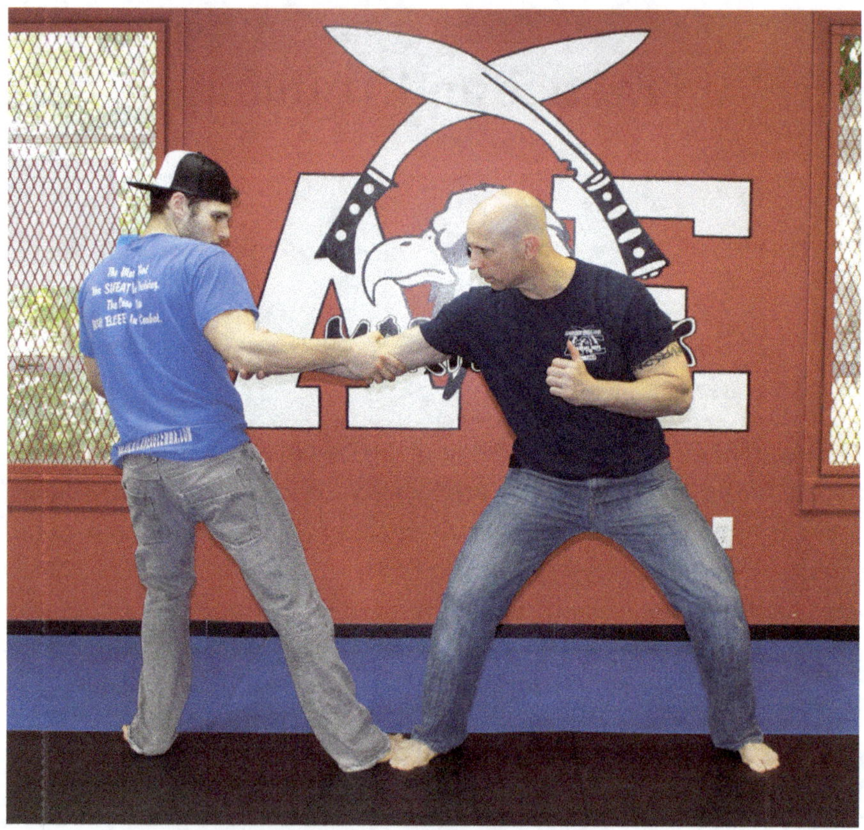

Push-pull drill.

3. **Inside-Control Balance Drill:** Inside control is essential to grappling success, especially on your feet. Assume the inside position with your hands on the inside of your partner's biceps and push and pull them in different directions: back, forward and side-to-side. Switch partners and then battle with each other for the inside-control position.

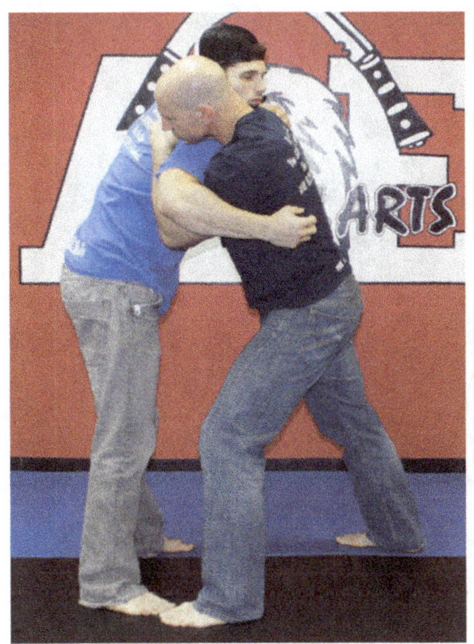 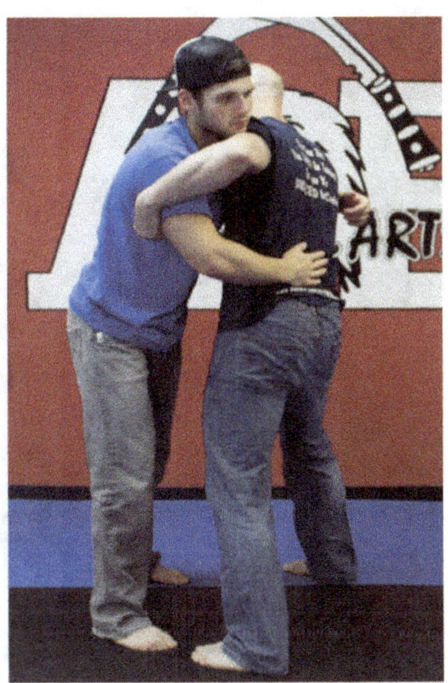

Pummeling drill.

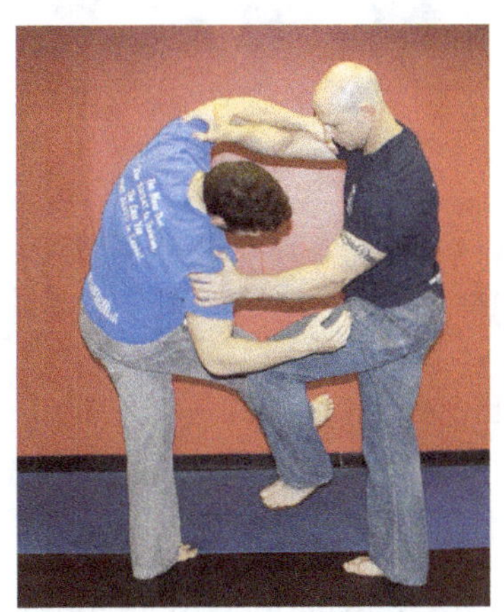

Outside sweep.

4. **Sweeps and Disruptions:** If you are wearing a kimono or a jacket, you may grab onto the sleeves and lapels. If not, start from the Inside Control position and employ the movement practiced in the previous drill, tapping their feet with yours as an additional step. Use the bottom of your foot to contact their foot. Use anticipatory movement knowing that if you pull them toward you, their foot will have to land for them to maintain their balance. Put your foot where their foot is heading. If they do not fall, immediately go in the other direction. This action will result in them falling or at least cause them to lose their balance, enabling you to secure a takedown or another advantageous position.

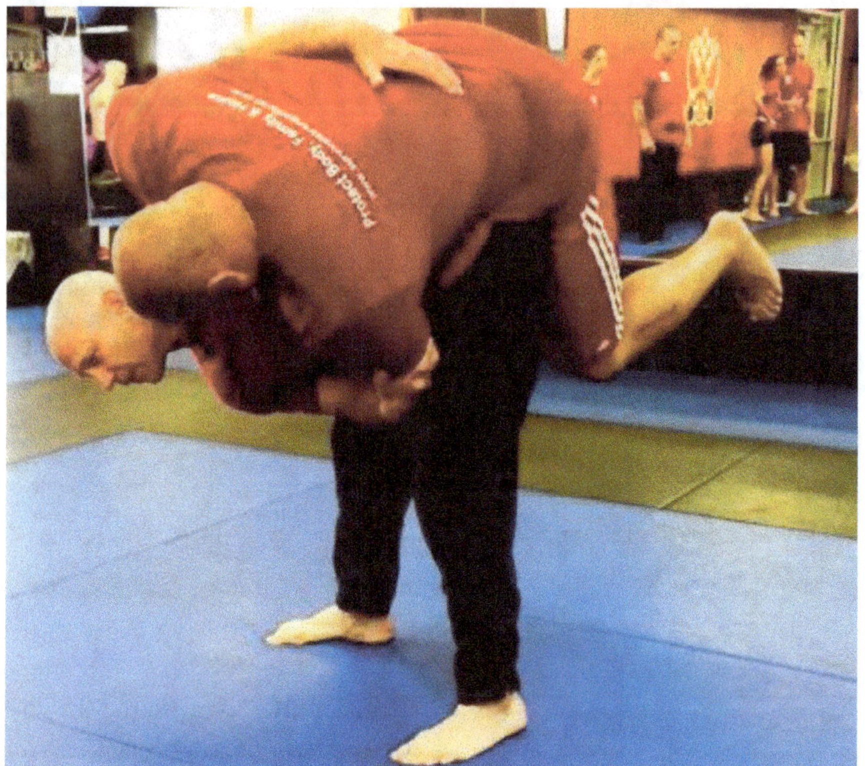

Hip toss.

5. **Throws:** Practice all of the throws you know. Practice them slowly for technique perfection and then work them harder. Do a "Throw-Around" by setting the timer for two to five minutes and go back and forth with your partner practicing your throws. Use pushing, pulling and movement. Remember that throws are dynamic and require movement to be executed.

6. **Ducks, Slips, Parries and Weaves:** Have your partner wear focus mitts or simply use each other's boxing gloves as targets. If you don't have gloves, use open palms and slaps. Have your partner throw strikes at you as you practice moving out of the way and positioning yourself to counterstrike. You should barely get out of the way of the strikes so

that you are closer, thus affording you a better opportunity to deliver your counterstrikes.

7. **Chi So (Single Side and Dual Hand):** Stand in front of your partner, with both of you having one palm up and the other down. Press the inside of your wrists to your partner's. Bend your knees, close your eyes and move around in small circles, shifting your weight. You are not trying to "beat" your partner per se, but rather trying to feel their energy and flow, moving and maintaining contact with them the whole time. Move and flow with each other, taking turns leading the action and following. This is a great drill for developing sensitivity.

8. **Partner Carries:** These drills can be used at the beginning of a workout as a means to warm up, or at the end as an overtime drill. Pick up your partner and carry them as you move quickly across the room. There are many different carries to use, such as the Double-Leg, Fireman's Carry, Marriage Carry, Piggy-Back and Dog-Stance Lifts. On the last one, your partner is on all fours and you are both facing the same direction. Wrap your arms around their waist, lift them and move them forward. They won't move too far, but it's a heck of a strength-developing drill nonetheless.

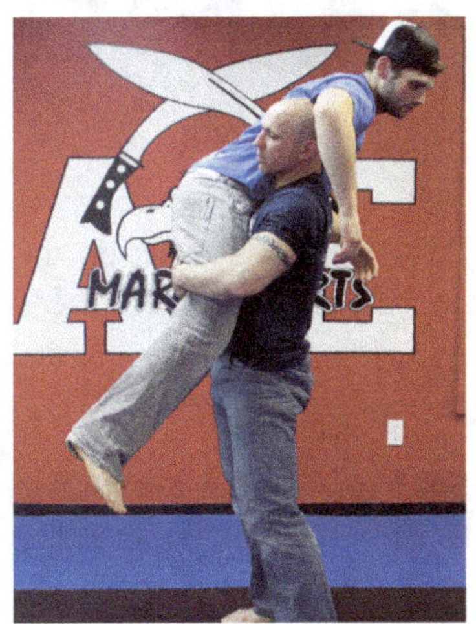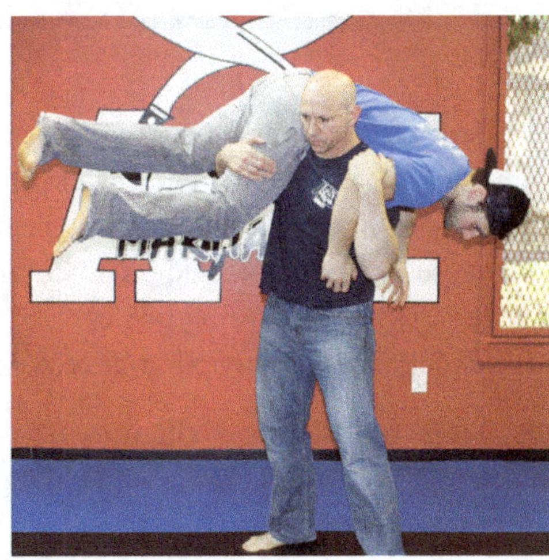

Double-leg lift | Fireman's carry.

9. **Stick Grappling:** One person holds the staff vertically and has their feet shoulder-width apart, knees slightly bent, and hands approximately a foot apart. The other person grabs the staff outside the stationary partner's hands and moves around them, pulling and yanking on the pole as the stationary partner tries to maintain their position. Don't twist the staff, this does not make the drill better and you may hit your partner or injure their wrists. Do this drill in spurts of 15 seconds on, 15 seconds rest and 15 seconds for the other partner. Repeat so that each person gets two to three rounds in as a warm-up drill.

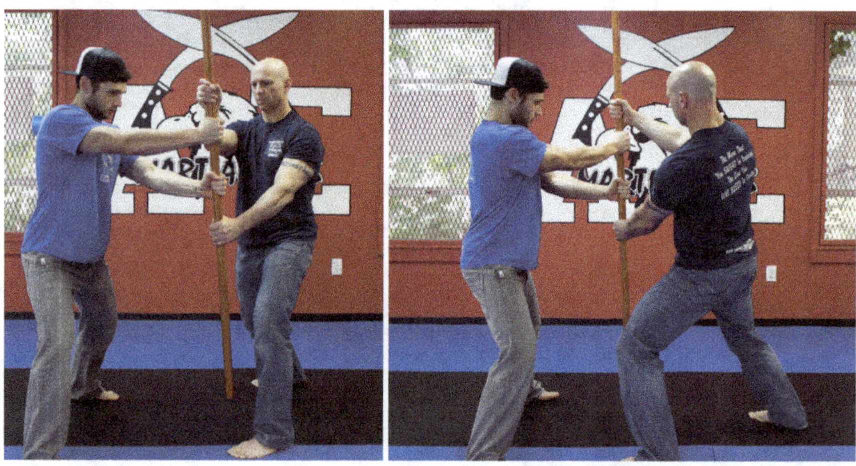

10. **Wall Drill (Slaps):** One partner starts in a very negative position with their knees bent and back against the wall. The other partner starts slowly and then builds to striking faster, trying to land slaps on the other's head, face, and body. Closed fists to the body are acceptable and even help to condition bodies. Don't try to smash your partner too hard, though, this is a reaction-developing drill.

11. **Defensive Boxing Drill into Dirty Boxing:** One partner throws punches, and the other takes an angle, gets inside and drives the other back onto their heels with strikes and shoves. The first partner will respond by grabbing the back of the other's neck or arm before delivering strikes.

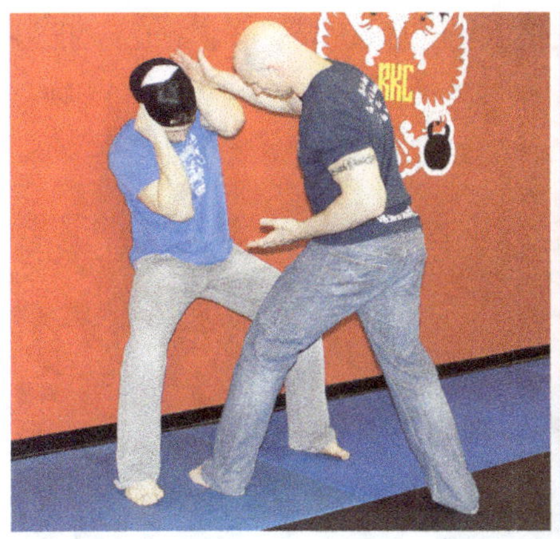
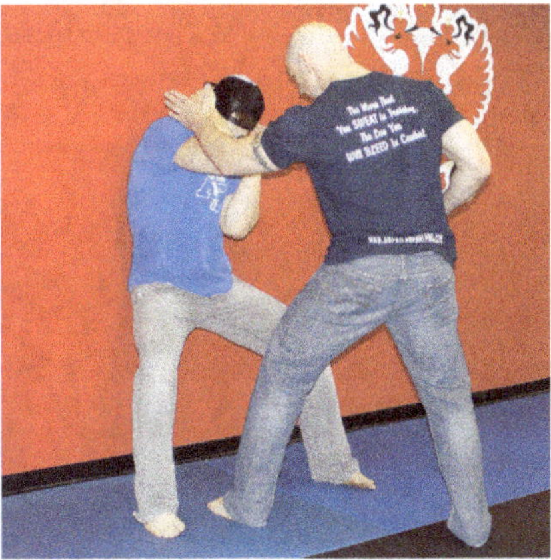

Wall drill slaps.

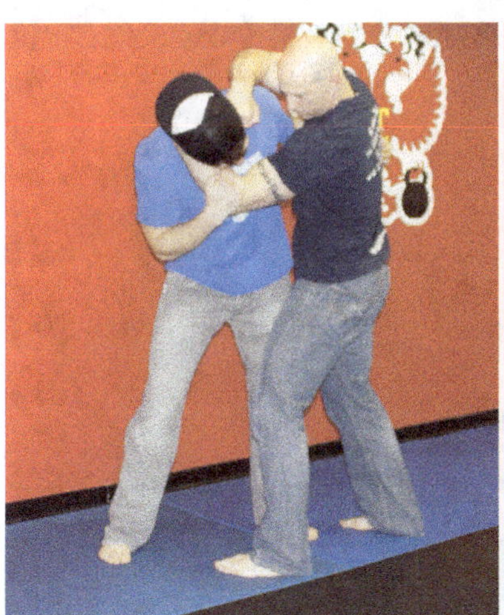
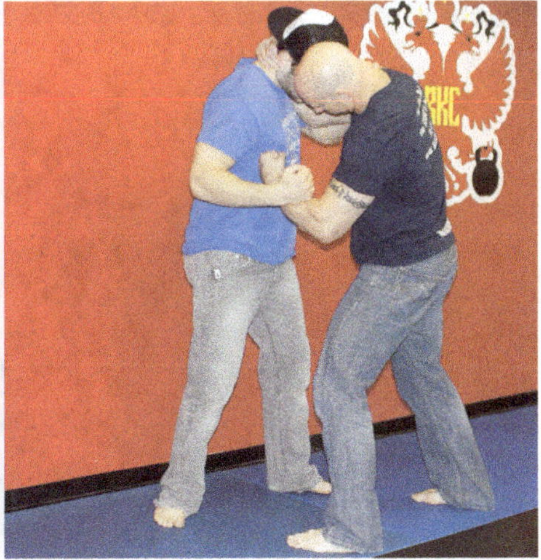

Wall drill, dirty boxing.

12. **Drop Out Balance Disruption-Game**: Both partners are on the floor facing each other in a push-up position. Using one hand (obviously), try to grab each other's hand and knock the other off-balance. If you fall or your knee hits the ground, you lose.

13. **Pop Shots:** With both partners facing each other in a good grappling stance, take both hands and pop your partner's shoulders as you lower your level, shoot a Double-Leg Takedown, and lift them into the

air. Put them down without completing the takedown so that they land on their feet. Repeat this move in sets of 10 repetitions for each partner.

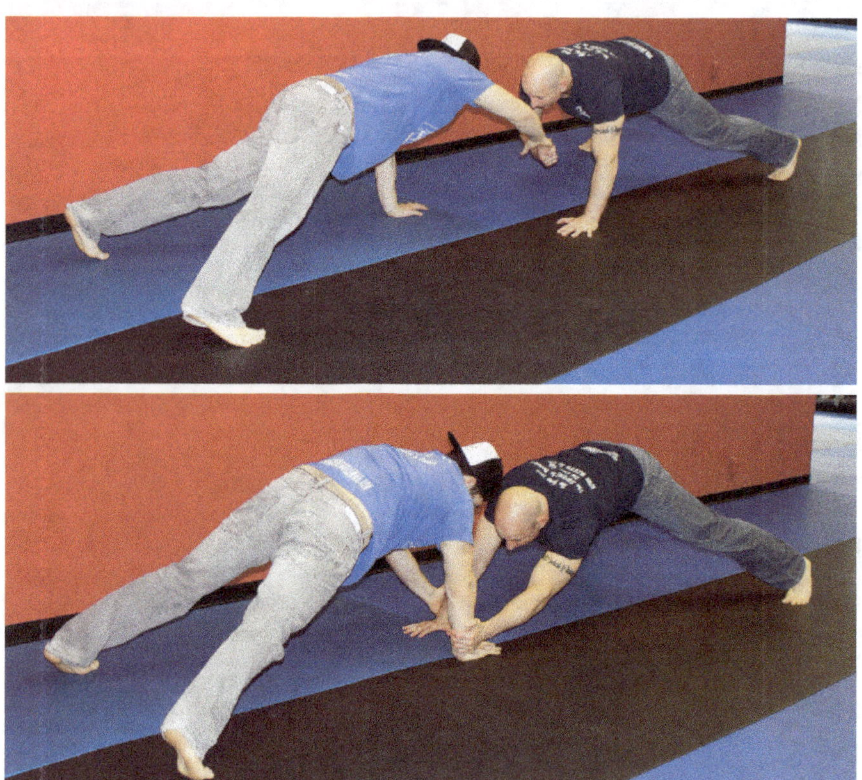

Drop Out Balance Disruption Game.

14. **Body Lifts:** Assume the Overhook/Underhook position and slide yourself to the side of the Overhook as you trap your partner's far arm, lock your hands around their waist and press the side of your head against their chest. You are now in a Single- Arm Bear-Hug. Pinch their leg between your knees, pop your hips and lift your partner toward the sky. Repeat this move in sets of 10 repetitions for each individual.

15. **Bridge Backs:** Be very careful when practicing this drill. This should be used only by the more experienced and conditioned practitioners. Have your partner stand on your side, grab each other's hands, and have them use their other hand to support your elbow. Bridge back as far as you are able to go. If you can touch the mat with your head, great, but I do not recommend that you start this way. Once you bridge backward as far as you can safely go, come back up. Your partner should assist you as much as needed on the way down and on the way up. Start with five repetitions per set and gradually increase to 10.

16. **Sticky Hands:** This is yet another great training technique advocated by Bruce Lee. The goal of this drill is to develop sensitivity and awareness of your opponent's movement. Stand in front of your partner with one palm up and one palm down. Place the inside of your wrists in contact with your partner's. Now begin to move in small horizontal circles and gradually make them larger and "flow" to the back of the arm while shifting your weight. Do not force any movement; go with 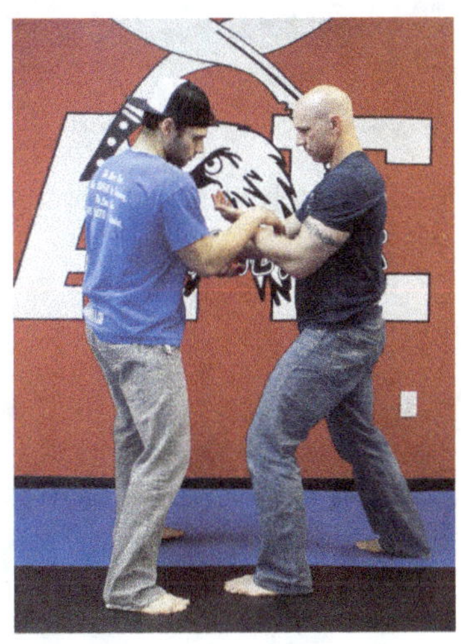 the flow of energy as you shift your weight and slide your arms against your partner's while moving and attempt to maintain contact throughout the drill. This is a fun drill, even though your goal is not to "win" per se but to learn how to follow the movements of your partner.

PUNCHES: 1 THRU 6 COMBINATIONS

You need muscle memory to successfully throw combinations in a stressful situation. Practice these combinations in a mirror, on focus mitts or on a heavy bag. Also, be sure to incorporate your bobs, weaves, slips and general movement when striking. Always try to make it "real."

1. 1, 2
2. 1, 3, 2
3. 2, 3
4. 1, 4, 3
5. 3, 6
6. 6, 3
7. 2, 3, 2
8. 1, 6, 3
9. 1, 1, 2
10. 1, 2, 1

ENDURANCE PUNCHING SEQUENCE

Do 20 repetitions of each sequence. Do both sides (right and left foot forward).

1. 1, 2
2. 2, 3
3. 3, 4
4. 4, 5
5. 5, 6
6. 6, 1

BAG WORK

There are many people who hang a heavy bag, turn on the theme to *Rocky*, and start wailing away on the bag as the tempo to *"Gonna Fly Now"* picks up. Are they getting some cardio and developing some muscle? Possibly. Are they tired at the end? Most likely. Have they developed their striking skills and created some useful muscle memory? Probably not.

When you hit the heavy bag, you want to make the best use of your time. You need to hit the bag with purpose. You should hit the bag while utilizing movement, just as if you were fighting. Practice moving in and out, slips, ducks, bobbing and weaving. Always bring your hand to your head or your head to your hand.

You have to develop *proper* muscle memory.

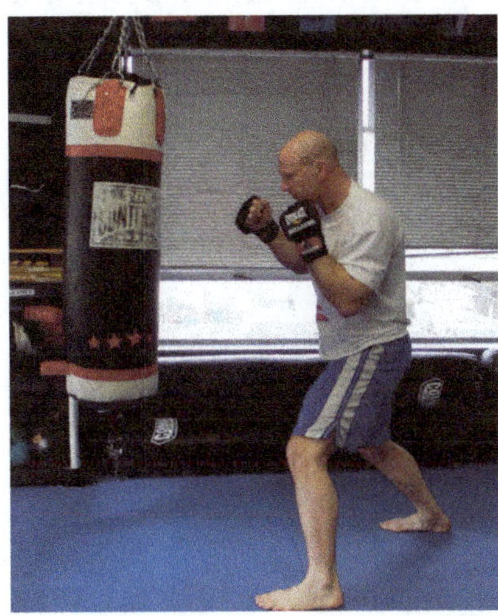 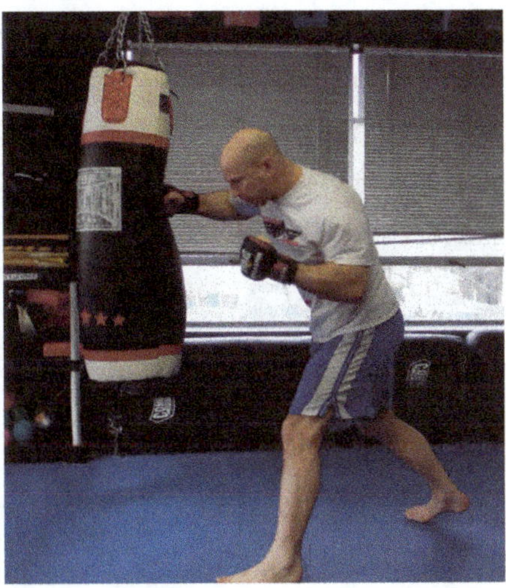

When you begin your training, you may be tempted to start with 10 rounds. I would not suggest that. Depending on your fitness level, start with three-to-five two-minute rounds and then build from there. Be sure to keep a straight wrist and tight fist while punching and a flexed foot while kicking.

GROUND AND POUND

There may come a time when you get someone on the ground and have successfully mounted them. It's time to unleash Hell! However, you'll want to be smart and not simply throw punches wildly at the downed assailant. You'll want to choose your strikes in a strategic manner.

To make sure you do this, you'll need to practice what you'd like to do on a heavy bag beforehand. Place your heavy bag on the floor and straddle it so that your knees are on the floor to either side of the bag. *DO NOT punch your assailant in the face.* The chances of you missing his face and punching the ground are quite good. Practice punching to the body and with open hand strikes and elbows to the head. You will want to rise up slightly, tilting your shoulders as you drop the elbows or make other strikes straight down.

If you wind up on their side, Knee Drives to the ribs, head and legs will be effective. Dropping elbows to the opposite side of the body and head will also cause damage. Just don't stay here too long, as it's better to have a full-mount position. It's also important to have a solid base. If your knees are too close together, you will be rolled over. Practice your mount position, striking from it and moving from side to side.

HANDS (BOXING DRILLS)

Our boxing coach, Joe Rubino, put together this incredible boxing training sequence for developing muscle memory and conditioning your hands for striking. If you want to develop more strength and conditioning, use 14-to 16-ounce gloves. To improve the conditioning of your hands, use thin bag gloves.

One essential component to working the heavy bag properly is to do so as if you were fighting. This means head movement, moving in and out on the bag, keeping your hands up, going head to hand or hand to head after you punch. Practice your bobs, weaves and slips as you move and strike. Stay on the balls of your feet and perform Herky-Jerky movements. The latter involves stomping the floor, feinting in and out of your opponent's range and throwing off their rhythm with your arhythmic motion. It's a great strategy to draw someone out and to get them to commit or to stop their movement, allowing you the opportunity to launch an attack.

COACH JOE RUBINO'S HEAVY BAG ROUTINE

- Round 1 – Working the jab around the bag.
- Round 2 – Working the 1-2 combination around the bag.
- Round 3 – Slipping, bobbing and weaving with combinations.
- Round 4 – Fast combinations around the bag (staying tall).
- Round 5 – Fast combinations up and down around the bag.

- Round 6 – Punching from angles (swing the bag).
- Round 7 – Short quick punches after working your way inside (for hand speed)/
- Round 8 – Power shot/s
- Round 9 – High-low combinations/
- Round 10 – Working the inside position (use elbows and forearms to control the bag).

Two-minute rounds with 30 seconds rest between rounds
Or
Three-minute rounds with one-minute rest between rounds

KICKBOXING: MIXING STRIKES OF THE HANDS AND FEET

Now we are going to add kicks to the mix.

Here's a routine that I have been using for quite a few years. Mind you, there are many other combinations and sequences that work, but this one is an old standard and a great place to start.

Our striking sequences are primarily done in a "Circle" fashion, as opposed to an X. To illustrate this point, we will consider the first combination. Start in your Orthodox stance and then throw a Right Cut Kick followed by a Right Jab, a Left Cross and finish with a Left Cut Kick. That would be an example of a Circle Striking configuration. An example of an X would be, starting in the Orthodox stance, a Left Jab, step across, and throw a Right Cut Kick. Another example would be a Left Jab, Right Cross and Left Roundhouse Kick. When in "Mirror Image" with an opponent, with both fighters either in an Orthodox or SouthPaw position, an X style of striking is recommended. When you are "Chest-to-Chest" with your opponent, both fighters in the same stance, "Circle Striking" works the best. These are not hard and fast rules but more like guidelines.

Please do not deliberate on the Circle versus the X for striking. Practice both and use what works best for you. However, understand that as a general rule the Circle is quicker and the X has more power. I have discovered that it's easier to put more power into my Circle attacks than it is to add more speed to my X's.

Additionally, when training in the kickboxing sequence, we work both Orthodox and Southpaw stances. In fighting and kickboxing, it's important to be able to switch your stances on the fly. Switch sides either halfway through the round or on every other combination.

KICKBOXING SEQUENCE

- Round 1 - Right Cut Kick, Right Jab, Left Cross, Left Cut Kick.
- Round 2 – Lead-Leg Roundhouse Kick, Jab and Cross.
- Round 3 – Lead-Leg Side Kick, Backfist, Cross.
- Round 4 - Full Leg (back one) Rapid-Fire Cut Kick, Round Kick, Round Kick, Lead Hook (hand), Cross and Lead Hook again. After your Full Cut Kick, your rear becomes your lead; you bounce your foot off the ground quickly as you deliver the next two kicks. After the kicks, execute a Lead Hook Punch with the same side.
- Round 5 - Piet a te, Lead Jab, Cross, Rear-Leg Cut Kick.
- Round 6 - Back Kick, Spinning Backfist, Stick Punch.
- Round 7 - Lead Jab, Spinning Backfist, Stick Punch, Double Knee.
- Round 8 - Double Jab, Body Shot (Rear Hook to the body), Cut Kick, Spinning Crescent, Hook or Wheel Kick (vary the kicks).
- Round 9 - Fake (Feint) the Jab, Slide the lead foot across and throw an Overhand Right, pivot on the lead foot and throw a Lead Hook followed by a Rear Elbow.
- Round 10 - Lunging Front Kick, side step and Shin Kick, Lead Hook, Rear Uppercut.

Two-minute rounds with 30 seconds rest between rounds
Or
Three-minute rounds with one-minute rest between rounds

THE FOUR RANGES OF COMBAT

Kicking Range: This is the distance where the feet are most effective. Closing the gap and covering distance are best accomplished with your feet. They are your first line of defense.

Punching Range: This is a range that you may begin at, depending on your proximity to your opponent. The Clenched Fist, Open-Handed Strikes, Finger Jabs, Axe-hands, Chops and Smashes are most effective at this distance. A good guard is essential here.

Trapping Range: Potentially the most ignored range in martial arts. This is an intermediary and a "gateway" from striking to grappling. At this distance, you "trap" your opponent's weapon (arm or leg) and deliver your Strike, Elbow, Knee or Head-Butt. There are a plethora of other targets you'll have available to you at this range. They include the hips, shoulders, thigh, forearms, neck, etc. Some styles break this range down into two distinct distances, but in practice I have found them to be one in the same. In this range, we also practice the art of "Dirty Boxing."

Grappling Range: If your confrontation lasts more than three to five seconds, you will be at this range, like it or not. At this distance, leverage, balance and knowledge of the body are most critical. All of your Takedowns, Choke-Outs, Submission Holds, Throws and joint manipulation occur at this distance. Please note that striking often occurs at this range as well. There is such complexity to body position and weight shifting that several arts focus solely on one or two aspects of this range.

HOW TO TRAIN

When you are in the fracas, get your hands up to protect your head. Keeping your hands up is the soundest advice I've been given.

It is best to start at one range before moving into another. Moving to a third and a fourth range is not helpful because you cannot effectively practice combinations to compensate for the variables which may occur.

We train in this manner:

Round 1: Start at range 1, then go to 2, then 3, then 4.
Round 2: Start at range 2, then go to 3, then 4, then 1.
Round 3: Start at range 3, then go to 4, then 1, then 2.
Round 4: Start at range 4, then go to 3, then 2, then 1.

Please note that you will not always be afforded the luxury of beginning in a range that is comfortable for you. However, through practice, you will be able to enter your most effective distance efficiently and rapidly.

Chapter 15
Dog Attacks

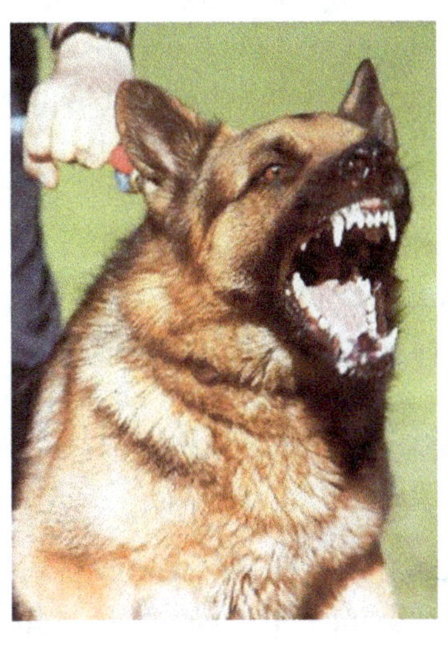

Man's best friend can also be his worst enemy. There are many large and powerful breeds that were created for fighting, crowd control and intimidation. Just imagine 125 pounds of fangs, fur and fury charging at you! These fierce animals are extremely difficult to deal with, but you are not without recourse.

As with all of the other chapters, this one also presents applications that have been utilized by me personally in the real world. There was one situation when I was in the front yard with my adult male boxer and six-month-old female shepherd. My dogs were trained to stay on my property. A gentleman and his wife were walking up the street with his 125-pound Akita. This would normally not be an issue, but he let go of the dog's leash and the dog made a bee-line for my yard. My six-month old shepherd was not quite as well trained as my boxer at this point, and chose to engage a dog that was more than twice her size at the end of the driveway. As they fought, the Akita grabbed her by the neck; normally, I would have booted the dog, but I did not want it to break my young pup's neck. So, I grabbed the dog by its tail and lifted it off the ground. As I hoisted it up off of the ground, the dog let go of mine, and I took one of my hands and grabbed its throat. By this time, my boxer, seeing me engaged, entered the fray.

This ended with me throwing the dog and the people finally grabbing their dog's leash and me getting my dogs under control. My wife at the time watched the whole encounter from the picture window and was amazed that I did not get bit. As I've stated, it's better to be lucky than good!

There are certain considerations to bear in mind. Chances are very good that you will suffer a bite in a confrontation with a dog. Know this going in. The bite pressure in psi (pounds per square Inch) of some domesticated dogs can be more than that of cougars (350 psi) and wolves (406 psi). These wild animals are able to crush the skulls and bones of their prey. Due to their massive heads and powerful neck and jaw muscles, the mastiff has the highest bite force of all domestic dogs, with a *psi of 556*. The Rottweiler comes in second with a psi of 328, third goes to the German Shepherd at 238 and then fourth is the American Pitbull at 235 psi. In contrast, the typical adult human male has a psi of just 150.

Awareness of the psyche of the dog is paramount to the success of your defense. There are postures and voice commands that can help you avoid the attack. A dog likes to have its feet planted on the ground. By lifting a dog off of the ground, you disrupt his ability to use his legs to drive off of the ground and significantly reduce his feelings of security. Many types of "guard" or "catch" animals have their tails docked to eliminate the tail becoming a handle. If they have a tail, use it to lift them off of the ground, thus rendering them unable to use their back legs to drive with. If they do not have a tail, grab their back legs.

The first line of defense is to use your voice command, and to make it loud, concise and pointed. This works very well in a surprisingly high percentage of instances. Next, position yourself to deliver a strong kick, aiming for the snoot, ribs, underbelly or hind quarters. If this does not work or you are not positioned to deliver a kick, offer up an arm and when the dog bites, lift the bitten arm up quickly and smash the dog's first vertebra where the skull meets the spine. Your goal will be to break the attacking canine's neck. If you have a knife, offer the arm and thrust the knife into the dog's throat.

Don't try to pull away from the dog once engaged. Shove your arm or fist deep into their mouth and attempt to knock them over. Stick your thumb in their eyes and deliver knee strikes to their ribs and underbelly. If there are multiple dogs, keep the fight standing delivering knee strikes and elbows as you move and position yourself so you are not engaged with more than one dog at once.

If the dog bites your hand, grasp the lower jaw firmly and pull down. Wrap your other arm around the dog's neck and apply a One-Armed Choke as you yank down on its jaw. A dog will bite and shake. Pulling down on its jaw makes it less able to bite down, and securing a Headlock-like Choke reduces its ability to thrash its head about. The dog may just try to get away from you at this point.

Different types of dogs attack in various manners. For example, German shepherds and Dobermans will repeatedly bite and release until they can gain a full mouth bite and then they will grab and shake. The bully breeds, pit bulls, bulldogs, mastiffs and the like tend to grab, hold and shake as opposed to biting and releasing. Your general defense to either type of attack will not vary, but I think it is worth mentioning, so you'll know what to expect during an encounter. You should also know that if a dog has had Schutzhund or "bite training," their approach will be in accordance with how they were trained.

It is comforting to know that most trained dogs will go after the first limb that gets presented and are generally trained to bite their oppo-

nent's arm once engaged. This doesn't make their bite any less dangerous, but it does make their behavior more predictable.

Chapter 16
Unconventional Weapons: Practice Is Essential

Practice with your weapon on a regular basis. There are many instances when a person is trying to defend themselves and the weapon gets taken away and used on them, and needless to say this is what you want to avoid. Get used to its weight, size and how it reacts when you use the weapon.

Unconventional Weapons, as with Conventional, require practice to become proficient. They are easy to travel with, and you will not get questioned by the TSA if you possess them. Some of these weapons are readily available in the environment.

Always consider all options and keep your wits about you, that is one important lesson that applies to any situation. Here is an real-life unconventional weapons story that I've chosen to relate which will illustrate the value of an intelligent approach:

One of my martial arts students, John Geraghty, was traveling abroad in India for business. The area that he visited was an exceptionally impoverished region. He was at a business dinner with a gentleman in his late 60s, and they were taking a cab back to the hotel. There was quite a bit of drinking at the dinner; wisely, John did not partake.

The arrangements for the cab were made by a third party. As they neared the hotel, which had barbed wire and armed guards at the gate, the cab drove past it. John was very aware of what had just happened, but his comrade was not. Traveling internationally with conventional weapons is frowned upon, but John did remember that in class we had learned how to use a rolled-up magazine as a weapon, which was a most unconventional choice to be sure. Fortunately, he had one in his hand.

The cab traveled past the secure entrance to the hotel, and John immediately began questioning the driver. This individual was not forthcoming, only telling them to "get out here." John got out of the cab with his slightly inebriated partner in tow and was almost instantly surrounded by a group of six or so assailants. The cab sped off.

John had taken his makeshift weapon from the back seat of the cab prior to getting out. As the group descended, he had to act quickly. The closest assailant was the recipient of the butt of the rolled-up magazine applied to the occipital region of his head. He dropped to the ground as John grabbed his compatriot by the belt and fled quickly to the hotel gate as the gang was in disarray.

In this harrowing scenario, John displayed his awareness skills while deploying an unconventional weapon. He listened to his survival voice and acted decisively with conviction, and knowing where to place a strike saved his life and that of his business associate. This all happened so quickly that the travel partner was in total shock and 100-percent unaware of what had just transpired until he witnessed the aftermath.

UNCONVENTIONAL WEAPONS CHOICES

A Pen, Towel, Brush, Sock with Batteries, Magazine, Chair, Umbrella, Garbage Can Lid, Change, Briefcase, Belt with Buckle, Chemical Deterrents, Hornet Spray and Air Horn, this is a preliminary list of choices. All can be used to deploy various strikes, parries, techniques and strategies that will really work. You can work a Diamond Defense with a chair, break a board with a magazine, or throw change into the eyes and face of the assailant. Creativity and imagination are an asset here.

PEN

A pen may be used to slash and stab an opponent. Both the Ice Pick and Fencing Grips may be used. The target areas for the slash are the eyes and throat. Thrusts are directed to the temple, eyes, neck and groin.

TOWEL

A towel may be used to wrap your hand in to battle a knife wielding assailant. You may also use it to ward off blows and offensively as a means to apply a choke or to tie up an assailant.

BRUSH

A hair brush may be used in two different applications. Rake the bristles across the eyes of an assailant or use the butt end of the handle to strike vital and semi-vital target areas.

SOCK WITH BATTERIES

Take an athletic tube sock or another calf-covering sports sock and place two Size D batteries in it. This may be used to swing and connect, causing pain when hitting vital and semi-vital target areas.

MAGLITE

A flashlight is a great emergency tool to have. Why not have one that doubles as an effective weapon? I recommend that you get the version that requires four or more size-D batteries. If you are defending yourself in a dark setting, hold the Maglite with your knuckles facing upward and the light section by your pinky. The long end is facing backward. Keep the light off until the last second. Turn it on and temporarily blind the assailant and then smash him over the top of the head with the long end of the light. Immediately turn your palm down and strike the side of their head with a backstroke. If necessary, turn your palm up on the follow-through and hit the other side of their head on the way back.

MAGAZINE

Procure a magazine, preferably a thicker one: *Cosmo*, *Muscle & Fitness*, *Glamour*, etc. Roll it up very tight and keep it in your hand at the ready, to be used as a club. Its primary effectiveness will be for Hammer Strikes downward or across to the neck, jaw, temple or nose. Thrusting may be used on the solar plexus, throat or groin.

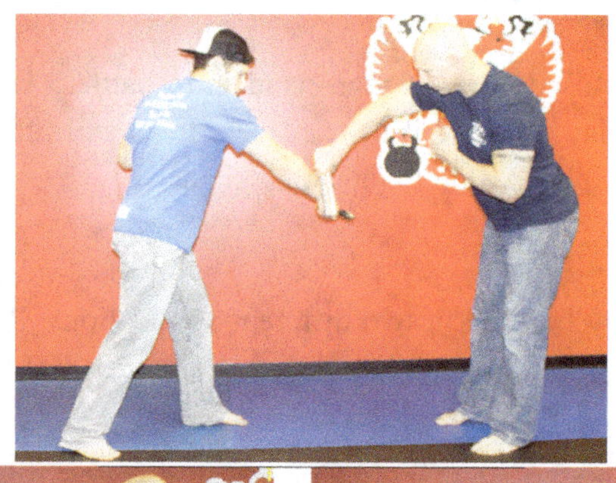

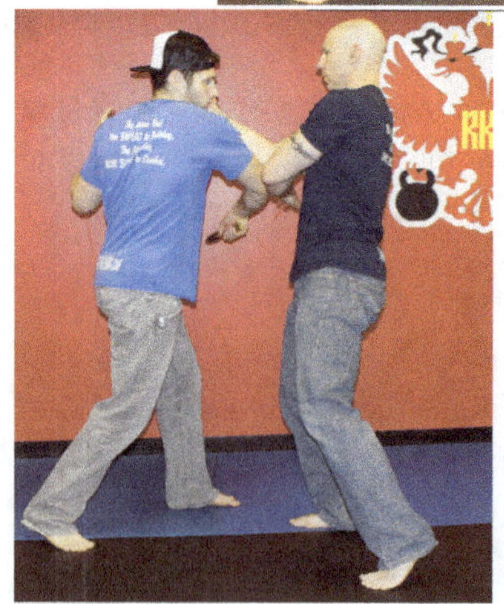

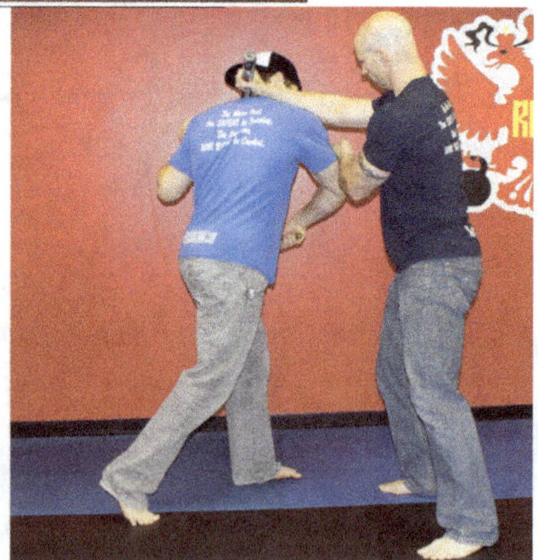

Magazine vs. knife.

CHAIR

Chairs are available in most places. Can you use a chair like they do in the WWE? Yes, you can grab a folding chair and hit someone over the head or across the back with it. However, there is a much more effective way to use a chair. Position the chair in your hands with the four points facing the opponent in a Diamond Formation. This will position the top and bottom points at your adversary's groin and face. The other two legs are to the outside, making it difficult for your attacker to hit you. The Chair Defense is good for defending against a knife attack. Be very aggressive with the chair and back the attacker up with jabs and thrusts.

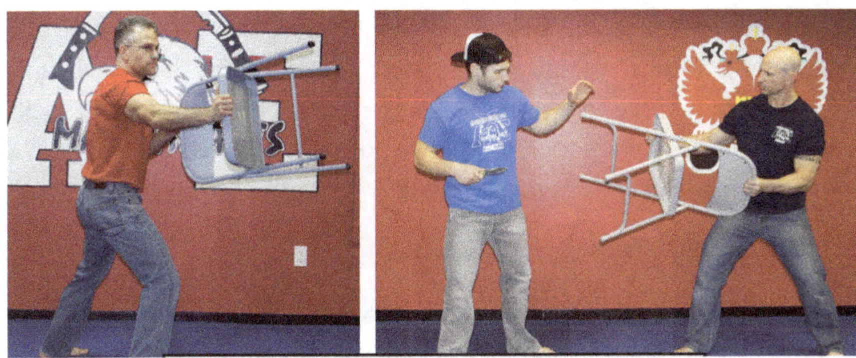

Diamond chair formation vs. knife.

UMBRELLA

The large golf umbrellas work best. Use the point to jab and thrust into the vital and semi-vital target areas. If the handle is hard plastic, that can be used to add power to your strikes as well.

GARBAGE CAN LID

Pick up a garbage can and hit the adversary with it. Grab a lid to block strikes and knife thrusts. Use the edge of the lid to administer strikes as counter-offensives. This is improvisation at its finest!

CHANGE

Have loose change available in your pocket. When faced with an assailant, throw it in their face as a distraction and follow immediately with your counterattack.

BRIEFCASE

Most of us don't carry a briefcase any longer, but you can still apply the principles here. Use the edge and corners of the case to strike the groin or knees, or drive it up into the chin of an assailant. You'd be surprised how effective this technique is!

BELT WITH BUCKLE

Having a good-sized belt buckle has its advantages. Pull your belt off quickly and wrap the strap around your hand, leaving a short length (approximately three to five inches) unwrapped before the buckle. The leather strap adds protection to your hand for punching and the buckle can be used to swing and cut the face of your target.

CHEMICAL DETERRENTS

There are a variety of chemical deterrents available on the market. The most well-known include pepper spray, or OC (oleoresin capsicum) spray and Mace, or Phenacyl chloride (CN/tear gas). The two are often referred to as one and the same; however, they are not. Pepper spray is more effective and legal in most states. Mace was proven ineffective when used in many situations when the assailant is intoxicated or under the influence of alcohol. Pepper spray irritates and inflames the mucus membranes resulting in breathing difficulties, temporary blindness and confusion. As a side note, the Mace brand still carries its *Triple Action Defense Spray*, which is claimed to be a combination of OC pepper spray, CN tear gas and UV-marking dye.

When using pepper spray, it is important not to be downwind, or you will risk having the spray blown back in your face. Also, employ the "sign of the cross" when spraying. By spraying in both the vertical and horizontal planes, your coverage of the assailant will be maximized.

This strategy will allow the fumes to travel upward toward their mouth and nose, making the impact more debilitating. It is easy to miss the attacker's face when aiming directly at it. As an aside, if the assailant is covered with vomit, feces or urine, it will nullify the effects of any chemical sprays. This tactic has been successfully employed by prison inmates.

HORNET (WASP) SPRAY

Depending on the laws in your jurisdiction, carrying a chemical deterrent may or may not be legal. There are no laws against hornet or wasp spray anywhere, though. The range of such a spray is up to 20 feet. This is quite a bit farther than the commercial chemical deterrents currently available on the market.

AIR HORN

This little device is readily available and 100-percent legal to carry. If you are confronted, literally shove the horn in the face of the assailant and then press the button. There will be a moment of "shock" that will afford you the opportunity to deliver a well-placed kick and escape to safety. Additionally, the horn is quite loud and will attract attention.

FIRE EXTINGUISHER

These items are available in virtually every building. These are particularly useful in active shooter situations and their location should be noted every time you enter any structure. The extinguishers can be used to spray and create a distraction, or be used as a blunt instrument to hit the assailant or be thrown at them. For the best results, use the extinguisher to attack the vital and semi-vital target areas of the perpetrator.

Chapter 17
Conventional Weapons

Practice with your weapon on a regular basis. There are many instances when a person is trying to defend themselves and the weapon gets taken away and used on them, and this is what you can prevent from happening if you've developed more comfort and a better feel when using it. You have to get accustomed to its weight, size and how it reacts when you strike or stab something with it, or when you fire it if it's a gun.

We are providing a simple overview of weapons use here. Whole books can and have been dedicated to each of the weapons listed below.

WEAPONS OF CHOICE

There are so many weapons to choose from. There will be laws to consider and they will differ from state to state, but we are not going to address the legality of weapons in-depth here. I am simply going to discuss my favorite weapons and how best to use them.

Some of the essentials for high-level self-defense include the Expandable Baton, Baseball Bat, Short Stick, 12-gauge shot-gun, Glock 9mm,

Special Ops folding knife, Ka-Bar and Sap gloves.

It is essential to practice drawing, shooting, striking, or cutting with your weapon. It should feel natural and familiar to your hand, its weight, shape and general "feel" all well known. You must be very comfortable with the weapon if you want to use it effectively in a stressful situation.

GUN

When using a gun, shoot to kill. Aim for the center mass and then to the head; two rounds in the body and one round in the head. The attacker may be wearing a bullet-proof vest. Wounding someone will only make them more enraged and increase the chance of them getting to you and causing serious injury or death. There is no such thing as "shooting someone in the leg to wound them." Shoot to kill, period.

I prefer a 12-gauge, pump action Remington 870 Express. When you lock and load and the intruders hear the "click, click"; they know that the "BOOM" is coming next and that they are in trouble. Often times the "click, click" sound will be enough to scare them off. If not, the intruder knows where you are, so be prepared to shoot.

As far as pistols go, I like the Glock, either a 9mm or 40-caliber. I have put close to 20,000 rounds through my Glock 19, and it still fires true. I found the pistol grip a little small for my hand, so I put a rubber grip sleeve over the handle. Since then, I have purchased the Glock 45 Gen 5. It's a Glock 19 with a Glock 17 handle. This one also has a red dot.

Join a shooting club, get some lessons and practice until you are comfortable. Make your shooting part of your training routine.

KNIFE

I love knives and carry one with me at all times. My house also has several knives strategically placed throughout for easy access in case of an emergency. Once you get used to carrying a knife, you'll feel naked without it. I have to purposely remind myself to take my knife off and leave it at home when I go to the airport. You should keep your knives sharp and available at all times.

The basic knife movements include the Thrust, Slash and Flick. The basic defensive maneuvers are Parries and Blocks. You also must consider how you grip your knife when holding it. If your knife has a hilt, practice pressing your thumb into the hilt. This will make your grip more stable.

Be certain to check the laws in your current municipality regarding what type of knife is legal to carry. Generally, a double-edged blade is illegal to have on your person.

Thrust: This is a straight and powerful attack. Aim for soft target areas, such as the abdomen, lower back and sides, groin, neck and throat. To inflict maximum damage, twist the knife upon exit. A Thrust is meant to finish an individual off.

Slash: You should slash primarily at downward angles, but upward works in some instances. Aim for the neck, wrists, arms, inner thighs or groin. Slashing is designed to make you bleed and set up the opponent for a finishing Thrust.

Flick: This is thrown as you would a Backfist. It's very quick and difficult to avoid or block. Flicks are thrown to the face and throat. They are designed as an entry technique to help you administer a more lethal attack.

Parry: Use the flat of the blade to redirect a Thrust or a Slash. Follow up with another redirect or Parry with your free hand and then counter-attack with your knife.

Block: The edge of the knife is best suited for blocking; the Block can also double as a slice used to cut the attacking limb. When facing an armed foe, it's better to go metal to metal when blocking a blade coming at you.

BATON

You may choose to work with several different types of batons. The Bando Short Stick, Expandable Baton, Police Billy Club, Baseball Bat and I would even include Rattan (Arnis) in this group. You want to focus on what works best for you. Personally, I keep an Expandable Baton with me and keep both a Baseball Bat and a Bando Short Stick at the ready in my house.

When you practice, mix your strikes, swings and thrusts. Set up a station where you can practice. Take a garbage can and flip it over. Next, place a piece of wood on top of the can's bottom and strike the split log, knocking it off. Another method is to find a dead tree in the woods or some pole. If the tree is alive, wrap it up with carpet. Practice your strikes. These methods will provide you with feedback on the effectiveness of your strikes, letting you evaluate the best grip and determine the best angles for maximum striking power.

There's a video on YouTube that I suggest you watch, called *Master Phil Minute: Baseball Bat Defense*. I review some of the best methods of training with a baseball bat for defensive purposes.

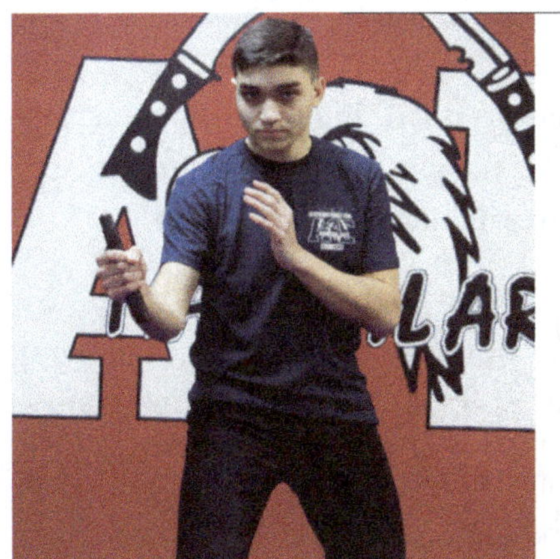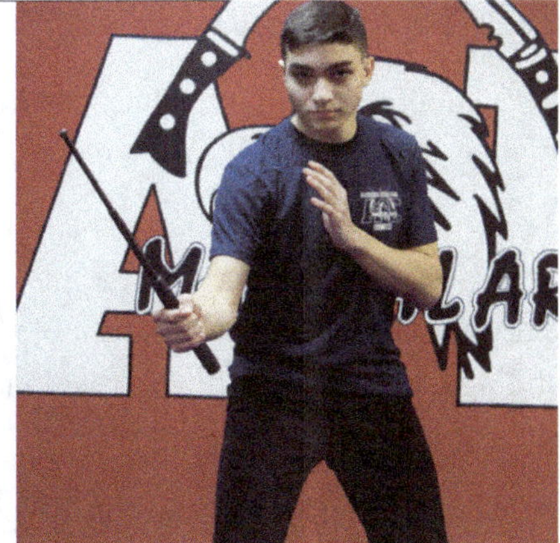

Expandable baton.

Chapter 18
Home-Preparedness

You should install some type of alarm or home warning system, and failing that you should at least have a window sticker that claims you've installed such a system. Some deterrent is better than none.

A dog is great for home protection. Most criminals will pass on a house with a large dog and move onto one without a canine. They will travel the path of least resistance.

You should have emergency numbers coded into your phone, but written down as well. Your electronic devices may be compromised, which is why you shouldn't become overly dependent on them.

Secure your windows and doors and keep them secure at all times. Keep them locked and place a pole or dowel in the floor track of your sliding glass door. A sturdy dowel makes for an effective weapon, too!

You should strategically place weapons in every section of your house. Firearms, clubs, knives, swords, baseball bats, saps, black jacks, expandable batons, etc., should be available to you in an emergency, in every room. However, they need to be secured so that no unauthorized family members, especially the very young, can access them. Also, be sure that you know who comes in and out of your house. More often than not, the friends of your children are very curious and will coax your young ones into "showing" them a weapon. That's how accidents happen.

Please use your best judgment when it comes to the accessibility of weapons and make safe decisions about who knows their locations. Nothing works better than common sense in action.

For every contingency, you should have a plan *and* a back-up plan. Murphy's Law usually doesn't apply to back-up plans. Make certain that everyone in the house knows both plans, inside and out.

"Man plans, and God laughs. When Man has a back-up plan, He smiles." Or so the saying goes.

In addition to your weapons, have a survival kit set up for natural disasters. Water, batteries, generator(s), canned goods, emergency food packs, first aid supplies, etc. should be included in your kit.

Never neglect fire safety. Window ladders, Smoke Detectors and Fire Extinguishers are essential, every floor should have a fire extinguisher and all upper floors a window ladder. Make sure that your smoke and carbon monoxide detectors are fully operational, strategically placed and with fresh batteries. A fire extinguisher can double as a great weapon, you can spray or strike with it.

The Door: Do not open the door for uninvited, unscheduled guests. Period. Have them make an appointment, THEN show identification and clearly state why they are there before you even entertain letting them in. Many home invasions occur without forced entry. People are often duped into letting unidentified strangers or people with false identities into their homes.

You should obtain a firearm and learn how to use it. A pump shotgun, preferably a 12-gauge, is the best weapon for home protection. The ammunition should be shells loaded with buckshot. Consult the NRA and/or your local gun shop for firearms-safety courses and lessons.

Know your weapon and how to handle it. Avoid accidental shootings and keep your weapon in a safe but accessible place.

To make sure you will be prepared when the time comes to act, you should practice moving about your home in darkness. Count the steps of your staircases; this will enable you to move more easily in the darkness without having to think. The assailant does not know your home like you do, so you should learn to exploit that "home field" advantage.

Chapter 19
Every-Day Public Places

No matter how much you fortify your home, you will need to venture out. Now don't be mistaken; I'm not advocating you become a hermit living on some mountain top with an electric fence, a pack of pit bulls in the yard, and an M60 mounted to your roof on a turret. But you will have to take precautions when you go out in public. Bring with you weapons, either standard or unconventional, that you are adept at using and that are legal to possess in your jurisdiction. Be alert and watchful. Forget walking around with your headphones or "air-buds" on and your eyes glued to your smartphone. Keep your eyes up, remember they are your first line of defense.

MALL SAFETY

The malls are a haven for criminals. Mall owners squelch their true crime statistics, and many crimes go unreported and/ or unrecorded. If the general population knew how much crime occurs at the mall, they would sit at home and do their shopping via Amazon! The mall is laden with predators. Look at the bounty they have to choose from! People have money on them, or at least credit cards. They are preoccupied with their shopping. The unsuspecting targets generally don't travel in groups of more than two. There are mothers with children in strollers, older folks looking to get out of the house, and others in a rush to get in and out. What a cornucopia of potential victims!

Trouble often starts in the mall parking lot. Shoppers are laden with too many bags as they fruitlessly search for their cars because they were too busy "updating their status" on Facebook and forgot to check where they parked. Huge mistake. They are a crime statistic waiting to happen.

Most crimes don't happen by chance. If you become a victim it is more likely that you were specifically targeted. Just like the lion looks for the slow, old or weak zebra, you were chosen as easy prey. Criminals, thugs, skells, hoodlums and dirtbags, whatever you choose to refer to them as, are purely predatory creatures. Know this and be aware of this at all times.

Do not be afraid to ask a salesperson to walk you to your vehicle. The retailers and the mall do not want to be responsible for a theft, injury or death of a customer, especially if they have asked for help. It's bad for business.

Look under and around your vehicle. Are there "unsavory characters" watching you? Is there someone under your vehicle waiting to slash your Achilles tendon as you open your car door?

Check your windshield and door handles. There are instances where criminals have poured honey or other sticky substances to door handles and windshields. Another set-up used is tying the windshield wipers together with wire ties. When the unsuspecting victim gets out of the vehicle – they are *attacked!* If you notice any of the listed – DO NOT GET OUT OF THE VEHICLE – CALL 911 IMMEDIATELY!

ELEVATOR

There are times when our "civilized upbringing" makes us vulnerable. If you are alone on an elevator and a group of rowdy youths enter, leave. When you are getting into the elevator, look at who is in there. If you feel strange passing it up and feel like saying something, say,

"Oops, wrong direction!" and then move on. We are so preoccupied with insulting perfect strangers that we compromise our own safety. It is always better to avoid a situation than it is to defend yourself physically; so many things can go awry.

Let us suppose that you are alone on an elevator, and you become surrounded by a rambunctious group of individuals. They begin to harass you and close in around you. Let us hope that you have a self-protection weapon at the ready. Most people do not have a concealed-carry firearm permit. If you are one of those lucky few, now it's time to have your hand on the weapon. Don't brandish it until it's necessary and don't ever point a gun at something that you don't intend to shoot.

But if you don't have a gun, and you're faced with four hostile individuals, what will happen to you? Ideally, you'll have prepared yourself with some good training and have one of your weapons of choice with you. If you don't have any weapons, you will need to make the first strike. Go for the vital and semi-vital target areas, throat, eyes, groins, etc. Hit and move! Strike and spin like an NFL running back as he cuts through the line. Keep moving. Do not allow yourself to be grabbed. You will have to hope for some good luck as well. As soon as the elevator door opens, get out!

PUBLIC BATHROOMS

As always, look around and see who is sharing the room with you. If you are a female and there's a man in the restroom with you, turn around and get out! Be astute when you are entering the restroom. Was anyone watching you when you went in? Did someone follow you in? Keep your eyes peeled.

Guys, look out for groups of people. And remember you are very vulnerable when you are at a urinal. Once you start urinating, place your other hand against the wall. This will make it more difficult for a perpetrator to sneak up on you and slam you into the wall.

RESTAURANTS

Once you arrive, scan the area. Look at the patrons and general layout, locate the restrooms and the exits. Have a plan in mind in the event that a robbery or assault occurs. Take a walk through the restaurant and scout it out. Even if you don't have to go to the bathroom, do so. Always sit so that the door is in plain view. While you are out to dinner or in a restaurant, you should never get too inebriated. You will not think clearly, and no matter what you think, your reactions will be slower and less precise. Don't get drunk and leave yourself and those you are responsible for exposed.

PARTIES AND BARS

This advice is primarily geared toward the younger set. The dangers that you may encounter when you are out trying to have a good time are many. Women are more often the target of drugging, but it may happen to guys well. Follow these rules, as well as all other safety rules and stay alert. If something feels wrong, remove yourself from the situation. Have a back-up plan and a means to leave.

1. Never take an open drink. Even if it's from someone you know. Do you trust that they had their eyes on the drink the whole time? No open drinks, even water. Only accept a closed beverage.
2. Keep your hand over the top of your glass and never set your drink down anywhere.
3. Know the people that you are attending the party with and have a designated meeting place.
4. DO NOT get uncontrollably drunk. There are far too many bad things that can happen to you if you are intoxicated or pass out.
5. Go in groups, especially if you are going to an unfamiliar location. There is safety in numbers.

Chapter 20
Mass Hysteria

The year was 2004, and I was part of a crew working a detail at an event hall. There were eleven of us working security and we were equipped with metal detectors and wands to check the attendees for weapons prior to entrance to the party. The establishment was located in Little Ferry, NJ, on Route 46 West and directly across the river from Paterson. This party was the last event to be held there. The hall was shut down after what transpired that night.

Steve Cirone (he's in this book) and I were both on the detail. Things started to go awry from the beginning. We found out that the party was a "Jeans and Boots" event; this was not a good thing. The people showing up would not be dressed well, and generally, people would act in accordance with their attire. Meaning that if one is dressed up and presentable, they will behave better. If they are wearing boots, jeans and sweatshirts, they don't care if their clothes get messed up. Call it profiling, call it stereotyping, call it what you want. I'll call it what it is: a fact.

As the night went on, the patrons became more intoxicated. The owner was selling full champagne bottles, even though we advised him not to. There were factions from two rival gangs in attendance as well. Soon, and unsurprisingly, things really started to heat up. Skirmishes were breaking out on and around the dance floor, and the DJ was calling for Security to intervene.

In one skirmish, one of the partiers raised his champagne bottle to strike someone, and I grabbed his hand. I directed him to relax and put the bottle down. His response was the opposite of compliance. He then came at me, which elicited my survival reaction. I punched him square in the face. All Hell broke loose.

Steve Cirone planted a boot in the back of a rioter and sent them to the ground. The three of us, Steve, Tony (Blandino) and I, then went back-to-back-to-back. We fought our way to the kitchen. People were screaming, running and fighting. The place was in total chaos. I have no idea how we did not get hurt or even hit (that I can remember). We were shoving, kicking, punching, bobbing and weaving as we extracted ourselves from the melee.

Normally, I don't remember exactly what happens with perfect accuracy during an altercation, until a witness fills me in. In this case, the witnesses that would have normally described my actions to me (Steve and Tony) were also wrapped up in the evolving chaos.

There were cops from fifteen towns there, but none dared to come in. They waited outside in the parking lot. Police will not enter a situation like this. The chance of losing their weapons is far too high. They generally wait until it dissipates or in extreme cases, administer tear gas to move people out. They didn't have to in this case; people came out on their own accord. Someone threw a chair through a wall mirror and a woman screamed "HE HAS A *GUN!*" Now the brouhaha had escalated to an even higher level! People started rushing for the door. We made certain that there was no gun and began to push and shove the crowd, "helping" them to get out of the door and into the parking lot.

Many of the rabble-rousers began to fight with the police. It was quite a scene! Police cars, ambulances, blood, fights, rock throwing, bottles being broken and throngs of people in conflict. The police wound up arresting a bunch, but most of them were simply "pushed" out of the area and toward the bridge heading to Paterson.

As security personnel, we succeeded in getting everyone out of the establishment. Nevertheless, mistakes were made and there were consequences. Had I been in charge, I would have briefed everyone on staff prior to the start of the evening so they would be on the lookout for trouble. With that type of crowd, there should have been a plan in place or some mechanism to keep certain people out.

Again, I was not in charge. When the fights began, the other eight bouncers were nowhere to be found. They scattered, and the three of us were left to deal with the situation. Also, a staff of eleven bouncers for over 600 people is far too small. There should have been at least double what we had.

The important thing to note is that we kept our heads, knew when to act, when to exit, and where to go when push came to shove. There was a great deal of confusion, and people could have easily been killed, although thankfully no one was. However, the situation was a total clusterfuck, and they were discussing it on the news for a couple of days afterward. The establishment was shut down by the town as a result of this debacle.

How does this story relate to you? You may never become a bouncer or a protection agent. However, you may find yourself in a situation where a crowd is in panic or is engaged in a riot. In this era of terror-istic threats, unruly protesters and out-of-control mobs, what can you do?

Needless to say, if you find yourself three feet away from an exploding backpack, you'll be out of luck. No method, thought process or training will help you then. The "stars" were not aligned in your favor. But barring something this dramatic, you will have time to react to protect yourself and your loved ones.

If you are caught in a terrorist attack, or encounter an uncontrolled mob, a lone assailant, a group of shooters, explosive devices detonated from a distance, or some type of chemical attack, the number one thing to remember is that ***COOLER HEADS PREVAIL!*** Keep your cool. You don't want to panic and run from the frying pan straight into the fire.

In all of these scenarios, ***mass hysteria*** will set in. People will be screaming and running wildly. I've been involved in a few of these incidents, and it's not a pretty sight. You have to be cognizant of not being trampled and not getting pushed in the wrong direction. Things get more complicated when you have a small child or otherwise less self-sufficient companion with you. Protect who you are with and try to have a wall to your back. Avoid getting knocked down and keep your sight on an exit.

We will consider several scenarios. For example, let us ponder an incident involving a lone shooter. This could occur *anywhere*. In a mall, a school, a movie theater, a parking lot, you name it. One must maintain vigilance at all times.

Look, you don't have to run around in a completely paranoid state like John Belushi sneaking into Dean Wormer's office in the classic 70s moving *Animal House*. But you do have to be aware. If you are walking around with your earbuds plugged in, or your headphones blaring the latest JZ rap song, how can you be in tune with your surroundings? You need to lose the headsets and anything else that will divert your attention. Be alert, at all times.

The first thing you do is to hit the deck and bring your loved ones down to the floor with you. Don't stay on the ground long, though; people will begin to run amuck, panicking and running wild. It will be frightening to see the look of abject fear on their faces and in their eyes as they scramble aimlessly, trying to flee. However, since you have been vigilant, you know where the closest exit is. Stay low and look for cover as you make your way to that location.

When considering the following scenarios, your course of action will not be much different, just more difficult. If there are several shooters or explosive devices being detonated, please realize that you are most likely in the middle of an organized attack. You are living on borrowed time, so every second you are alive is bonus time … so use it wisely. Immediately hit the deck and seek cover. Stay low.

Try to determine where the shooters are. In an organized attack, the perpetrators may have set up diversions that will "funnel" the crowd into an even worse situation, so be cognizant of the options and don't follow the most obvious escape route without considering that it might be a set-up.

Terrorists count on hysteria to maximize their death totals. You can only hope Lady Luck will be on your side.

There are other situations to consider, where safety is the prime issue. If you are in a public place and a fight breaks out - MOVE! Exit the area post-haste. There are far too many incidents of innocent bystanders getting injured or killed when a fight breaks out.

Picture this scene: two or more guys get into a scuffle. Tempers flare, and one of these boneheads pulls out a gun and begins to fire. You have no control over where the bullets go. You only have control over how you react to a situation. React by removing yourself from harm's way. As we have discussed before, you can avoid over 95 % of danger situations simply by not being there. Exit the area post-haste. Don't let curiosity do to you what it did to the cat.

Chapter 21
Car Safety

Make it a habit of being able to see the rear tires of the car in front of you when at a stop light. If you are able to see those rear tires, you will be able to pull around them.

This will prevent someone from boxing you in. Typically, if you are being set up, criminals will "box" you in by having a car in front and one in back of you. Once you are boxed in, they will converge on your vehicle from both sides. If there is a car in front of you and one behind you, and you notice the tail lights of the car ahead of you illuminating, MOVE! You are most likely being set-up and you had best remove yourself from the area.

Criminals will stoop to the lowest levels imaginable in order to relieve you of your money and property. There have been incidents of these deviants feigning distress by posing with a "baby" next to a "disabled" vehicle. There have been other occurrences of an attractive woman standing by a car looking helpless and forlorn. In both of these cases, their accomplice was hiding nearby, waiting for their opportunity to pounce on the hapless good Samaritan. Do not stop. Keep driving and call 911 to alert them of the person in need of roadside assistance. If you don't have a cell phone or service, wait until you come to a location that has a phone and then call.

When driving you should have at your immediate disposal an expandable baton, club, or some other type of blunt instrument, a knife with a serrated edge and a chemical spray. Not only are these great defensive weapons, but the blunt instrument and the knife can be used to help you extract yourself from a compromised vehicle in the case of an accident. The blunt club or baton may be used to break a window. The serrated knife can serve as a means to cut loose a malfunctioning seat belt.

Make certain that you have an emergency kit in your car. Mine includes a compass, pocket fishing pole, fishing lures, water purifying kit, handheld chainsaw, fire starters, matches, flint, lightweight thermal blankets, MRE's, a Leatherman, a sharpening stone, a collapsible eating utensil kit and a survival knife. You never know how long you are going to be stuck and who you might run into. There are several very good disaster survival books and courses to read or take. These are written by or conducted by others more qualified than me in these matters, and I will defer the details of disaster preparation to these experts.

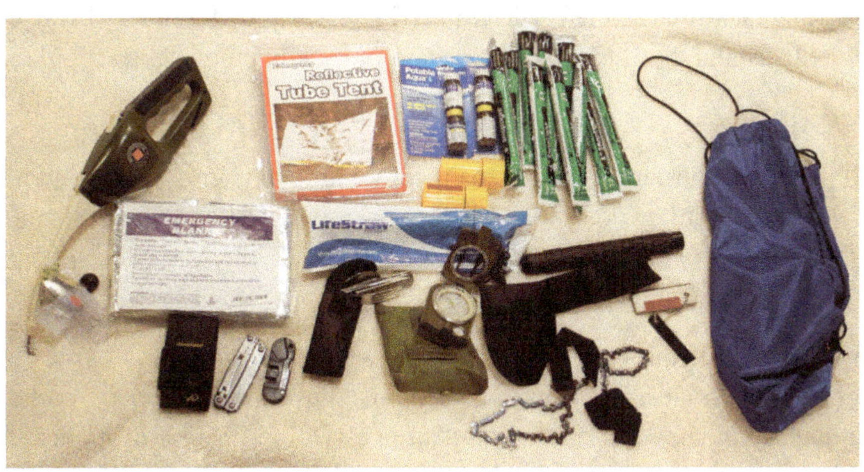

UNMARKED POLICE CARS

Do not pull over if an unmarked police car tries to pull you over. Immediately call 911, especially if you were not speeding. Just because you are a guy, don't be all "macho" and think that nothing can happen to you. It can and it will. Call 911, and if you do get pulled over, don't open the car door or window until you are absolutely certain this is a real police officer.

ROAD RAGE

As stated before - *cooler heads prevail*. Always keep this in mind.

Yes, there are a lot of bad drivers and complete fools out on the road. But are any of them worth more than your life? Don't ever pull over and get out of your car to "teach this guy a lesson." Too many times people have been hurt or killed in this fashion. You may even get run over by an oncoming car. There could be more than one person in the vehicle. He or she could have a weapon. Yes, I said *she*. There are prisons full of women, and the rate is rising. Maybe they want you to pull over so they can rob you. Whatever the case is, stay in your car.

At a stop light, always leave enough room in front of you to be able to see the back tires of the car in front. This ensures that you will be able to pull around the vehicle. If they begin to back up, move quickly!

OBSTACLES

If there are obstacles in the road, move around them. Do not stop. Disregard flaming tires, road-blocks or crowds out and about on the street in a rough neighborhood late at night. Keep your windows up and keep moving.

Know where you are going. Knowing where you are going avoids a great many issues. Use your GPS, but also have printed directions and a map. Remember that a backup plan is essential. Familiarize yourself with your route prior to embarking on your journey.

Have weapons available. Keep some type of weapon in your car. You should have at your immediate disposal an expandable baton, club or some other type of blunt instrument, a knife with a serrated edge, and a chemical spray. If you carry a baseball bat with you, be sure to have a glove and ball in the car as well. You could simply state that you use it in the park to shag fly balls with your friends if questioned.

Not only are these great defensive tactics weapons, but the blunt instrument and the knife can be used to help you extract yourself from a compromised vehicle in the case of an accident. An expandable baton or metal pipe/club may be used to break a window in case of a crash, either underwater or if the doors malfunction. A knife with a serrated edge may be used to cut you out of a jammed safety belt in case of a malfunction after an accident. A chemical deterrent won't help you escape following an accident, but you should have one with you in your car as well.

Always abide by this axiom: ***It's better to have it and not need it than it is to need it and not have it.*** These are words to live by.

Chapter 22
The Importance of Training

The saying goes: Victory does not favor the righteous or the wicked; *Victory favors the prepared.* The benefits and the transformation of your mind and body you will enjoy from regular training will surpass what you'd imagined was possible. Do not set limits on yourself, and do not think that you are unable to develop the reflexes necessary to defend yourself adequately.

Consider the sport of baseball. It takes 400 milliseconds for the pitcher to deliver a baseball across home plate. The minimum human reaction time is 200 milliseconds. A batter must make his decision to swing at a ball by the time it's less than halfway from the pitcher's hand to crossing home plate.

You may be asking yourself why this is important. What does it have to do with self-defense training? It has everything to do with it. Please note that I stated, "minimum human reaction time." That is distinct from an "elite-level athlete's reaction time."

Scientists have been studying human reaction times for over 40 years. After decades of administering tests, it was determined that there was zero difference between an elite athlete's reaction time and the reaction time of your accountant. You may still be asking why this is important.

The point of this passage is to make apparent that you have the ability to develop quick reactions by training and training often. The only way a professional baseball player is able to hit a ball traveling 95 mph is due to his ability to predict where the ball will cross the plate. He is able to predict this because he has seen thousands upon thousands of pitches over many hours through many years of training. You can do the same thing.

You have the ability to develop IT, or Instinctive Technique, once you have trained yourself and remove thought from the process. You have the equipment, and now you have the knowledge. It's all up to you to practice and practice properly. In order to give yourself the best chance of victory, you must be PREPARED!

Excuses for not training are far too common. Avoid the temptation to make them, which you will need to do to succeed.

There is no way on earth you will be able to practice all of the techniques, defensive tactics and strength and conditioning movements in this book on a daily basis. There is far too much volume and too many variations. So what you need is a plan that will add variety and diversity to your exercise and training routines over the course of many days and weeks, so everything is covered.

While training, you will need to warm-up sufficiently with your jump rope and your mobility and flexibility routines for five to seven minutes. Spend 20 to 25 minutes on strength and conditioning and use the remainder of your session on your defensive tactics. How much time you spend on the different aspects of the training will depend upon what else you do. For example, if you train at a BJJ (Brazilian Jiu Jitsu) Academy, you will not want to spend too much time grappling. If you are a kickboxer, you'll want to spend less time on your striking combinations. If you are extremely fit and work out at a gym a great deal, you will spend more time working on your strikes, self-defense and grappling and less time on the fitness aspects provided in this book.

If you'd like to train in the program five or six days a week, split it up. Spend an hour every other day on fitness, and do your bag work, body conditioning, striking and grappling on the alternate days. You also have to consider when a training partner is available or not. If you are training solo, focus on your strength and conditioning, body conditioning (toughening) and your bag work. When you do have a partner, work on the defensive tactics, grappling and partner drills.

Below we have listed a guide to aid you in your training rotation.

SURVIVAL STRONG TRAINING ROTATION

1. Push-Ups, Abs and Bridges. Pad Work: Station Rotation.
2. Handstands, Pull-Ups and Squats. Four Ranges of Combat.
3. Walk the Plank, Ab Crawls and Lunges. Ground-Up Fighting.
4. Dips, Cossacks and Planks. Zones and Herky Jerky.
5. Plyometric (Leap up, Thrusters, Push-Ups). Body Conditioning.
6. Push-Ups, Squats and Bridges. Power Strikes.
7. Primal Move, Walk the Plank, Ab Crawls. Unconventional Weapons
8. Handstands, Bridges, Lunges. Get up from the ground with an attacker on you, prone and supine. Body Conditioning
9. Push-Ups, Pull-Ups, Abs, Squats. Multiple Attackers
10. Push-ups, Abs & Jump Rope, Handstands. Knife Attacks.
11. Pull-Ups, Hanging Abs, Squats and Lunges. Power Strikes, Slaps, and Punch Defense.
12. Handstands, Pull-Ups, Bridges, Break Falls, Roll-Outs, and Upkicks
13. Push-Ups, Dips, Abs. Power Strikes, and Quick Strike Defense.
14. Push-Ups, Squats, Bridges. Movement, Punch Defense, and Baseball Bat Defense.

15. Handstands, Lunges, Back Pressure Abs. Cut Kicks, Slaps, and Knife Defense.
16. Push-Ups, Squats, Bridges, Dips, Knee Drives, Elbows, and Bear Hugs.
17. Pull-Ups, Dips, Abs, Bridges, Side and Front Kicks, Axehands, and Wrist Locks.
18. Push-Ups, Squats, Planks, and Four Ranges of Combat.
19. Handstands, Bridges, Lunges. Throws and Sweeps.
20. Dips, Hanging Abs, Squats. Ground Fighting and Knife Defense, Menacing.
21. Handstands, Bridges, Push-ups. Takedowns, Gun Defense.
22. Squats, Pull-Ups, Planks. Dog Attacks, Knife at the throat.
23. Handstands, Dips, Lunges. Chokes: Three and Four Point, Front, with entries.
24. Bridges, Handstands, Ab Crawls. Power Strikes: Hands and Elbow with entries.
25. Pull-Ups, Push-Ups, Hanging Abs. Knife and Knife Versus Gun.
26. Partner Bodyweight: Push-Ups (hold ankles or on back), Abs (Standing or Dog Stance), Bridge Back (Greco Drill) and Squats (on back). Wrist Locks.
27. Dips, Plyo Squats/Box Jumps, Levers and "Phil-Ups". Club attacks.
28. Push-Ups, Bridges, Lunges. Four Ranges of Combat.
29. Handstands, Abs and Squats. Open hand strikes.
30. Pull-ups, Dips (rings, too), Bridges. Kick Defense.
31. Push-ups, Lunges, Abs. Choke and Guillotine Defense.
32. Pull-ups, Bridges, Squats. Ground Attacks
33. Handstands, Hanging Abs, Plyo Squats. Wrist Locks.
34. Push-Ups, Bridges, Squats. Knife Attacks, held to the neck.
35. Plyometrics – Push-Ups and Squats. Kicks
36. Handstands, Abs, Elbows, and Bear Hugs.
37. Bridges and Squats. Body Conditioning, Quick Strike Defense.

38. Push-Ups and Abs. Ground-Up defense and Arm Drags to take down.
39. Pull-Ups, Lunges, Dips. Kicks, Combos, Choke from behind
40. Dips, Plyometric Squats, Lying Abs. 1-6 Punches and Combinations.
41. Bridges, Handstands, Lunges. Power Strikes, Elbows, and Knees
42. Terrorist Attacks: 1) Holstered, 2) Reloading, 3) From behind & 4) From the Front, you will need to drop and bear crawl or forward roll.
43. Dynamic Tension with Push-Ups, Squats, and Bridge and Hold. Ground Defense with arms pinned. Takedown and Mount.
44. Plyo Push-Ups, Spilt-Squats, and Table-Top Bridge. Defense from the ground while being choked. Ground and Pound from the top, once you reverse.
45. Handstands, Pull-Ups. Knife Basics.
46. Push-Ups, Abdominals. Throws: Hip Toss, Body Lock and Head Locks.
47. Squats (One and/or two legs), Bridges. Body Conditioning and Pad Work.
48. Lunges, Dips, and Plyo Push-Ups. Choke defense, standing and on the ground.
49. Bridges, Plyo Squats or Box Jumps. Four Ranges of Combat.
50. Handstands, Hanging Abs (or Abs), Push-Ups. Car scenarios, Multiple Attackers.

The beauty of this plan of action is that you can customize it to fit your needs, ability and time constraints. The most important aspect to bear in mind, though, is to train on a consistent basis. Once a month or once a week is not enough; three times a week is the *minimum*, but four or five times a week is recommended.

Chapter 23
Breathing and Meditation

Breathing will help calm you and reduce anxiety during a stressful situation. When we experience an adrenaline dump, our breathing becomes shallow. If you are "chest breathing," you will run out of air quickly and become exhausted. This is NOT conducive to effectively defending yourself.

Make certain to practice breathing in through your nose, to the bottom of the lungs, and using the diaphragm to push the air out through your mouth. Breathe into your abdomen and practice this breathing not only when you are meditating, but also while you are training or simply walking around. This type of breathing promotes relaxation and quick, explosive movements.

Get into the habit of doing your breathing exercises and meditating. There are many effective methods to employ. I developed a meditation CD, *Powerful Spirit*; it is 23 minutes long and based on Self Hypnosis and Positive Imagery, as is taught at the West Point Military Academy. I've had significant success with my fighters and wrestlers using the CD. Even my mother's friends use it to fall asleep!

While practicing meditation, use this time to address the mindset that is necessary for success in defense of yourself or loved ones. Review the movements and scenarios as you visualize how you will respond. Through training and visualization your confidence will increase, and your response time will be diminished as IT takes over.

Focusing on your intended target will yield victory. There are two types of animals in the wild kingdom: predators and prey. Prey are vigilant and look out for danger. Mimicking prey behavior, try to avoid dangerous situations if at all possible and run if you are able to run. A dead hero is of no use to anyone. However, there comes a point when the prey must transform into the predator, and that's how it should be with you. When that time comes, act with great focus and extreme violence, and permit yourself to be what you are designed to be – The Apex Predator! This is your mindset. Be certain that you are able to "flip the switch" from lamb to lion at a second's notice.

I would recommend that you read some books on the powers of Zen and meditation. This knowledge will prove helpful in your training and will boost your overall mental health.

Chapter 24
Recommended Training Aids

There are a certain minimum number of items that you will need to maximize your training efforts. Listed below are some equipment, books and videos that I have found extremely beneficial to my mindset and physical conditioning.

EQUIPMENT

- Focus Mitts
- Rubber Knife & Gun
- Clubs or Baseball Bats (Wiffleball Bats acceptable for training)
- Jump Rope
- Kicking Shields
- Various Unconventional Weapons as previously listed
- Body Conditioning (Hardening) Tools
- Staff or Dowel, 6 feet
- Martial Arts Belts
- Towel
- Abdominal Wheel (Wheel of Death)

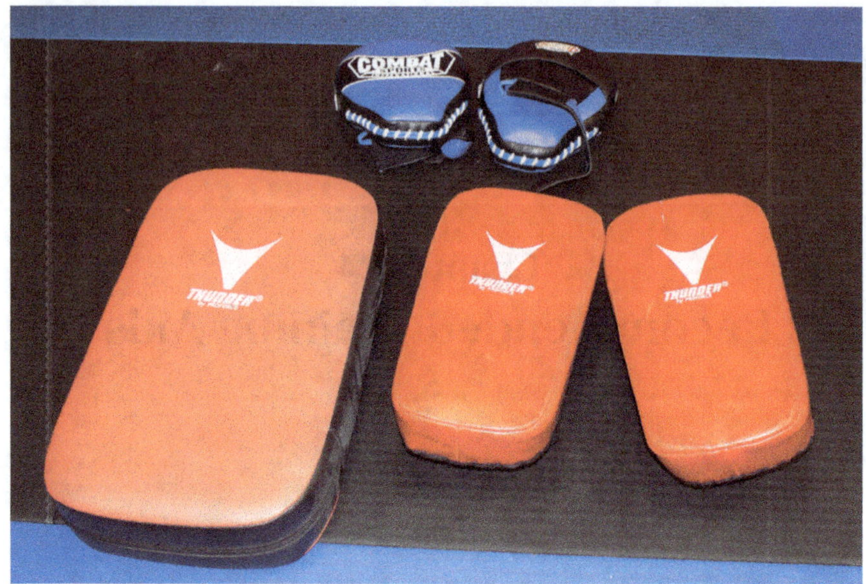

RECOMMENDED TRAINING MATERIAL

The Convict Conditioning Series (1, 2 & 3)

Available on the Dragon Door Site:

www.dragondoor.com/?apid=4640

In addition to the books, the Gold Standard in Kettlebells, The RKC Kettlebell are available here as well.

Main Site: www.philross.com
Survival Strong Virtual Training:
www.survivalstrong.philross.com/
Included are six educational videos on proper execution of technique and 20 workout videos to make and keep you sharp!
Enjoy a ten% discount by using code: SSBook2E

The 23 Lethal Knife Movements:

Knives are readily available, that's good news and bad news. Good news, they're available to you, bad news, they're available to criminals and thugs. Our concise, precise and effective system will equip you with the knowledge to know how to use a knife properly and what to expect when facing one.

Available on video and in-person seminars.

Phil Ross' S.A.V.E. Video Training Series

Complete Set, 4 videos and Audio CD Mental Preparation CD. This video series was Rated #1 by two separate organizations, besting Bruce Lee's System and Krav Maga. Beginner, Intermediate, Advanced Levels as well as a fitness video are included. Each video is approximately one hour. The 24-minute audio CD guides you through the mental preparation process preparing the mind for victory in a conflict.

To increase your Strength and Conditioning, delve into Hardstyle Kettlebell and Bodyweight Training. My Patreon Channel, Master Phil Ross (www.patreon.com/MasterPhilRoss) has over 150 workouts including the Survival Strong video training, The Kettlebell Workout Library, The Secrets of Kettlebells, as well as weapons training, heavy bag workouts and more.

OTHER SOURCES

SUGGESTED READING MATERIALS:

I have read a multitude of books over the years and several of them have had a profound impact on my thinking and training. Either by reaffirming what I had already experienced or by enhancing my training in a positive direction.

The Way and The Power: Secrets of Japanese Strategy

by Frederick J. Lovret

This book was incredibly instrumental in re-enforcing that I was on the right path with my training and mindset. When I read this book, I was already doing 95 percent of what the author espoused. This was enlightening.

Kill or Get Killed

by Col. Rex Applegate

I was introduced to Art of Close Quarters Trench Warfare tactics in 1988 by a Carl Cestari, a former U.S. Army Green Beret, mercenary and judo champion. This system is brutal to the point, relatively simple to learn and extremely effective. This method changed my approach to defensive tactics.

Ferocious Fitness: A Fighter's Proven Action Plan to Develop Blazing Power, Animalistic Strength and Killer Conditioning

by Phil Ross and Marty Gallagher

Kettlebells, bodyweight and guidance through strength and conditioning throughout a fight camp. You don't have to be a fighter to train like one. True to life stories and rankings of the most bad-assed fighters through history. Develop the strength and explosive power to help you to "become your own bodyguard".

MMA for Dummies

by Frank Shamrock

Frank Shamrock was the first ever Five-Time Undefeated UFC Middleweight Champion and the prototype for the modern MMA Fighter. He guides you though the training and philosophies necessary to train like a successful fighter and provides incredible insight to the specifics of the sport. Having worked with Frank as an assistant to him in many workshops and a few fight camps, I can assure you that his knowledge and experience are unsurpassed.

Infinite Insights into Kenpo

by Ed Parker

Master Parker was an incredible martial artist with a great deal of street fighting experience. His tenets of fighting and his techniques make the practitioner "Street Ready." I never trained directly with him, but did train with his disciple Grand Master Mike Klier, and found the system and teachings to be exceptionally effective and congruent to my training.

A Book of Five Rings

by Miyamoto Musashi

Single Mindedness and training with extreme purpose. This book helps the reader understand the importance of purposeful training to develop cat-like reflexes and respond without thinking.

Ultimate Athleticism

by Max Shank

www.ultimateathleticism.com/

This is another great book on a system developed by one of the strongest people I have ever met. A strength competitor, feat performer and martial artist, Max's approach to strength training is applicable to developing the strength and power to defend oneself in the street.

Develop the Predator Mindset: Win in Sports and Life

by Gene Zannetti

There comes a point when the predicament is unavoidable and the switch needs to be flipped. You are no longer prey – but you are now the predator and your total focus is on the assailant. Confidence, focus and mental exercise prepare you for success in the task at hand. Not only do I believe in the system, but I'm one of the Certified Mindset Coaches!

Exercise Snacks: Fitness Five Minutes at a Time

by Phil Ross

The number one objection to not adopting a fitness regimen is the perceived lack of time. Who does not have five minutes? There are 54 workouts that are approximately five minutes long each. Kettlebell, dumbbells, bodyweight, dynamic tension and martial arts are all included. Move daily and move often to keep the weight down and the skills sharp.

A Guide to Martial Arts Training with Equipment

by Dan Inosanto

Proper training gear is essential to success in fighting. Review this list of equipment and incorporate it's use to develop power, speed and accuracy.

Epilogue

There are no shortcuts to self-defense, strength development and honing your survival skills. You must make your training a lifestyle and adopt a mindset of vigilance and preparedness.

When I first launched this book project, the dangers of terrorism and social unrest were already on the rise, and I observed the ever-growing constraints placed upon law enforcement and the general population. People, on the whole, are good-hearted and simply want to live their lives in peace and freedom. Unfortunately, there are factions, whether they be radical religious fanatics, sociopaths, or hardened criminals, determined to take what's rightfully yours and bring undeserved harm to you and your loved ones. We must realize that the police and the government will not be there to provide protection at all times and that protecting ourselves is ultimately our responsibility. *The police are there in minutes when seconds count.*

This book includes an incredible amount of advice, techniques and other information you should know. The movements and strategies you have been introduced to must be practiced on a regular basis, and there is no substitute for hands-on instruction by a qualified instructor. If you cannot find a suitable instructor in your area, we conduct Survival

Strong Seminars and Workshops and we can come to your facility. We also have a video training series, as referenced in the previous chapter.

The movements and exercises in this book are relatively basic and can be learned and executed by virtually anyone. Weapons-centric training will be covered more in-depth in future publications.

No matter what your level of training, nothing can replace good judgment and sound decision-making. At the beginning of the book, I discussed a situation where I fought six guys and lost, very badly. The group that I was with got in a scuffle with a group of other guys. I was friends with the bouncers, and this group of six was shoved out of the side door of the bar with one of my friends. I was 5'10", 202 pounds, heavily muscled, and filled with testosterone and a good measure of beer. Alone, I bolted out through the unlocked front door to come to the aid of my friend, while leaving the rest of my crew inside. I thought that I was an invincible superhero.

Wrong. I recall asking my buddy if he was okay. He said all was good, so I turned my back to go back to the bar. When I did this I was hit in the back of the head with a beer bottle. My initial response was to turn and shoot a double-leg takedown on the assailant. Upon lifting him in the air and smashing him on the pavement, the remaining five guys began to kick me. When a fight goes to the ground, the winner is usually the one with more friends. As I was lying there, I buried my face close to his to protect my face as much as possible and squeezed my knees around his hips to protect my groin. I was getting kicked and stomped.

It's funny what goes through one's mind in situations like this. I thought of watching a show where a guy was on the ground getting kicked and stomped like I was. IT SUCKED, and I wanted it to end! People claimed that I let loose with a mighty yell, pulled myself up, dropped two of the guys and then got hit in the back of the head again. I have no idea if it was with a bottle or a fist.

Everything went black. When I came to, the ambulance was there and I was covered in blood. I told one of my friends that I was going to get those guys. Well, my friends got them that night and I later found out that I was set-up. No worries, though, I "settled the score," when I went face-to-face, one-on-one with the ringleader.

So what's the point of all of this? Here's what I'd like you to know and consider:

1. Street fights and crime have a zero element of fairness. I got my ass handed to me, and every shot I got hit with was from behind.
2. Don't let your ego get in the way. Street fights are not worth it. Who really won this confrontation? We all lost.
3. Cooler heads prevail. Keep your cool and pay attention to what's happening around you. I did neither.
4. No matter how tough you are or how good of a fighter you are, if someone wants to take you down, they will – if you leave yourself exposed.

I want to wish you good luck in your training, and other than the strength and conditioning in this book, I hope that you never have to use any of the techniques in a real-life situation. If you do, let's hope it's the avoidance strategies you have the opportunity to use, and that they enable you to prevent conflicts from actually occurring. If it doesn't work out that way, I'm confident that if you have practiced hard and often and developed your "IT," you will react properly and secure a positive result. Remember to act concisely, decisively and with great fervor.

Strength and Honor,

Master Phil

Acknowledgments

I would like to thank my parents for providing me with the solid mental and emotional foundation that is the basis for my vision, indomitable spirit and belief in myself.

There are many people who have had a positive influence on my life, especially regarding my training in the martial arts. I have had the great fortune of having some incredible instructors, coaches and training partners over the years. I also have trained and worked with war veterans, police officers, security professionals and "street guys." I would like to thank them for their knowledge and influence and for being part of my journey.

Major Influences: My grandfather Cosmo Ferro, my father Phil Ross, wrestling coach Rich Witte, Tim and Chris Catalfo (wrestling), Sensei James Martin (karate), Instructor Bill Timmie Taekwondo), Dr. Mike Evangel (Taekwondo), Professor Jon Collins (Bando), Dr. Pat Finely (Arnis, Jun Fan, Bando), Dr. Tony Palminteri (Japanese jiu jitsu), Brendan Behr (student & training partner), Steve Cirone (security, bodyguard, martial arts, defensive tactics instruction, firearms instruction), Joe Rubino (boxing, kickboxing), Frank Shamrock (MMA & submission fighting), Robert Smith (martial arts student and training partner),Tom Patire (bodyguard & security, defensive tactics, firearms instruction), Carl Cestari (defensive tactics and Combato Defendo), Mitch Coats (Brazilian Jiu Jitsu), Khyl Farrisson (Brazilian Jiu Jitsu), Jay Hayes (Brazilian Jiu Jitsu), Percy Alston (security and martial arts and strength training partner), Brian Ebersole (MMA, grappling, former UFC Fighter), Rusty Read, NCAA D1 All American

(Wrestling, Grappling & MMA training partner), John Robert (Bob) Pierson (student and martial arts training partner, weapons instruction, security details), Damian Ross (brother, student, training partner, wrestling, martial arts) and John Holster (student of mine for over 30 years, training partner). There have been others along the way, but these people have had the most profound influence on me and what I've done in the street, on the mat and in the ring.

My students and family members who helped me with the photographs, Drew Donofrio, Scott Crisanto, Matt and Andres Burgos, Zack Fox, and my family, Amy, Nicole, Spencer and Adrienne Ross. Thank you for taking the time to pose for and take pictures. I'd also like to thank Max Shank, who is not only the strongest person that I know, pound for pound, but also one of the strongest people I've ever met, period. His consultation on the bodyweight training sections in this book made this system complete.

About the Author

Phil Ross, M.S., is known on the world stage for his accomplishments in martial arts and fitness. He has successfully competed on the national level in submission fighting, kickboxing, full contact karate, taekwondo and Olympic style wrestling. He has also held several titles in bodybuilding and powerlifting and is a Master Kettlebell instructor as well as a college professor in the field of exercise science and sports management. More important than his personal accomplishments are the many benefits that his students have gained from his coaching in physical and mindset training. His training methods have produced champions in the sports of karate, submission fighting, MMA, kickboxing, both collegiate and Olympic wrestling, football, volleyball, soccer, and track and field, just to name a few. In addition to this Second Edition of *SURVIVAL STRONG*, he has also published *FEROCIOUS FITNESS* and has a new project, *EXERCISE SNACKS: Fitness Five Minutes at a Time*. He is also the creator of *S.A.V.E.*, a top-rated self-defense and fitness video series (2007), and *The Kettlebell Workout Library*, a 20-hour video set consisting of 104 kettlebell and bodyweight-based workouts, and the developer of The BodyBell Method® of kettlebell, body weight and dynamic tension and the Survival Strong certifications.

Master Phil, as he's known in film and on TV, has appeared on History Channel's *Knife or Death* and *Forged in Fire: Bladesgiving*, Newsmax TV and infomercials for the Trusted Butcher Chef Knife and Commando Light. His film work includes being a featured master in the *Warrior Island* series, *M23 Cargo/Mechanical* and *Diamond Caskets*, to name a few.

Train hard, train smart and train often!
Strength and Honor!